Diagnostic Imaging: Point-of-Care Ultrasound

Editors

GREGORY R. LISCIANDRO
JENNIFER M. GAMBINO

VETERINARY CLINICS
OF NORTH AMERICA:
SMALL ANIMAL PRACTICE

www.vetsmall.theclinics.com

November 2021 • Volume 51 • Number 6

ELSEVIER

1600 John F. Kennedy Boulevard • Suite 1800 • Philadelphia, Pennsylvania, 19103-2899

http://www.vetsmall.theclinics.com

VETERINARY CLINICS OF NORTH AMERICA: SMALL ANIMAL PRACTICE Volume 51, Number 6

November 2021 ISSN 0195-5616, ISBN-13: 978-0-323-89752-5

Editor: Stacy Eastman

Developmental Editor: Axell Ivan Jade Purificacion

Veterinary Clinics of North America: Small Animal Practice (ISSN 0195-5616) is published bimonthly by Elsevier Inc., 360 Park Avenue South, New York, NY 10010-1710. Months of issue are January, March, May, July, September, and November. Business and Editorial Offices: 1600 John F. Kennedy Blvd., Ste. 1800, Philadelphia, PA 19103-2899. Customer Service Office: 3251 Riverport Lane, Maryland Heights, MO 63043. Periodicals postage paid at New York, NY and additional mailing offices. Subscription prices are $358.00 per year (domestic individuals), $933.00 per year (domestic institutions), $100.00 per year (domestic students/residents), $451.00 per year (Canadian individuals), $998.00 per year (Canadian institutions), $488.00 per year (international individuals), $998.00 per year (international institutions), $100.00 per year (Canadian students/residents), and $220.00 per year (international students/residents). To receive student/resident rate, orders must be accompanied by name of affiliated institution, date of term, and the *signature* of program/residency coordinator on institution letterhead. Orders will be billed at individual rate until proof of status is received. Foreign air speed delivery is included in all *Clinics* subscription prices. All prices are subject to change without notice. **POSTMASTER:** Send address changes to *Veterinary Clinics of North America: Small Animal Practice*, Elsevier Health Sciences Division, Subscription Customer Service, 3251 Riverport Lane, Maryland Heights, MO 63043. Customer Service (orders, claims, online, change of address): Elsevier Periodicals Customer Service, Elsevier Health Sciences Division Subscription **Customer Service 3251 Riverport Lane Maryland Heights, MO 63043. Tel: 1-800-654-2452 (U.S. and Canada); 314-447-8871 (outside U.S. and Canada). Fax: 314-447-8029. E-mail: journalscustomerservice-usa@elsevier.com (for print support); journalsonlinesupport-usa@elsevier.com (for online support).**

Reprints. For copies of 100 or more of articles in this publication, please contact the Commercial Reprints Department, Elsevier Inc., 360 Park Avenue South, New York, NY 10010-1710. Tel.: 212-633-3874; Fax: 212-633-3820; E-mail: reprints@elsevier.com.

Veterinary Clinics of North America: Small Animal Practice is also published in Japanese by Inter Zoo Publishing Co., Ltd., Aoyama Crystal-Bldg 5F, 3-5-12 Kitaaoyama, Minato-ku, Tokyo 107-0061, Japan.

Veterinary Clinics of North America: Small Animal Practice is covered in *Current Contents/Agriculture, Biology and Environmental Sciences, Science Citation Index, ASCA, MEDLINE/PubMed (Index Medicus), Excerpta Medica,* and *BIOSIS*.

Contributors

EDITORS

GREGORY R. LISCIANDRO, DVM
Diplomate, American Board of Veterinary Practitioners; Diplomate, American College of Veterinary Emergency and Critical Care; Hill Country Veterinary Specialists, FASTVet.com, Spicewood, Texas, USA

JENNIFER M. GAMBINO, DVM
Diplomate, American College of Veterinary Emergency and Critical Care; Vet-CT, Philadelphia, Pennsylvania, USA

AUTHORS

SØREN R. BOYSEN, DVM
Diplomate, American College of Veterinary Emergency and Critical Care; Professor, Faculty of Veterinary Medicine, Veterinary Emergency and Critical Care, Department of Veterinary Clinical and Diagnostic Sciences, University of Calgary, Calgary, Alberta, Canada

JANE CHO, DVM, DACVO
Veterinary Eye Specialists PLLC, Thornwood, New York, USA

LAURA COLE, MA, VetMB, MVetMed Cert, VPS Cert, AVP(ECC), MRCVS
Diplomate, American College of Veterinary Emergency and Critical Care; DECVECC, Clinical Science and Services, The Royal Veterinary College, University of London, London, United Kingdom

TERESA C. DEFRANCESCO, DVM
Diplomate, American College of Veterinary Internal Medicine (Cardiology); Diplomate, American College of Veterinary Emergency and Critical Care; Department of Clinical Sciences, College of Veterinary Medicine, North Carolina State University, Raleigh, North Carolina, USA

SAMUEL A. DICKER, DVM
Diplomate, American College of Veterinary Emergency and Critical Care; Veterinary Emergency & Referral Group, Brooklyn, New York, USA

HELEN DIRRIG, BVetMed(Hons), MVetMed(Hons), MRCVS
Diplomate, American College of Veterinary Radiology; Diplomate, European College of Veterinary Diagnostic Imaging; Clinical Science and Services; The Royal Veterinary College, University of London, London, United Kingdom

ROBERT M. FULTON, DVM
Residency Trained Theriogenology, Clarividus Veterinary Ultrasound and Education, Southern Veterinary Partners

KAREN HUMM, MA, VetMB, MSc CertVA, FHEA, MRCVS
Diplomate, American College of Veterinary Emergency and Critical Care; DECVECC, Clinical Science and Services, The Royal Veterinary College, University of London, London, United Kingdom

GREGORY R. LISCIANDRO, DVM
Diplomate, American Board of Veterinary Practitioners; Diplomate, American College of Veterinary Emergency and Critical Care; Hill Country Veterinary Specialists, FASTVet. com, Spicewood, Texas, USA

STEPHANIE C. LISCIANDRO, DVM
Diplomate, American College of Veterinary Internal Medicine (SAIM); Hill Country Veterinary Specialists and FASTVet.com, Spicewood, Texas, USA; Medical Director, Oncura Partners, Fort Worth, Texas, USA

KERRY LOUGHRAN, DVM, DACVR-EDI,
Resident, Cardiology, University of Pennsylvania, Philadelphia, Pennsylvania, USA

ERIN MAYS, DVM
Diplomate, American College of Veterinary Emergency and Critical Care; Godfrey, Illinois, USA

KATHRYN PHILLIPS, DVM
Diplomate, American College of Veterinary Radiology; UC Davis, Davis, California, USA

SUSANNE STIEGER-VANEGAS, Dr med vet, PhD
Department of Clinical Sciences, Carlson College of Veterinary Medicine, Oregon State University, Corvallis, Oregon, USA

JESSICA L. WARD, DVM
Diplomate, American College of Veterinary Internal Medicine (Cardiology); Department of Veterinary Clinical Sciences, College of Veterinary Medicine, Iowa State University, Ames, Iowa, USA

Contents

Section I: Respiratory

 Video content accompanies this article at http://www.vetsmall. theclinics.com.

Vet BLUE, a standardized and validated rapid lung ultrasound examination, includes 9 acoustic windows: 4 transthoracic bilaterally applied named Caudodorsal, Perihilar, Middle, and Cranial Lung Regions plus the Diaphragmatico-Hepatic view of AFAST/TFAST. Moreover, Vet BLUE has a B-line scoring system (weak positives—1, 2, and 3 and strong positives—>3 and infinite) that semiquantitate degree of alveolar-interstitial syndrome and a visual lung language for signs of consolidation (Shred Sign [air bronchogram], Tissue Sign [hepatization], Nodule Sign, and Wedge Sign [pulmonary infarction]). Using its regional, pattern-based approach, a respiratory working diagnosis may be rapidly developed point-of-care and followed serially.

Lung ultrasound (LUS) has high sensitivity for the rapid and reliable diagnosis of pulmonary contusions (PC) in patients who have sustained trauma. LUS diagnosis of PC exceeds that of thoracic radiographs in multiple animal and human studies. The sonographer should understand potential caveats and confounding variables for proper diagnosis of PC with LUS. LUS does not replace conventional radiography or computed tomography, especially in the polytrauma patient. LUS should be used concurrently with other point-of-care ultrasound trauma protocols to rapidly optimize patient assessment before movement to the radiology suite.

 Video content accompanies this article at http://www.vetsmall. theclinics.com.

A sonographic diagnosis of pneumothorax (PTX) traditionally relies on excluding the presence of lung sliding, lung pulse, and/or B lines/lung consolidations, and identifying the lung point. However, these criteria can be difficult to identify, particularly in critically ill patients with respiratory disorders, and the lung point is infrequently used. Newer sonographic findings, such as mirrored ribs, reverse lung sliding, and abnormal curtain signs, have been identified to try to increase the accuracy of diagnosing PTX. This article describes and discusses the lung ultrasonography criteria used to diagnose PTX in both human and small animal patients.

Section II: Non-pulmonary Thoracic and Cardiac Ultrasound

Gregory R. Lisciandro

 Video content accompanies this article at http://www.vetsmall. theclinics.com.

TFAST, a standardized and validated thoracic point-of-care ultrasound examination, includes 5 acoustic windows: bilaterally applied chest tube site and pericardial site views plus diaphragmatico-hepatic view, also part of AFAST/ Vet BLUE. TFAST is used for rapid detection of pneumothorax and pleural and pericardial effusion. By following a set of TFAST rules, image interpretation errors are avoided, including mistaking cardiac chambers for effusion. Moreover, TFAST echocardiography is used as a screening test for chamber size and soft tissue abnormalities, volume status and contractility, and intracardiac abnormalities.

Kerry Loughran

 Video content accompanies this article at http://www.vetsmall. theclinics.com.

Heart disease is a common cause of morbidity and mortality in cats. Focused cardiac ultrasonography (FCU) is a useful diagnostic tool for identifying heart disease in symptomatic and asymptomatic cats when performed by trained veterinarians. When used in conjunction with other diagnostics such as physical examination, blood biomarkers, electrocardiography, Global FAST, and other point-of-care ultrasonographic examinations, FCU may improve clinical decision making and help clinicians prioritize which cats would benefit from referral for complete echocardiography and cardiac consultation. This article reviews the definition, advantages, clinical indications, limitations, training recommendations, and a protocol for FCU in cats.

Teresa C. DeFrancesco and Jessica L. Ward

Focused cardiac ultrasound (FCU) is a useful point-of-care imaging tool to assess cardiovascular status in symptomatic dogs in the acute care setting. Unlike complete echocardiography, FCU is a time-sensitive examination involving a subset of targeted ultrasound views to identify severe cardiac abnormalities and is performed as part of an integrated thoracic ultrasound including interrogation of the pleural space and lungs. When integrated with other clinical information, FCU can be helpful in the diagnosis of left-sided and right-sided congestive heart failure, pericardial effusion and tamponade, and severe pulmonary hypertension, and can provide estimates of fluid responsiveness in hypotensive dogs.

Video content accompanies this article at http://www.vetsmall.
theclinics.com.

Point-of-care ultrasonography as part of the physical examination is
becoming considered a core skill. AFAST includes 5 acoustic windows
over the abdomen and serves as a rapid screening test for free fluid (ascites, retroperitoneal, pleural and pericardial effusion) and soft tissue abnormalities (target-organ approach), and has an abdominal fluid scoring
system (semiquantitating volume). Moreover, add-on skills are possible
without additional views that include characterizing the caudal vena
cava and hepatic veins (volume status), measuring the urinary bladder
(volume estimation and urine output), screening for free air (pneumoperitoneum,   pneumoretroperitoneum),   and   assessing   gastrointestinal
motility.

 Video content accompanies this article at http://www.vetsmall.
theclinics.com.

This article discusses the usefulness of ultrasound examinations in the
management of the patient with an emergency urinary tract disorder. It discusses the use of previously described point-of-care ultrasound protocols
such as the abdominal focused assessment with sonography for trauma,
triage, and tracking protocol in the unstable azotemic patient. Point-of-
care ultrasound examination can help direct investigations and expedite
the diagnosis of specific causes of azotemia. The limitations of point-of-
care ultrasound assessment of the kidneys, ureter, bladder, and urethra
are also addressed, emphasizing that point-of-care ultrasound examination should complement and not replace a complete urinary tract ultrasound examination.

Add "in dogs and cats"? This article covers image acquisition of the fetus
and the reproductive organs of the female (cervix, gravid and nongravid
uterus, and ovaries) and male (testicles and prostate) reproductive tracts.
This article is a brief overview of normal sonographic anatomy and important clinical conditions for each sex using point-of-care ultrasound as a
screening test. In addition to normal sonographic appearance and common conditions of the scrotum and testes, prostate, uterus, and ovaries,
this article discusses the use of ultrasound for diagnosis of and evaluating
pregnancy, fetal maturation, and fetal stress during dystocia.

In small animals, point-of-care ultrasound can be used by nonradiologist sonographers to identify thrombosis at several anatomic sites. Dogs and cats are well-suited for vascular interrogation using ultrasound because of their small body size. Ultrasound can be used to investigate targeted vessels based on clinical signs. The safety and tolerability of the examination makes this a useful modality to evaluate critical patients for evidence thromboembolic disease. Once vascular imaging techniques are learned they can be easily coupled with other point-of-care examinations such as focused cardiac ultrasound, Vet Blue, AFAST, and TFAST.

Soft tissue swellings, masses, and fluid collections commonly occur in small animal patients and can be the main reason for the clinical examination of the patient or an incidental finding. Several of these masses are likely benign or nonneoplastic, and ultrasound can help further evaluate these lesions to guide treatment planning. Careful attention to optimizing the ultrasound technique and Doppler settings is necessary to ensure that the vascularization of a mass is assessed correctly.

Indications for, technique, and findings for normal and abnormal ocular ultrasound are discussed, with specific sonographic findings, images, differential diagnoses, and other considerations. Because the eye is a fluid-filled structure, ultrasound can be used as a screening test when pathology prevents direct examination. Structural abnormalities, such as lens luxation, retinal detachments, and intraocular and orbital masses, also may be defined better using point-of-care ultrasound. Details on additional ophthalmic diagnostics, treatment, and prognosis are not covered.

Please verify if FAST should be expanded at first use – "focused assessment with sonography for trauma"?: Global FAST consists of abdominal FAST, thoracic FAST, and Vet BLUE combined as a single point-of-care ultrasound examination used as an extension of the physical examination. By applying its unbiased set of 15 data imaging points, information is gained while avoiding image interpretation errors, such as satisfaction of search error and confirmation bias error, through selective POCUS imaging. Moreover, Global FAST is used for integrating information from both cavities, rapidly screening for the Hs and Ts of cardiopulmonary resuscitation, and staging localized versus disseminated disease, helpful diagnostically and prognostically for patient work-up. By seeing a problem list, patient care is improved.

VETERINARY CLINICS OF NORTH AMERICA: SMALL ANIMAL PRACTICE

SERIES OF RELATED INTEREST

Veterinary Clinics of North America: Exotic Animal Practice
https://www.vetexotic.theclinics.com/

THE CLINICS ARE NOW AVAILABLE ONLINE!
Access your subscription at:
www.theclinics.com

Preface

Point-of-Care Ultrasound: —The Awakening of a Sleeping Giant

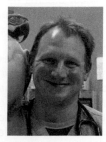   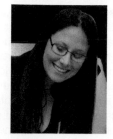

Gregory R. Lisciandro, DVM   Jennifer M. Gambino, DVM
Editors

In 1999, as a general practitioner, I declared my first attempt at learning ultrasound a failure after taking an abdominal ultrasound course. Thus, 7 years later as a resident in emergency and critical care (2005-2007), I was resistant to making FAST ultrasound part of my clinical research requirement. The phrase by my Intern Director (1991), the late Dr Michael Garvey, has always been part of my daily practice since: "never send a patient out the door (home) with something you could easily have diagnosed." Shortly after learning and routinely applying AFAST and TFAST as an extension of the physical exam in 2005 (and later Vet BLUE, 2010), these FAST ultrasound examinations became part of my quick assessment tests.

In our original study, case number 7 of 101 dogs, a dog named Zeke, presented collapsed and in hypovolemic shock after having been hit by a car 45 minutes earlier. With traditional training, I would have fallen for the obvious radiographic pneumothorax (and only a slight decrease in abdominal serosal detail ruling against a hemoabdomen) being the cause of his clinical signs. However, on AFAST, Zeke had the highest abdominal fluid score of 4, and the abdominocentesis and fluid testing confirmed his hemoabdomen. Also, of note, he was the first pneumothorax case I diagnosed using TFAST knowing of the pneumothorax *before* the radiograph.

The hemoabdomen was the major player contributing to his shock along with a co-morbidity of pneumothorax. I was completely misled by radiography and clinical impression without ultrasound. Zeke survived. All this information that allowed a more accurate clinical course was acquired on presentation with point-of-care AFAST and TFAST within a few minutes. From this case, I not only was hooked but also had the epiphany that I could do ultrasound and was also convinced of the need to always look in both cavities to best evaluate the patient. AFAST and TFAST were initially called Combo FAST until Vet BLUE was developed, which led to the examination being named Global FAST.

Vet Clin Small Anim 51 (2021) xi–xiii
https://doi.org/10.1016/j.cvsm.2021.08.001
0195-5616/21/© 2021 Published by Elsevier Inc.

We created AFAST after the original FAST study by Dr Søren Boysen and colleagues out of Tufts, published in 2004. AFAST changed the direction of the scanning plane more strategically into gravity-dependent pouches. It also added the umbilical view and took on a new mindset of not only a target-organ approach for soft tissue abnormalities but also an abdominal fluid scoring system to better categorize patients with ascites. At the same time, we created TFAST for a rapid assessment of the thorax not only for pleural and pericardial effusion but also for pneumothorax and brief echocardiography. In 2010, we created Vet BLUE, and never in my wildest dreams had I thought that proactive lung ultrasound would be so impactful for improving patient care (and easy to learn). This has become one of our proudest achievements, as so many colleagues had underestimated the value of what we had begun.

As a resident, I can still remember reading "Ultrasound in the management of thoracic disease" by Daniel Lichtenstein, in the journal *Critical Care Medicine* (2007). Lichtenstein concluded that we (point-of-care sonographers) had awakened the "sleepy giant" in terms of its applications and potential to improve patient care. Thus, we too in veterinary medicine have awakened its potential with an explosion of applications in the past few years. In veterinary medicine, we have been handed a rare opportunity to be ahead of our physician colleagues in making standardized goal-directed point-of-care ultrasound (POCUS) a core skill.

Dr Jennifer Gambino, a board-certified veterinary radiologist, and I met over a decade ago during her tenure at Mississippi State University, while doing the first issue of our textbook. She cowrote with Dr Søren Boysen an article on Focused Gastrointestinal and Pancreas Ultrasound and contributed input on some of the other abdominal organ articles. She saw the immediate value in more abbreviated structured training (FAST and Focused examinations) of nonradiologist veterinarians over comprehensive ultrasound examinations, the latter a difficult skill to gain proficiency.

Moreover, she saw the potential for these abbreviated FAST and Focused formats to serve as an important and valuable screening test that could capture significant disease that would have otherwise been missed without ultrasound use early in the triage process. Not only were cases with significant disease captured, but also treatment was more evidence based with the potential to keep patients alive for later gold-standard imaging (her area of expertise). Of special note, Dr Gambino's preference for alcohol-based hand sanitizer gel as an excellent coupling medium for ultrasound (over coupling gel) came to my attention, a brilliant discovery.

Which brings us to our next point: the development of this issue came to fruition during a time perhaps when hand sanitizer was a scarce commodity: the COVID 19 pandemic. We all felt the impact of the pandemic (eg, surging case numbers, curbside appointments, and busier-than-ever schedules). Never before has goal-directed POCUS been more relevant, and never before has our profession been as ready to adapt its principles for better patient care and improved outcomes.

So, let's define veterinary POCUS! It includes FAST ultrasound examinations, defined as a goal-directed ultrasound examination performed by a veterinary health care provider "cage side" (or bringing imaging to the patient) to answer a specific diagnostic question or questions or guide performance of an invasive procedure (**Fig. 1**). Global FAST, a term coined in 2010, is the combination of AFAST (abdomen), TFAST (thorax), and Vet BLUE (lung). Focused or POCUS exams are interchangeable terms that refer to target imaging of specific organs or systems.

There are some important features of POCUS that the reader should be aware of. First, these should be considered screening tests that are user-dependent founded on proper training. Second, recording findings on goal-directed templates (data entry forms) and archiving studies with good image acquisition make it clear to our

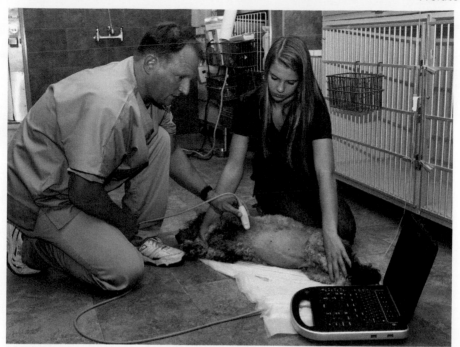

Fig. 1. Veterinary POCUS allows for cage-side (or at the patient's side) imaging. (*Courtesy of Dr Gregory Lisciando, Hill Country Veterinary Specialists and FASTVte.com.*)

colleagues what the objectives of the POCUS examination were, while keeping the sonographer disciplined and on task. Third, targeted or focused POCUS can lead to image interpretation errors, such as satisfaction of search error, stopping at the first major abnormality, and confirmation bias error through selective imaging (picking and choosing what will be imaged). Global FAST is an approach in which an unbiased set of data imaging points is acquired of both the abdomen (AFAST) and the thorax (TFAST and Vet BLUE) from which the sonographer may do additional POCUS examinations. Thus, Global FAST helps eliminate such image interpretation errors.

We are excited about this issue and the article authors who have generously given their time and expertise as leaders in this new frontier of veterinary medicine that undoubtedly is a game-changer for patient care. We also want to recognize all those in the radiology community who have spent untold numbers of hours of due diligence and time studying ultrasound. By publishing their research, they have created the foundation for the nonradiologist sonographer.

Gregory R. Lisciandro, DVM
Hill Country Veterinary Specialists
FASTVet.com
Spicewood, TX, USA

Jennifer M. Gambino, DVM
Vet-CT
Philadelphia, PA, USA

E-mail addresses:
FastSavesLives@gmail.com (G.R. Lisciandro)
Jennifer.Gambino@vet-ct.com (J.M. Gambino)

Section I: Respiratory

Lung Ultrasound Fundamentals, "Wet Versus Dry" Lung, Signs of Consolidation in Dogs and Cats

Gregory R. Lisciandro, DVM, DABVP, DACVECC[a],*,
Stephanie C. Lisciandro, DVM, DACVIM (SAIM)[a,b]

KEYWORDS

• Lung ultrasound • B-lines • Shred sign • B-line scoring system

KEY POINTS

• Vet BLUE is a standardized regional, pattern-based lung ultrasound examination with exact clarity to its 8 transthoracic views plus the Diaphragmatico-Hepatic View.

• Dry lung artifacts are expected all Vet BLUE acoustic windows with uncommon single B-lines.

• Wet lung may be scored using the Vet BLUE B-line scoring system of 1, 2, 3 as weak positives and greater than 3, and infinity (∞) as strong positives.

• Dry lung in all views rules out all common wet lung conditions including cardiogenic and noncardiogenic lung edema, pneumonia, lung hemorrhage, and lung contusions.

• Consolidation is categorized as Shred Sign (air bronchogram), Tissue Sign, (hepatization), Nodule Sign (nodular diseases), and Wedge Sign (pulmonary thromboembolism).

• 8 discreet regional transthoracic views and a pattern-based approach may be used

  ○ to formulate a working diagnosis in patients with suspected respiratory compromise in less than 2 min

  ○ as a tool to serially track (improvement, deterioration, static) respiratory patients in less than 2 min

  ○ plus the use of the Diaphragmatico-Hepatic view for lung surface along the pulmonary-diaphragmatic interface inaccessible from transthoracic views.

• Using its transthoracic views bilaterally, pneumothorax and the location of the lung point is searched for automatically.

[a] Hill Country Veterinary Specialists and FASTVet.com, Spicewood, TX, USA; [b] Oncura Partners, Fort Worth, TX, USA
* Corresponding author.
E-mail address: FastSavesLives@gmail.com

Vet Clin Small Anim 51 (2021) 1125–1140
https://doi.org/10.1016/j.cvsm.2021.07.012
0195-5616/21/© 2021 Elsevier Inc. All rights reserved.

Video content accompanies this article at http://www.vetsmall.theclinics.com

INTRODUCTION

In 2004, the first translational study of focused assessment with sonography for trauma (FAST) from humans to small animals documented that minimally trained non-radiologist veterinarians could proficiently recognize ascites, and that hemoperitoneum was far more common than previously reported.[1] Moreover, pleural and pericardial effusion could be detected via the subxiphoid view by looking cranial to the diaphragm and lung abnormalities during TFAST at the Chest Tube Site view.[1,2,3,4] As a result, Vet BLUE was created in 2010 as a more comprehensive screening test and has been evaluated in clinically normal adult dogs, adult cats, and puppies and kittens aged over 6 weeks.[5,6,7,8]

Vet BLUE is unique in that its regional views were developed to mimic the manner in which most veterinarians interpret lung findings on thoracic radiography helping to rapidly and in real-time develop a working differential list for respiratory small animals.[5,9,10,11,12] Moreover, Vet BLUE has its B-line scoring system and its visual lung language that are "all or none" ultrasonographic phenomenon, meaning its findings are either present or they are not.[5,6,7,8,9,10,11,12] In comparative imaging studies, Vet BLUE and lung ultrasound have been shown to exceed the sensitivity of thoracic radiography and fare favorably with computed tomography (CT) for various respiratory conditions.[13,14,15,16,17] The use of lung ultrasound has clear visual advantages over the subjective nature of lung auscultation and is rapidly becoming the screening test and monitoring tool of choice for pneumonia and congestive heart failure in human medicine and small animals.[18,19,20,21,22,23,24,25,26,27,28,29] The time is here—the ultrasound probe is our new stethoscope![18,19,30,31]

Although Vet BLUE may be used as a standalone ultrasound examination, through the standardized approach of Global FAST, sonographers avoid common imaging mistakes such as "satisfaction of search error" and "confirmation bias error" through selective POCUS imaging. As an example, Vet BLUE may show dry lung in all views with thoracic radiography being unremarkable, and the patient being sent home with a conservative plan for upper airway disease or occult lower airway disease (ie, bronchial disease). However, by incorporating the Global FAST approach that includes TFAST echocardiography, the patient is found to have left ventricular enlargement and poor contractility with a working diagnosis of dilated cardiomyopathy confirmed with complete echocardiography thereafter. The thoracic radiograph was interpreted as unremarkable. This is one of many examples of how integrating Global FAST information leads to a more accurate diagnosis with similar strategies being advocated for human medicine.[32,33,34]

VET BLUE OVERVIEW
Gator Sign Orientation

The fundamental orientation for all lung ultrasound is the Gator Sign.[5,6] The Gator Sign is composed of 2 ribs with its interposing intercostal space (ICS) much like a partially submerged alligator peering at the sonographer (**Fig. 1**) (Videos 1–3). The interposing ICS is where the lung surface is expected to be immediately against the thoracic wall. We refer to this as the "Lung Line" over the parietal and visceral pleura interface because when pleural space abnormalities exist, the "Lung Line" better describes the location of the lung surface.[9] Without the Gator Sign orientation, it becomes easy to mistake fascial planes, flat bones, air reverberation artifact for the "Lung Line," and thus errors in interpretation will occur.[9] In instances where the probe is

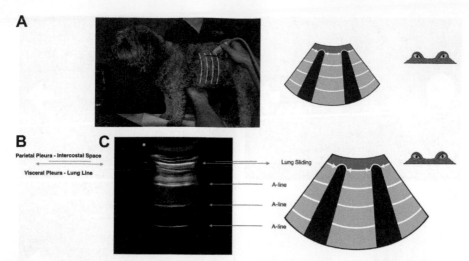

Fig. 1. The gator sign orientation is the fundamental orientation for all lung ultrasounds. Without it, the sonographer cannot be certain they are identifying the correct bright white line (*hyperechoic line*) representing the lung surface, which we refer to as the lung line. In (*A*), the scanning plane is perpendicular to the long axis of the ribs to create the gator sign appearance of rib, intercostal space, and rib, like an eye, bridge of the nose or forehead, and eye. In (*B*) is the schematic showing that lung sliding (arrows) is created by visceral and parietal pleural on a micro level sliding over one another or on a macro level the lung sliding over the intercostal space compared to C) with the correlative B-mode ultrasound still image. This is a real-time phenomenon and cannot be shown on still images. A-lines are maximized when the angle of insonation is at 90° to the aerated and thus reflective lung line. (© 2021 Gregory R. Lisciandro.)

rotated from longitudinal to transverse orientation along the lung surface, the Gator Sign should be periodically checked, making sure that the "Lung Line" is being properly followed.[9]

Curtain Sign

Air reflects ultrasound and borders of aerated structures cast a linear border at margins of the respective aerated structure. This linear air-associated border is likened to a curtain covering and uncovering the structures in that immediate area (Video 4 and 5). "Curtain Sign" was first used to describe the curtain sign of pleural effusion.[35] However, with lung ultrasound, the "Curtain Sign" similarly covers and uncovers the transition zone between the pleural and abdominal cavities (**Fig. 2**).[9,36]

Vet BLUE Standardized Methodology—Names, Views, Order, and Probe Maneuvering

Vet BLUE has bilaterally applied transthoracic views named Caudodorsal, Perihilar, Middle, and Cranial Lung Regions plus the Diaphragmatico-Hepatic (DH) view, providing a deeper acoustic window along the pulmonary-diaphragmatic interface inaccessible from transthoracic views with the updated methodology described here (**Fig. 3**).[9,37] The Caudodorsal view is located by identifying the "Curtain Sign", the "Transition Zone" between the pleural and abdominal cavities, and then sliding 3 ICSs cranially *away* from the abdominal cavity. This is the starting point for the Caudodorsal view and referred to as its "primary" ICS. From this primary ICS, slide

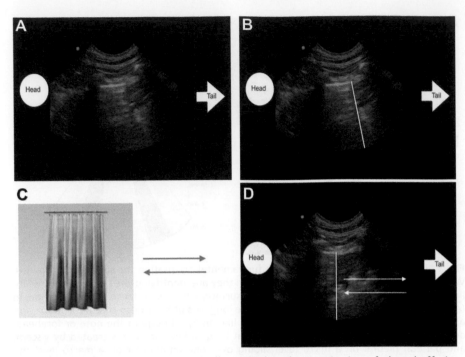

Fig. 2. The curtain sign is a term originally applied to the curtain sign of pleural effusion. However, it is a basic principle. When air moves over any structures, it has a linear border. In the thorax, the curtain sign created by air-filled lung, covers and uncovers the adjacent regions because of the movement during phases of respiration. In (A), (B), and (D), that linear border is shown with overlays and shows the curtain sign transition zone of the pleural and abdominal cavities. The arrows in (D) represent the sliding to and fro of the curtain sign with phases of respiration. In (C) is a picture of window curtain to emphasize the curtain sign. The importance in recognizing this area during Vet BLUE is to not mistake abdominal structures for pulmonary or other intrathoracic pathology. Note that the head is to the left of the screen and the tail to the right so that abdominal structures are always expected to enter the view from the right. (© 2021 Gregory R. Lisciandro.)

caudally one ICS, return to the primary ICS, and then slide cranially for a third ICS (Video 6). Each Vet BLUE regional view surveys a minimum of 3 ICSs at that respective regional view. Sliding caudally first from the primary ICS should be made a habit because the question is asked, "where is the abdominal cavity?" In haste and with improper training, the stomach, liver, and gallbladder are easily mistaken for lung pathology such as pseudo B-lines, pseudo shred sign, and pseudo tissue sign (Video 4 and 5).[9] By understanding the "Curtain Sign" of the "Transition Zone," the sonographer is better able to differentiate the pleural from abdominal cavities at the Caudodorsal, Perihilar, and Middle Lung Regional views.

The Perihilar view is next imaged by drawing a line, called "the Vet BLUE Line," with acoustic coupling medium from the primary ICS of the Caudodorsal view to the patient's elbow. Approximately halfway to the elbow is the Perihilar Lung Region view. The same methodology of evaluating an ICS cranial and caudal to this site is repeated. Slide caudally first and ask, "where is the abdominal cavity (and is the curtain sign identified)?" Then, return to the primary ICS, and then slide cranially for the minimum

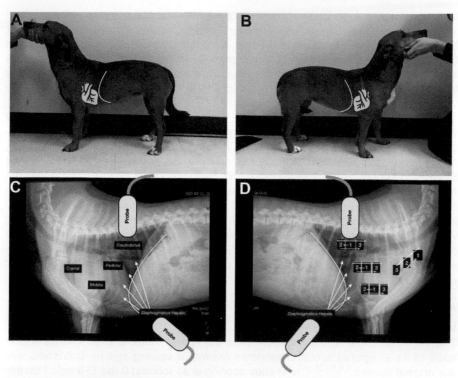

Fig. 3. The Vet BLUE shown on a standing dog with external anatomy in (*A*) and (*B*) and then overlays in (*C*) and (*D*). The lung regions are named as caudodorsal, perihilar, middle, and cranial. The caudodorsal view is located by finding the transition zone, curtain sign, and sliding 3 intercostal spaces cranially away from the abdominal structures. At each respective view, a minimum of 3 intercostals spaces are surveyed by sliding first caudally and then cranially (numbers and *arrows*). The cranial lung region is found by flexing and abducting the foreleg so that the probe may be placed in the axillary area over the thoracic inlet and then the first 3 ribs. The DH view is part of Vet BLUE because it provides a window of the lung along its pulmonary-diaphragmatic interface that is not accessible via transthoracic views. (© 2021 Gregory R. Lisciandro.)

of 3 ICSs (Video 6). Moving on to the Middle Lung Region, slide ventral over heart along "the Vet BLUE Line" to the elbow. Slide dorsally to eliminate the heart from view and identify the Gator Sign orientation. Then slide caudally from the primary ICS, back to the primary Middle Lung Region ICS, and then cranially as the previous 2 regional views. In many small animals and exotic companion mammals, you may be at the "Curtain Sign" of the "Transition Zone" at the start of the Middle Lung Region. In these cases, slide over the first 3 ICSs as you move cranially away from the "Curtain Sign" and count those IVCs as the middle lung region. Even though the sonographer slides 3 ICSs from the caudodorsal "Transition Zone" and follows "the Vet BLUE Line," the respirophasic dynamics of the Caudodorsal, Perihilar, and Middle lung regions often still bring the abdominal structures into the field of view.

The final transthoracic view is the Cranial Lung Region performed by gently flexing the foreleg and working the probe dorsal and cranially into the patient's axilla heading for the middle of the first rib. The "Transition Zone" is now to the left of the screen and is the transition between the lung within the pleural cavity and the thoracic inlet. The thoracic inlet is best recognized by the pulsating of the Costocervical trunk and carotid arteries. The probe is then slid caudally over Gator Sign orientations of the first rib, first ICS, second rib, second ICS, and third rib, third ICS (Video 7). Of note, the cupula of the lung in some small animals extends cranially to the first rib and in the author's experience, the first ICS is much smaller than the subsequent ICSs. The author prefers to start with the left Vet BLUE and then move to the DH view, before completing the Vet BLUE examination on the right side.

The advantages here are that the TFAST right Pericardial Site echocardiography views, generally the most time-consuming and most challenging for many sonographers, are left for last when doing TFAST and Vet BLUE simultaneously. Moreover, much information has been already gained with this recommended order of Vet BLUE and Global FAST. The Global FAST Fallback Views of Vet BLUE/lung, the AFAST-TFAST DH view, and the characterization of the caudal vena cava and hepatic veins have already been assessed. Thus, the sonographer advantageously knows if there is wet versus dry lung, if there are abnormalities with the caudal vena cava and hepatic veins, and if there is pericardial and pleural effusion (or pneumothorax) *before* performing the TFAST echocardiography views. Furthermore, the sonographer has a better idea of safe degrees of physical and chemical restraint.

Pitfalls and Limitations

Vet BLUE B-line scoring system

The Vet BLUE B-line scoring system takes the highest number over a single ICS at each of its 9 regional acoustic windows (views), a scoring system published with our original studies.[6,7,10,38] The B-lines scoring is as follows: 0 (no B-lines), 1 (single B-line), 2 (2 B-lines), 3 (3 B-lines), greater than 3 (more than 3 B-lines, however, not confluent over an entire ICS), and infinity (confluent over an entire ICS) (Videos 8

Vet BLUE B-line Scoring System

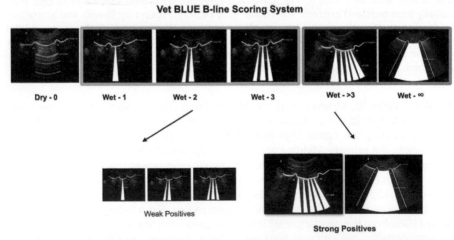

Dry - 0   Wet - 1   Wet - 2   Wet - 3   Wet - >3   Wet - ∞

Weak Positives

Strong Positives

Fig. 4. The Vet BLUE B-line scoring system is performed by taking the highest number of B-lines over a single intercostal space at each respective Vet BLUE view. The scoring is 0 for no B-lines (dry lung). The wet lung scores are 1, single B-line, 2, 2 B-lines, 3, 3 B-lines, greater than 3, more than 3 B-lines but not confluent, and infinite, B-lines that are confluent over the entire intercostal space. Scores of 1 to 3 are considered weak positives and those of greater than 3 and infinite as strong positives. (© 2021 Gregory R. Lisciandro.)

and 9).[6,7,10,38] These may be further broken down into weak (1–3) and strong (>3 and infinity) positives, which helps with placing a severity score on each patient through B-line scoring combined with positive regions (**Fig. 4**).[38]

B-lines and pseudo B-lines

B-lines are primarily created by the cuffing of aerated alveoli around fluid or soft tissue. The echoes enter this reflective chamber and then exit back to the transducer and are cast through the far field as a tight band of reverberation.[38,39] Most commonly B-lines represent types of alveolar-interstitial edema and when doing so are referred to as alveolar-interstitial syndrome. The cuffed fluid is most commonly water (cardiogenic and noncardiogenic pulmonary edema), blood (hemorrhage and contusions), or exudate pus (pneumonia). However, we have described "pseudo B-lines" created by aerated alveoli cuffing nodules and air surrounding gastric ingesta (Video 10).[38] Lung fibrosis also may be placed in this category because the term "pseudo B-lines" differentiates "true B-lines" caused by alveolar-interstitial syndrome from these non–fluid-related causes.[38]

Vet BLUE Sign of Consolidation

When enough air has been displaced by pulmonary parenchymal disease, the echoes can penetrate past the pleural margin imaging deep to the lung surface (Lung Line).

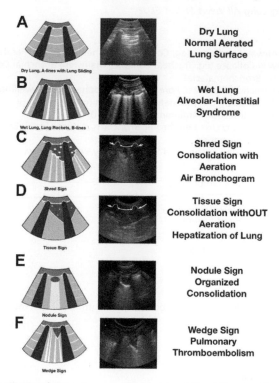

Fig. 5. The Vet BLUE Visual Lung Language consists of the following from most normal to most abnormal lung ultrasound signs as follows: (*A*) dry lung (A-lines with lung sliding), (*B*) B-lines most commonly representing forms of alveolar-interstitial edema, (*C*) shred sign representing air bronchograms, (*D*) tissue sign representing hepatization of lung, (*E*) nodule sign, and (*F*) wedge sign representing pulmonary thromboembolism. (© 2021 Gregory R. Lisciandro.)

Signs of lung consolidation sonographically include the Shred Sign (air bronchogram) and Tissue Sign (hepatization of lung), terms used in human medicine (Videos 11 and 12).[5,38,40] We have added the Nodule Sign and Wedge Sign (**Fig. 5**).[5,15,38,41]

The Shred Sign is hallmarked by hyperechoic foci (bright white) within the consolidation with generally irregular borders along its far field. These hyperechoic foci represent air bronchograms that may be dynamic or static. In dynamic air bronchograms, air can be seen wisping through the hyperechoic foci (bronchi).[42] However, these 2 forms of air bronchograms are often difficult to differentiate in spontaneously breathing patients. As a general rule, static air bronchograms represent atelectasis and dynamic air bronchograms represent types of pneumonia.[42]

The Tissue Sign represents a complete lack of aeration within the consolidated lung. Thus, the tissue sign appears ultrasonographically hepatized or like the liver.[5,35,38] In fact, it can be difficult to tell the difference between the Tissue Sign of the lung and the actual liver. This is why we have Vet BLUE sonographers understand and be able to recognize the "Curtain Sign" at the transitions zones of the Caudodorsal, Perihilar, and Middle Lung Regions.[9,38]

Box 1
Differentials for the finding of dry lung all views during Vet BLUE

Differentials for Dry Lung All Views on Vet BLUE

Respiratory
　Pneumothorax
　Dynamic Upper Airway Conditions (eg, Collapsing Trachea, Laryngeal Paralysis)
　Intrathoracic Airway Collapse (eg, Tracheal Collapse, Mainstem Bronchial Collapse, Lobar Bronchial Collapse, Bronchomalacia)
　Upper Airway Obstruction (eg, Mass, Foreign Body, Oropharyngeal Swelling, Inflammation, Nasopharyngeal Polyp [cats], Granulomatous Laryngitis [cats])
　Tracheobronchitis (eg, Infectious, Inflammatory, Irritant)
　Inflammatory Lower Airway Disease (Chronic Bronchitis, Asthma [cats], Eosinophilic Bronchitis [dogs], Bronchiectasis)
　Lung Pathology not Located at the Lung Surface at any Vet BLUE view

Cardiac
　Pericardial Effusion/Cardiac Tamponade
　Cardiac Arrhythmia
　Dilated Cardiomyopathy (DCM)
　Right-sided Congestive Heart Failure

Pulmonary Vascular Disease
　Pulmonary Thromboembolism (PTE)
　Pulmonary Hypertension

Undifferentiated Hypotension
　Canine Anaphylaxis
　Cavitary or Spatial Bleeding (eg, Hemoabdomen, Hemothorax, Hemoretroperitoneum, Hemopericardium, Fracture Site)
　Gastric Dilatation-Volvulus/Bloat
　Sepsis

Other Nonrespiratory
　Pyrexia/Heat Stroke/High Fever
　Severe Metabolic Acidosis
　Severe Anemia
　Neurologic Disease
　Pain

© 2021 Gregory R. Lisciandro.

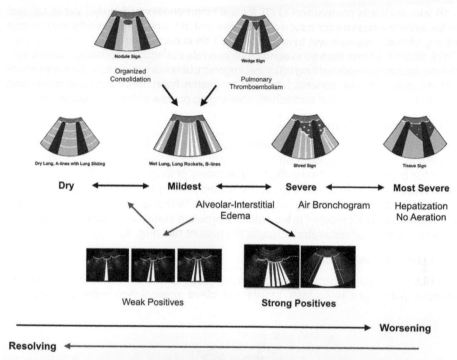

Fig. 6. Vet BLUE may be used as a monitoring tool dependent on the type of respiratory disease. However, the concept is that dry lung progresses to wet lung and B-lines that may be further differentiated by weak vs strong positives followed by signs of consolidation including shred sign which is less severe than a tissue sign. Nodule sign and wedge sign represent additional categories of consolidation. By understanding the basic gist of this schematic, the clinician performing Vet BLUE has a monitoring tool for tracking in a low impact manner, point-of-care that fares well with other imaging modalities of thoracic radiography and computed tomography. (© 2021 Gregory R. Lisciandro.)

The Nodule Sign is created by aerated alveoli cuffing soft tissue and is characterized by a hypoechoic or anechoic oval or circle with a hyperechoic far border and a pseudo B-lines extending from the far border through the far field (Video 13).[5,15,38] Lastly, the Wedge Sign is an amalgam of the Shred and Tissue Signs and represents lung infarction.[41,43–45] When the Wedge Sign is found in non–gravity-dependent Vet BLUE regions (Caudodorsal and Perihilar), its finding supports the presence of pulmonary thromboembolism (lung infarction) (Video 14).[41] In gravity-dependent regions, the wedge sign is difficult to differentiate from a Shred Sign and pneumonia.[38,41] Note all the Vet BLUE lung findings may be recognized along the pulmonary-diaphragmatic interface at the DH view (Video 15).

Vet BLUE Rules Out Wet Lung Conditions

The major strength of Vet BLUE is the finding of dry lung, A-lines with lung sliding, in all views. Dry lung in all Vet BLUE views effectively rules out in less than 60 seconds all wet lung conditions (those with B-lines) including cardiogenic and noncardiogenic pulmonary edema, pneumonia, pulmonary hemorrhage, and contusions (**Box 1**).[6,7,11,12,14,16,17] In veterinary studies, Vet BLUE has shown its superiority over

TXR with favorable comparison to CT for wet lung conditions.[13,14,16,17] Vet BLUE provides evidence-based information of a negative test (dry lung in all views) for the absence of any clinically relevant wet lung conditions. This is hugely impactful for patient care. Think about it. In less than 60 seconds, one can rule out acute respiratory distress syndrome, transfusion-related lung injury, neurogenic pulmonary edema, pulmonary hemorrhage in coagulopathic patients, left-sided congestive heart failure and volume overload, and aspiration pneumonia; traditionally challenging or time-consuming diagnoses.

Vet BLUE Patient Monitoring

The echelon of lung ultrasound findings ranges from normal lung surface to most abnormal loosely follows dry lung (A-lungs with lung sliding), wet lung (B-lines), Shred Sign (air bronchogram), Tissue Sign (hepatization of lung), Nodule Sign, and Wedge Sign (supportive of PTE) (see **Fig. 5**). By understanding this, echelon Vet BLUE may be used for patient monitoring and answering the clinical question in real-time, cageside (at the patient's side)—"Is the patient's problem static, worsening, or resolving?" dependent on what respiratory disease the patient has (**Fig. 6**).

Vet BLUE Lung Metastasis Check

Vet BLUE is hugely impactful as a quick lung metastasis check because by ruling out obvious pulmonary metastasis makes the client presentation more positive than

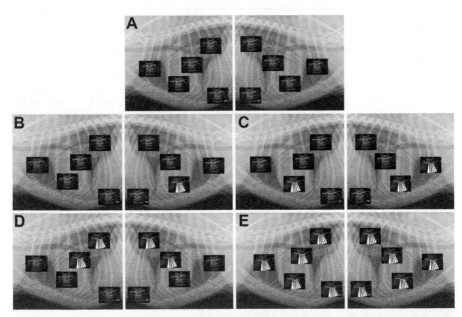

Fig. 7. Some examples of Vet BLUE illustrating its regional, pattern-based approach showing B-lines. Its greatest power may be the finding of dry lung all views as in (*A*) because all clinically relevant dry lung conditions are ruled out in a matter of 1 to 2 minutes. In (*B*) and (*C*), patterns that are gravity dependent and asymmetrical commonly represent types of pneumonia. In (*B*), you would expect wet lung in the right middle lung region in a dog for classic aspiration pneumonia. Wet lung in pneumonia could be replaced with signs of consolidation like shred sign and tissue sign. In (*D*) and (*E*), patterns are more non–gravity-dependent or generalized and symmetric commonly supporting the presence of cardiogenic and noncardiogenic pulmonary edema. (© 2021 Gregory R. Lisciandro.)

when nodules are found.[15,37] Care should be taken to not over-interpret abnormalities along the lung surface. A true nodule should have a pseudo B-line extending through the far field (see **Fig. 4**).[9,37,38] From our preliminary studies, true sensitivity and specificity for Vet BLUE in detecting metastatic nodules is unclear. In one study comparing Vet BLUE, TXR, and CT, Vet BLUE was found to be similar in sensitivity and specificity of TXR with CT outperforming Vet BLUE.[37] The study design, however, did not have consistency in imaging order and Vet BLUE was often performed after anesthesia and CT, confounding interpretation. Moreover, the time interval between imaging modalities was up to 2 weeks. In a pilot study published as an abstract, Vet BLUE clearly outperformed TXR.[15] At this time, the author's conclusion would be that Vet BLUE should be used as a rapid pulmonary metastasis check as part of the initial patient evaluation. A negative Vet BLUE examination for nodules should help move the client to a continued work-up including 3-view TXR and CT when indicated for a more comprehensive evaluation.

Case Examples

Vet BLUE's unique regional, pattern-based approach helps rapidly develop a working diagnosis in respiratory suspects and patients. For example, cardiogenic and noncardiogenic lung edema will involve upper regional views and generally is symmetric in contrast to pneumonia that would be more gravity-dependent and asymmetrical. A dog with classic aspiration pneumonia would be wet or consolidated in the right middle lung region. Examples are shown (**Fig. 7**). Differentiating wet lung due to cardiogenic or noncardiogenic pulmonary edema requires incorporating TFAST echocardiography views and Global FAST findings. Algorithms may be used for the

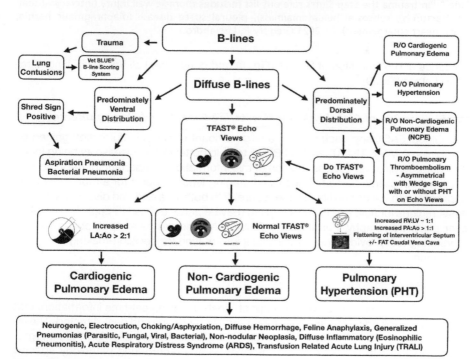

Fig. 8. Algorithm for the differential diagnoses of B-lines during Vet BLUE. (© 2021 Gregory R. Lisciandro.)

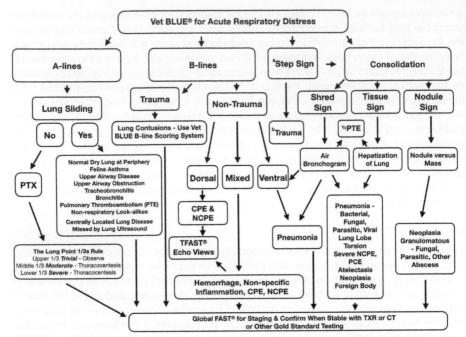

Fig. 9. Algorithm for Respiratory Patients Using Vet BLUE Lung Ultrasound Signs. [a]Step Sign is a deviation from the linear expectation of the pulmonary-pleural interface and the "Lung Line." [b]In trauma the Step Sign's rule out list includes thoracic wall injury (intercostal tear, rib fracture(s), subcostal hematoma/mass), pleural space disease (diaphragmatic hernia, mass, heart enlargement). (© 2021 Gregory R. Lisciandro.)

presence and distribution of B-lines (**Fig. 8**) and considering all Vet BLUE lung ultrasound signs (**Fig. 9**).[38]

Vet BLUE as Part of Global FAST for Monitoring Patients and Staging Disease

The Global FAST approach obtains a large amount of clinical information gained by combining AFAST, TFAST, and Vet BLUE to help better define disease as being localized or disseminated. The assimilation of this information is important for the initial discussion with clients being that localized staging lends support for a more optimistic approach with the possibility of patient cure.[46] In both localized and disseminated disease, regions for fluid and tissue sampling may be better defined through Global FAST over plain radiography. Furthermore, Global FAST serves as a rapid, cost-effective, monitoring tool providing real-time clinical information for decision-making and guiding therapy.

SUMMARY

Vet BLUE is minimally invasive, low impact, cost-effective, real-time information, that is rapidly gained point-of-care while being radiation-sparing and goal-directed. The ultrasound probe has clear advantages over lung auscultation, allowing the sonographer to "see" with evidence-based information and record lung pathology specific to the described Vet BLUE lung regions. The standardized regional, pattern-based Vet BLUE approach allows clinicians to better direct diagnostic plan and serves as an effective monitoring tool. Vet BLUE's greatest strength may prove to be in *ruling out* wet lung conditions with the finding of dry lung all views, use as a monitoring tool, and its ability to detect the smallest of lung surface pathologies that are sometimes unclear on TXR and perhaps not temporally evident on CT. Its major limitation is the requirement for lung pathology to be present at the lung surface at one of its acoustic windows and the cranial dorsal thorax is limited by the foreleg and its associated musculature. Global FAST, which includes Vet BLUE, should be used as an extension of the physical examination on a daily basis for nearly all patients in the clinical setting and should preempt add-on POCUS examinations to optimize a correct patient assessment and prevent imaging interpretation errors.

CLINICS CARE POINTS (VET BLUE)

- Vet BLUE serves as a regional, pattern-based approach to lung ultrasound that allows for the development of a working diagnosis for respiratory conditions.
- The sonographer should expect absent to rare single B-lines in normalcy in adult dogs and cats, and puppies and kittens over 6-weeks of age.
- Vet BLUE dry all views effectively rules all out all clinically relevant wet lung conditions in minutes including cardiogenic and non-cardiogenic edema, pneumonia, lung hemorrhage, and lung contusions.
- The combination of Vet BLUE and its B-line scoring system and numbers of positive regional views allows for a severity score for wet lung conditions.
- Vet BLUE serves as a real-time, point-of-care, radiation-sparing and low risk (minimal restraint) tracking tool for congestive heart failure and all other respiratory conditions.

DISCLOSURE

The authors are the owners of FASTVet.com, a private corporation that provides veterinary ultrasound training to practicing veterinarians. Ultrasound companies sponsor Global FAST Courses and include Oncura Partners, Universal Imaging, El Medical, and Sound; and El Medical and the Veterinary Medical Network have licensed Global FAST education materials. Stephanie Lisciandro, is a veterinarian and Medical Director at Oncura Partners, Fort Worth, Texas. The authors have no funding sources to declare for this article.

SUPPLEMENTARY DATA

Supplementary data to this article can be found online at https://doi.org/10.1016/j.cvsm.2021.07.012

REFERENCES

1. Boysen SR, Rozanski EA, Tidwell AS, et al. Evaluation of a focused assessment with sonography for trauma protocol to detect free abdominal fluid in dogs involved in motor vehicle accidents. J Am Vet Med Assoc 2004;225(8):1198–204.

2. Lisciandro GR. The use of the diaphragmatico-hepatic (DH) views of the abdominal and thoracic focused assessment with sonography for triage (AFAST/TFAST) examinations for the detection of pericardial effusion in 24 dogs (2011-2012). J Vet Emerg Crit Care 2016;26(1):125–31.

3. Lisciandro GR, Lagutchik MS, Mann KA, et al. Evaluation of a thoracic focused assessment with sonography for trauma (TFAST) protocol to detect

pneumothorax and concurrent thoracic injury in 145 traumatized dogs. J Vet Emerg Crit Care 2008;18(3):258–69.

4. Lisciandro GR. Abdominal and thoracic focused assessment with sonography for trauma, triage and monitoring in small animals. J Vet Emerg Crit Care 2011;21(2): 104–22.

5. Lisciandro GR. Chapter 10: The Vet BLUE Lung Scan. In: Lisciandro GR, editor. Focused ultrasound techniques for the small animal practitioner. Ames IA: Wiley Blackwell; 2014.

6. Lisciandro GR, Fulton RM, Fosgate GT, et al. Frequency of B-lines using a regionally-based lung ultrasound examination (the Vet BLUE proto Lisciandro GR, Fosgate GT, Fulton RM. Frequency of ultrasound lung rockets using a regionally-based lung ultrasound examination named veterinary bedside lung ultrasound exam (Vet BLUE) in 98 dogs with normal thoracic radiographic lung findings. Vet Radiol Ultrasound 2014;55(3):315–22.

7. Lisciandro GR, Fulton RM, Fosgate GT, et al. Frequency of B-lines using a regionally-based lung ultrasound examination (the Vet BLUE protocol) in 49 cats with normal thoracic radiographical lung findings. J Vet Emerg Crit Care 2017;27(3):267–77.

8. Lisciandro GR, Romero L, Fosgate GT. The frequency of B-lines and other lung ultrasound artifacts during Vet BLUE in 91 healthy puppies and kittens. Abstract. J Vet Emerg Crit Care 2018;28(S1):S16.

9. Lisciandro GR, Lisciandro SC. Chapter 22: POCUS: Vet BLUE-introduction and image acquisition. In: Lisciandro GR, editor. Point-of-care ultrasound techniques for the small animal practitioner. 2nd edition. Ames IA: Wiley Blackwell; 2021. p. 425–58.

10. Ward JL, Lisciandro GR, Keene BW, et al. Accuracy of point-of-care lung ultrasonography for the diagnosis of cardiogenic pulmonary edema in dogs and cats with acute dyspnea. J Am Vet Med Assoc 2017;250:666–75.

11. Ward JL, Lisciandro GR, Ware WA, et al. Lung ultrasound findings in 100 dogs with various etiologies of cough. J Am Vet Med Assoc 2019;255(5):574–83.

12. Lisciandro GR, Ward JL, DeFrancesco TC, et al. Absence of B-lines on lung ultrasound (Vet BLUE protocol) to rule out left-sided congestive heart failure in 368 cats and dogs. Abstract. J Vet Emerg Crit Care 2016;26(S1):S8.

13. Ward JL, Lisciandro GR, DeFrancesco TD. Distribution of alveolar-interstitial syndrome in dogs and cats with respiratory distress assessed with lung ultrasound versus thoracic radiographs. J Vet Emerg Crit Care 2018;28(5):415–28.

14. Dicker SA, Lisciandro GR, Newell SM, et al. Diagnosis of pulmonary contusions with point-of-care lung ultrasonography and thoracic radiography compared to thoracic computed tomography in dogs with motor vehicle trauma: 29 cases (2017-2018). J Vet Emerg Crit Care 2020;30(6):638–46.

15. Kulhavy DA, Lisciandro GR. Use of a lung ultrasound examination called Vet BLUE to screen for metastatic lung nodules in the emergency room. Abstract. J Vet Emerg Crit Care 2015;25(S1):S14.

16. Vezzosi T, Mannucci A, Pistoresi F, et al. Assessment of lung ultrasound B-lines in dogs with different stages of chronic valvular heart disease. J Vet Intern Med 2017;31(3):700–4.

17. Rademacher N, Pariaut R, Pate J, et al. Transthoracic lung ultrasound in normal dogs and dogs with cardiogenic pulmonary edema: a pilot study. Vet Radiol Ultrasound 2014;55(4):447–52.

18. Lichtenstein DA, Meziere GA. Relevance of lung ultrasound in the diagnosis of acute respiratory failure: the BLUE protocol. Chest 2008;134(1):117–25.

19. Volpicelli G, Elbarbary M, Blaivas M, et al. International evidence-based recommendations for point-of-care lung ultrasound. Intensive Care Med 2012;38: 577–91.

20. Balk DS, Lee C, SchaferJ, et al. Kung ultrasound compared to chest X-ray for diagnosis of pediatric pneumonia: a meta-analysis. Pediatr Pulmonol 2018; 53(8):1130–9.

21. Nouvenne A, Zani MD, Milanese G, et al. Lung ultrasound in COVID-19 pneumonia: correlations with chest CT on hospital admissions. Respiration 2020; 99(7):617–24.

22. Vetrugno L, Bove T, Orso D, et al. Our Italian experience using lung ultrasound for identification, grading and serial follow-up of severity of lung involvement for management of patients with COVID-19. Echocardiography 2020;37(4):625–7.

23. Chavez MA, Shams N, Ellington LE, et al. Lung ultrasound for the diagnosis of pneumonia in adults: a systematic review and meta-analysis. Respir Res 2014; 15(1):50.

24. Stadler J, Andronikou S, Zar HJ. Lung ultrasound for the diagnosis of community-acquired pneumonia in children. Pedriatr Radiol 2017;47(11):1412–9.

25. Soldati G, Smargiassi A, Inchingolo R, et al. Proposal for international standardization of the use of lung ultrasound for patients with COVID-19: A simple, quantitive, reproducible method. Ultrasound Med 2020;39(7):1413–9.

26. Cardinale L, Priola AM, Moretti F, et al. Effectiveness of chest radiography, lung ultrasound and thoracic computed tomography in the diagnosis of congestive heart failure. World J Radiol 2014;6(6):230–7.

27. Lichtenstein DA. BLUE-protocol and FALLS-protocol: two applications of lung ultrasound in the critically ill. Chest 2015;147(6):1659–70.

28. Gargani L, Pang PS, Frassi F, et al. Persistent pulmonary congestion before discharge predicts rehospitalization in heart failure: a lung ultrasound study. Cardiovasc Ultrasound 2015;4(13):40.

29. Murphy SD, Ward JL, Viall AK, et al. Utility of point-of-care ultrasound for monitoring cardiogenic pulmonary edema in dogs. J Vet Intern Med 2021;35(1):68–77.

30. Filly RA. Ultrasound: the stethoscope of the future, alas. Radiology 1988;167:400.

31. Moore CL, Copel JA. Point of care ultrasonography. N Eng J Med 2011;364: 749–57.

32. Tavares J, Ivo R, Gonzales F, et al. Global ultrasound check for the critically ill (GUCCI) – a new systematized protcol unifying point-of-care ultrasound in critcally ill patinets based on clinical presentation. Emerg Med 2019;10(11):133–45.

33. Narasimhan M, Koenig SJ, Mayo PH. A whole body approach to point of care ultrasound. Chest 2016;150(4):772–6.

34. Lichtenstein DA. Chapter 19: Basic applications of lung ultrasound in the critically ill -A bedside alternative to CT and other irradiating techniques. In: Lichtenstein DA, editor. Whole body ultrasonography in the critically ill. Verlag Berlin Heidelberg: Springer; 2010. p. 181–8.

35. Neelis DA, Mattoon JS, Nyland TG. Chapter 7: Thorax. In: Small animal diagnostic ultrasound 2014. Mattoon JS and Nyland TG, editors. Elsevier Saunders: Philadelphia PA, pp. 188–216.

36. Boysen S, McMurray J, Gommeren K. Abnormal curatin signs identified with a novel lung ultrasound protocol in 6 dogs with pneumothorax. Front Vet Sci 2019;6:291.

37. Pacholec C, Lisciandro GR, Masseau I, et al. Lung ultrasound nodule sign for detection of nodule pulmonary lesions in dogs: comparison to thoracic

radiography using computed tomography as the criterion standard. Vet J, in press 2021.

38. Lisciandro GR, Lisciandro SC. Chapter 23: POCUS: Vet BLUE-Clinical Integration. In: Lisciandro GR, editor. Point-of-care ultrasound Techniques for the small animal practitioner. 2nd edition. Ames IA: Wiley Blackwell; 2021. p. 459–508.
39. Demi M, Prediletto R, Soldati G, et al. Physical mechanisms providing clinical information from ultrasound lung images: Hypotheses and early confirmations. IEEE Trans Ultrason Ferroelectr Freq Control 2020;67(3):612–23.
40. Lichtenstein DA. Should lung ultrasonography be more widely used in the assessment of acute respiratory disease? Expert Rev Resp Med 2010;4(5): 533–8.
41. Lisciandro GR, Puchot ML, Gambino JM, et al. The wedge sign: a possible lung ultrasound sign for pulmonary thromboembolism. J Vet Emerg Crit Care, in press 2021.
42. Lichtenstein DA, Meziere G, Seitz J. The dynamic air bronchogram. A lung ultrasound signs of alveolar consolidation in ruling out atelectasis. Chest 2019;135(6): 1421–5.
43. Copetti R, Cominotto F, Meduri S, et al. The "survived lung": an ultrasound sign of "Bubbly Consolidation" pulmonary infarction. Ultrasound Med Biol 2020. https://doi.org/10.1016/j.ultrasmedbio.2020.04.036.
44. Reissig A, Heyne J, Kroegel C. Sonography of lung and pleura in pulmonary embolism: sonomorphologic characterization and comparison with spiral CT scanning. Chest 2001;120(6):1977–83.
45. Reissig A, Kroegel C. Transthoracic ultrasound of lung and pleura in the diagnosis of pulmonary embolism: a novel non-invasive bedside approach. Respiration 2003;70:441–52.
46. Lisciandro GR, Lisciandro GR. Chapter 36: POCUS: Global FAST-patient monitoring and staging. In: Point-of-care ultrasound Techniques for the small animal practitioner. 2nd edition. Ames IA: Wiley Blackwell; 2021. p. 685–728.

Lung Ultrasound for Pulmonary Contusions

Samuel A. Dicker, DVM, DACVECC

KEYWORDS

- Lung ultrasound • Pulmonary contusions • Thoracic trauma • Motor vehicle trauma
- Vet BLUE • Alveolar-interstitial syndrome

KEY POINTS

- Lung ultrasound has high sensitivity for rapidly detecting pulmonary contusions.
- Multiple veterinary and human studies suggest that lung ultrasound is more sensitive for pulmonary contusions than thoracic radiography.
- Lung ultrasound is portable, safe, and radiation-sparing.
- Lung ultrasound does not replace conventional radiography, especially for the diagnosis of skeletal trauma.
- Diagnosis of pulmonary contusions with lung ultrasound, like any imaging modality, has limitations, including pneumothorax, pleural effusion, atelectasis, subcutaneous emphysema, and concurrent pulmonary disease.

INTRODUCTION

Rapid and reliable diagnosis of pulmonary contusions (PC) is essential to any veterinarian treating trauma patients. PC occur commonly in dogs, cats, and humans that have sustained blunt force thoracic trauma.[1–9] In dogs, severity of PC on thoracic radiographs (TXR) has directly correlated with oxygen supplementation duration and hospitalization time.[1] In humans, severity of PC on thoracic computed tomography (TCT) is highly predictive of the need for mechanical ventilation and the development of acute respiratory distress syndrome.[2,3,10]

Lung ultrasound (LUS) has been documented to effectively and safely diagnose PC in multiple prospective animal and human studies with high sensitivity and high specificity. LUS relies on ultrasonographic artifacts to diagnose normal lung or lung with increased extravascular lung water (B-lines and signs of consolidation, including shred sign, tissue sign, nodule sign, and wedge sign) at the pulmonary-pleural surface.[6–9,11–23]

Portable ultrasonography has become standard of care in most small animal veterinary practices treating emergencies, and its increased prevalence is largely due to

Veterinary Emergency & Referral Group, 196 4th Avenue, Brooklyn, NY 11217, USA
E-mail address: dicker.sam@gmail.com

Vet Clin Small Anim 51 (2021) 1141–1151
https://doi.org/10.1016/j.cvsm.2021.07.001
vetsmall.theclinics.com

marked improvements in technology, image quality, as well as increased portability, affordability, and ubiquity of operator skill. The diagnosis of PC with LUS allows the clinician to obtain rapid and reliable information about the status of the patient's lungs. Point-of-care ultrasound (POCUS) can rapidly diagnose PC as well as concurrent injury to allow for ongoing resuscitative efforts without the immediate need for transporting the potentially unstable patient to the radiology suite. Furthermore, TXR requires patient positioning in various recumbencies, potential for worsened alveolar ventilation, increased patient stress, and potential staff exposure to radiation. Although TCT imaging times are shortening and image quality continues to improve, TCT is typically limited to referral practices and commonly uses some degree of patient restraint or sedation.

IMAGING FINDINGS

Most aspects of LUS remain the same regardless of imaging protocol. In brief, with normal lung, the pulmonary-pleural line is identified, which is where the visceral pulmonary pleura contacts the costal parietal pleura. As the animal breathes, the pulmonary-pleural line "slides" to and fro; this "lung sliding" or "pleural glide" sign indicates lack of pneumothorax (PTX). With PTX, the pulmonary-pleural lung sliding sign is absent. It should be noted that LUS diagnosis of PTX is highly correlative with sonographer experience and skill and is discussed later in the article.[7,8,24–26] A-lines are horizontal lines that originate from the pulmonary-pleural line and are air reverberation artifacts. A-lines are present with normal aerated lung and with PTX. When alveoli begin filling with edema, this creates an ultrasonographic artifact called B-lines (**Fig. 1**). B-lines are created by the ultrasound waves interacting with the fluid-air interface in the alveoli on the surface of lung that creates a hyperechoic, nonfading, laser-like, vertical line originating from the pulmonary-pleural line and extending to the bottom of the ultrasound screen. These B-lines move in synchrony with phases of respiration and obliterate A-lines. B-lines can be quantified and increase as pulmonary edema increases.[7,9,11–22] With an increasing amount of pulmonary edema, alveoli become devoid of air; the lung parenchyma can now be sonographically visualized, and it appears more tissuelike, similar to liver. LUS signs of consolidation have been termed "shred sign," representing an air bronchogram, and "tissue sign," representing hepatization.

Collectively, any fluid in the lung is termed alveolar-interstitial syndrome (AIS).[6–9,11–23] LUS identification of AIS is not necessarily diagnostic for PC because AIS may indicate any type of pulmonary edema. The cause of AIS in a particular patient must be correlated with anatomic locations of edema and patient signalment, history, as well as other physical examination and diagnostic imaging findings.[7] Because previous studies determined that small numbers of B-lines are occasionally seen in healthy dogs and cats with radiographically normal lungs, most studies suggest that there must be greater than 3 B-lines (or signs of consolidation) present in order to be considered positive for increased extravascular lung water (edema) on LUS.[15]

IMAGING PROTOCOLS
Veterinary Brief Lung Ultrasound Examination

The Veterinary Brief Lung Ultrasound Examination (Vet BLUE) protocol was adapted from the Bedside Lung Ultrasound Examination in people and was first described in dogs and cats by Lisciandro and colleagues.[12,15] The Vet BLUE protocol was used to study PC in a study of motor vehicle trauma in dogs.[7] The Vet BLUE protocol consists of 4 bilaterally applied thoracic acoustic windows (8 total acoustic windows),

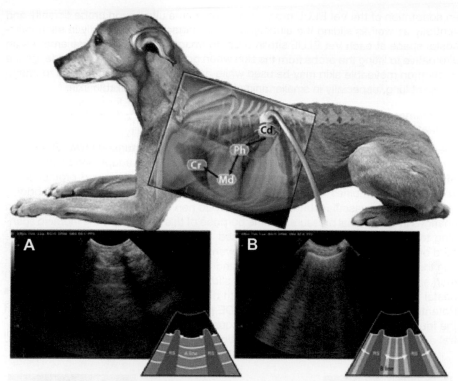

Fig. 1. The Vet BLUE. The patient may be in sternal recumbency or standing. The ultrasound probe is held horizontally (perpendicular to the long axis of the ribs) at 4 specific acoustic windows on each hemithorax. Lung pathologic condition is noted in real time. Ideally, video images are recorded for post hoc review ability. Below the illustration, still B-mode images with corresponding illustrations depict (*A*) normal LUS with no B-lines (*left*) compared with (*B*) abnormal LUS with B-lines (*right*). (Reproduced with permission from Ward JL, Lisciandro GR, Keene BW, et al. Accuracy of point-of-care lung ultrasonography for the diagnosis of cardiogenic pulmonary edema in dogs and cats with acute dyspnea. *J Am Vet Med Assoc* 2017;250(6):666-675.)

referred to as the caudodorsal (Cd), perihilar (Ph), middle (Md), and cranial (Cr) lung regions (see **Fig. 1**). Dogs are best imaged standing or in sternal recumbency to avoid atelectasis.[19,27] Hair is not clipped; the fur is parted to the skin, and a small amount of 70% isopropyl alcohol is applied at each acoustic window. If wounds are present, sterile ultrasound gel may be applied in lieu of alcohol. The ultrasound probe marker is directed cranially, and the probe is placed between 2 ribs, yielding the "gator sign," also described as the "bat sign" in human medical literature.[12,13,18,19] The ultrasound probe is fanned dorsally and ventrally to optimize visualization of the pulmonary-pleural line as well as to record the maximum number of B-lines at each acoustic window.[7,15]

A potential downfall of the Vet BLUE protocol is that the entire lung surface is not imaged, and acoustic windows are limited to 4 acoustic windows per hemithorax. However, the Vet BLUE protocol was designed to be rapid and easily repeated.[7] In addition, more recent adaptations of the Vet BLUE protocol include imaging at least 1 intercostal space cranial to and 1 intercostal space caudal to the initial acoustic window, limiting the amount of lung surface left unimaged.[20] The author typically performs an adaptation of the Vet BLUE protocol by fanning the ultrasound probe dorsally and ventrally as well as sliding the ultrasound probe dorsally and ventrally in each intercostal space at each Vet BLUE site in order to image more lung surface area. As an alternative to lifting the probe from the skin when good contact has been made, gentle traction on moveable skin may be used while moving the ultrasound probe to image adjacent lung, especially in smaller animals and animals with pliable skin.

Veterinary-Focused Assessment with Sonography for Trauma–Airway, Breathing, Circulation, Disability, and Exposure

The Veterinary-focused Assessment with Sonography for Trauma–Airway, Breathing, Circulation, Disability, and Exposure (VetFAST-ABCDE) is an adaptation of the FAST-ABCDE protocol used in human point-of-care emergency ultrasound protocols.[8,28] This protocol combines multiple POCUS techniques to assess thoracic and abdominal injury, cardiovascular status, as well as optic nerve diameter to assess presumed changes in intracranial pressure. For the purpose of this article, only the thoracic scanning technique (Breathing) will be discussed. For LUS, hair is clipped in the middle third of the thorax from the fourth to the seventh rib bilaterally (**Fig. 2**). In order to image the thorax, the skin is gently grasped and moved in several directions. The probe marker is directed cranially. The probe is slid dorsally and ventrally along the intercostal spaces between the fourth and ninth ribs on the left and right hemithoraces.[8] Potential downsides of the VetFAST-ABCDE protocol include only imaging between the fourth and ninth ribs (leaving certain acoustic windows, particularly the cranioventral and para-axillary regions, unimaged), time required to clip the patient's hair, and

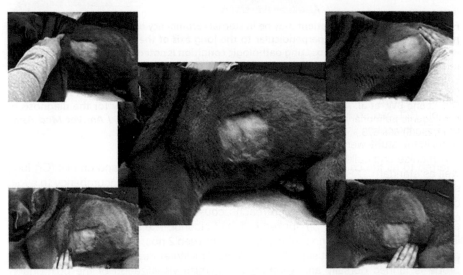

Fig. 2. Clipping fur is typically not required to perform a diagnostic LUS study. Parting of the fur usually provides an adequate acoustic window. The VetFAST-ABCDE protocol involves clipping fur in the center of each hemithorax and gently grasping and moving the skin to allow for visualization of all possible acoustic windows on the lateral aspects of the thorax. The ultrasound probe marker is directed cranially, and the probe is slid between the fourth and ninth intercostal spaces. (Reproduced with permission from Armenise A, Boysen RS, Rudloff E, et al. Veterinary-focused assessment with sonography for trauma-airway, breathing, circulation, disability and exposure: a prospective observational study in 64 canine trauma patients. J Small Amim Prac 2019;60:173-182.)

potentially unnecessarily clipping hair, which may be aesthetically unappealing to animal owners, especially in animals with minor injury that are ultimately not admitted to the hospital. An accurate LUS image is typically achievable without clipping hair.[7,15,17–25]

VETERINARY STUDIES

The study by Dicker and colleagues[7] was a prospective observational study examining the utility of LUS for diagnosing PC. The case population consisted of 29 dogs that sustained blunt force motor vehicle trauma and had thoracic imaging within 24 hours of presentation. Comparative imaging included LUS (Vet BLUE protocol), TXR, and TCT, and all 3 imaging modalities were completed within 30 minutes of one another. TCT was used as the gold standard. If PTX was identified on LUS, thoracocentesis was performed before full Vet BLUE protocol image acquisition. Dogs were considered positive for PC if greater than 3 total B-lines were identified. Twenty-one of 29 dogs were positive for PC on gold-standard TCT (72.4% prevalence). Vet BLUE was 90.5% sensitive (19/21 dogs) and 87.5% specific (7/8 dogs) for PC, whereas TXR was only 66.7% sensitive (14/21 dogs) and 87.5% specific (7/8 dogs) for PC. This study concluded that Vet BLUE had high sensitivity for diagnosis of PC, higher than TXR, and provided a reliable diagnosis of trauma-induced PC. Of the 32 dogs enrolled in the study, 3 dogs were excluded from statistical analyses. One dog had severe subcutaneous emphysema (SQE), and 2 dogs had large-volume pleural effusion (PE) (hemothorax). The Vet BLUE protocol used was an older protocol that surveyed only a single intercostal space at each Vet BLUE acoustic window; it is possible the newer, updated Vet BLUE protocol (imaging 1 intercostal space cranial and caudal to each Vet BLUE acoustic window) may have yielded higher sensitivity. Additional limiting factors for Vet BLUE are later discussed in this article.

LUS is limited to imaging the pulmonary-pleural surface and therefore only lung pathologic condition that reaches the lung periphery. Thus, LUS cannot detect deeper pulmonary pathologic condition. In this study, the radiologist examined if PC extended to the pulmonary-pleural interface on TCT. Interestingly, all 21 dogs true positive for PC on TCT had some degree of PC reach the pulmonary-parietal pleural interface on TCT, indicating that LUS *should* identify these as PC-positive dogs (**Fig. 3**). Two dogs in the study were falsely negative for PC on Vet BLUE for unexplained reasons.[7]

Armenise and colleagues[8] performed LUS using the VetFAST-ABCDE protocol as well as standard TXR on 64 dogs with blunt and/or penetrating trauma and reported similar findings. AIS consistent with PC were identified in 30/64 dogs (47% cases) on LUS and only 19/64 dogs (29.7% cases) on TXR. All of the dogs positive for PC on TXR were positive for PC on LUS. TCT was not used.[8] Both studies indicate that LUS has high sensitivity for diagnosis of PC, higher than TXR.[7,8]

HUMAN STUDIES

Multiple human trauma studies demonstrated the high sensitivity of LUS compared with the TCT "gold standard," and that LUS outperforms TXR for detecting PC.[6,9] In a study purely aimed at determining the diagnostic accuracy of PC, Soldati and colleagues[9] determined that LUS was 94.6% sensitive and 96.1% specific for identifying PC when compared with TCT, and TXR were 27% sensitive and 100% specific for PC. This study excluded patients with "PTX of any size or subcutaneous emphysema (SQE) large enough to compromise the quality of the examination, in the examiner's opinion."[9] However, SQE may be less problematic in dogs than in people. In the

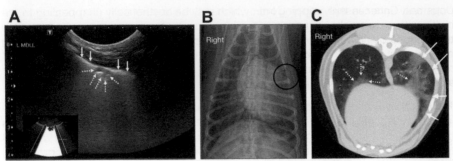

Fig. 3. A 2-year-old male neutered Chihuahua mix that was positive for PC on Vet BLUE, TXR, and TCT. (*A*) LUS image at the left Vet BLUE middle lung region with signs of consolidation (*dashed arrows*) and confluent B-lines (scored as infinite) (*solid arrows*). (*B*) Ventrodorsal TXR (combined with lateral radiographs, not shown) scored as positive for PC with an alveolar pattern in the right Vet BLUE caudodorsal and left Vet BLUE middle lung regions (*circle*). (*C*) Thoracic CT image of PC in both the left and the right lungs. Some degree of PC (*solid arrows*) reaches the pulmonary-pleural surface, and other regions of PC are more central (*dashed arrows*), the latter which are not visible with LUS. (Reproduced with permission from Dicker SA, Lisciandro GR, Newell SM, Johnson JA. Diagnosis of pulmonary contusions with point-of-care lung ultrasonography and thoracic radiography compared to thoracic computed tomography in dogs with motor vehicle trauma: 29 Cases (2017-2018). J Vet Emerg Crit Care. 2020;1–9.)

original Thoracic Focused Assessment with Sonography for Trauma (TFAST) study, 5% (7/138) of dogs had SQE, none of which were disqualified from TFAST imaging.[24] The investigators stated that gentle probe pressure displaced the SQE in order to identify the pulmonary-pleural line, allowing for PTX and LUS assessment.[24]

LUS has the ability to diagnose multiple manifestations of thoracic trauma, including PC, PTX, and hemothorax in human trauma patients. Hyacinthe and colleagues concluded that LUS had greater sensitivity than combined clinical examination and chest radiography for the diagnosis of PC.[6] LUS was 61% sensitive and 80% specific for diagnosis of PC, whereas clinical examination and TXR were 29% sensitive and 94% specific for diagnosis of PC. The investigators postulated that LUS achieved a lower sensitivity compared with previous studies (such as Soldati and colleagues[9]) because these studies excluded certain patients, such as those with SQE or those who required mechanical ventilation.[6,9] Furthermore, the investigators emphasized that PTX or hemothorax may have prevented a diagnosis of PC. The study findings highlight that multiple manifestations of thoracic trauma are often present in a single patient, and PC are often accompanied by limiting confounding variables, such as PTX, PE, and SQE (see next section, Limitations and Confounding Variables).[6]

LIMITATIONS AND CONFOUNDING VARIABLES
Pneumothorax

Because ultrasound poorly penetrates air, PTX precludes ultrasonographic visualization of the lung parenchyma and renders is it impossible to assess for PC at affected acoustic windows. Therefore, the clinician's proper identification of PTX via LUS is of utmost importance as to not mistake lack of pulmonary pathologic condition with normal aerated lung surface. Ultrasonographic evidence of PTX is diagnosed by lack of "lung sliding" and identifying the "lung point" along with other LUS imaging strategies (see Søren R Boysen's article, "Lung Ultrasound for Pneumothorax in

Dogs and Cats," in this issue). Correct ultrasonographic identification of PTX varies highly with sonographer experience and study protocol. These studies suggest and the author's opinion is that experienced sonographers infrequently misidentify clinically relevant PTX.[8,24–26] Therapeutic thoracocentesis allows for visualizing the pulmonary parenchyma; however, an indeterminate amount of time may be required for atelectasis to resolve (see the later section Atelectasis).[7,27]

Pleural Effusion

PE may be identified with any imaging modality, and LUS is no exception. Hemothorax is not an uncommon manifestation of thoracic trauma. PE can cause pressure atelectasis, causing an increased "fluid-air" artifact as seen with pulmonary AIS. Thus, PE may lead to B-lines or even signs of lung consolidation deep to the PE on the ultrasound screen, making a true diagnosis of PC confounded.[6,7] Large volumes of PE may require therapeutic thoracocentesis if clinically indicated. Serial LUS may help differentiate pressure atelectasis from true PC postdrainage techniques with atelectasis likely to resolve more quickly than PC.

Subcutaneous Emphysema

SQE is not uncommon with trauma. In the case of SQE, air artifact in the subcutaneous space potentially creates "E-lines," which are vertical hyperechoic beams similar to B-lines.[23] These E-lines do not move synchronously with respiration and originate from the subcutaneous tissue rather than the pulmonary-pleural line. As a general rule, if the pulmonary-pleural line (ie, gator sign) cannot be identified, then LUS cannot be performed accurately. Moreover, SQE may be noted on physical examination. SQE is generally surmountable with gentle ultrasound probe pressure that displaces the subcutaneous air so that the pulmonary-pleural line may be accurately identified.[24] In patients with SQE over rib fractures, the sonographer can avoid additional ultrasound probe pressure to avoid patient discomfort.[7]

Cutaneous Wounds

In cases of open wounds or degloving injuries, the clinician must make a judgment as to whether ultrasound imaging may cause more harm, such as causing pain or nosocomial wound contamination. If wounds are small, isopropyl alcohol may be substituted with an aqueous-based sterile ultrasound gel. The ultrasound probe should either be clean or covered with a sterile probe cover (or surgical glove).

Underlying Comorbidities

Although increased numbers of B-lines in trauma are likely PC, they are not pathognomonic and may indicate increased extravascular lung water of various causes, including acute or chronic pulmonary conditions. LUS serves as an excellent screening and monitoring tool for lung surface pathologic condition in traumatized dogs, but the presence of AIS does not necessarily indicate PC.[7,8,11–23] Dogs who sustain trauma, particularly those involved in motor vehicle trauma, are typically young dogs unlikely to have pulmonary or cardiac disease.[17,18,20–22] In an epidemiologic study in the United Kingdom, the median age for dogs in road traffic accidents was 2.5 years.[29] In 1 study, dogs with motor vehicle trauma had a mean age of 3.3 years (±3.0 years, standard deviation).[7] Another study describes the median age of trauma patients was 4 years.[8] Thus, younger dogs having recently sustained trauma with AIS on LUS likely indicate PC, but other manifestations of trauma, such as neurogenic pulmonary edema (eg, head trauma), negative pressure pulmonary edema (eg, strangulation or drowning), or nontraumatic causes of AIS, should be considered. Patient history, signalment, and the entire clinical profile are necessary when diagnosing PC on any imaging modality for accurate interpretation.

Atelectasis

Areas of lung atelectasis may yield a false positive for AIS or PC on any imaging modality. Atelectasis causes an increased "fluid-air" artifact as seen with AIS. Atelectasis is typically affected by recumbency, sedation, and patient ventilatory capability.[30] An advantage of LUS compared with TXR or TCT is that sedation is not required, and patients are typically imaged in sternal recumbency or standing to avoid atelectasis.[7] Examples of trauma patients that may have atelectasis on presentation include patients in lateral recumbency for a prolonged period of time, those hypoventilating, or those having received sedation.[30–32]

OTHER IMAGING MODALITIES

LUS for diagnosis of PC in conjunction with other POCUS protocols (ie, AFAST [Abdominal Focused Assessment with Sonography for Trauma], TFAST) is an excellent triage tool for rapid, reliable, and real-time results.[25,33] Although most trauma patients are destined for radiography, LUS is particularly useful for initial and serial assessment of hospitalized trauma patients without the delay in imaging and potential risk of transportation to the radiology suite. LUS, however, does not replace conventional TXR or advanced imaging, such as TCT, for thoracic trauma patients, especially for assessing skeletal fractures, diaphragmatic hernia, and mediastinal injuries. Additional imaging, such as TXR and TCT, when indicated, should be used in conjunction with LUS and other FAST findings.[34,35]

USE OF ACOUSTIC COUPLING MEDIUM

Large amounts of acoustic coupling medium are seldom needed and should be avoided. Isopropyl alcohol, ultrasound gel, and sterile saline are often used as acoustic coupling medium for ultrasound. The author rarely uses ultrasound gel for LUS because only certain acoustic windows are imaged. The patient's skin can often be gently moved to image multiple acoustic windows. The hair can most often be parted to the skin at the intended acoustic window, and isopropyl alcohol can be applied in a small quantity. Many animals being screened for PC are in shock or respiratory distress. Application of large volumes of isopropyl alcohol is unnecessary for most LUS imaging and may cause or worsen hypothermia. Alcohol fumes may be noxious to both the operator and the animal, especially if the animal is then placed into a confined oxygen kennel. Furthermore, isopropyl alcohol is flammable and thus serves as a fire hazard if electrical defibrillation is subsequently needed.[36]

SUMMARY

LUS is a rapid and reliable way to diagnose PC in patients who have sustained trauma, especially in young dogs with low probability of preexisting pulmonary comorbidities. LUS diagnosis of PC exceeds that of TXR in multiple animal and human studies. Diagnosis of PC with LUS is an essential tool for any small animal emergency clinician, and it may be easily learned. The sonographer should understand potential caveats for proper diagnosis of LUS with PC, including PTX, PE, atelectasis, and SQE. LUS does not replace conventional TXR or TCT, especially for diagnosis of skeletal trauma and deeper pulmonary pathologic condition. LUS should be used concurrently with other POCUS trauma protocols to rapidly optimize the clinician's assessment of the patient's clinical picture.

DISCLOSURE

The author discloses no conflicts of interest.

REFERENCES

1. Powell LL, Rozanski EA, Tidwell AS, et al. A retrospective analysis of pulmonary contusions secondary to motor vehicle accidents in 143 dogs: 1994–1997. J Vet Emerg Crit Care (San Antonio) 1999;9(3):127–36.
2. Hamrick MC, Duhn RD, Ochsner MG. Critical evaluation of pulmonary contusion in the early post-traumatic period: risk of assisted ventilation. Am Surg 2009; 75(11):1054–8.
3. Wang S, Ruan Z, Zhang J, et al. The value of pulmonary contusion volume measurements with three-dimensional computed tomography in predicting acute respiratory distress syndrome development. Ann Thorac Surg 2009;92(6):1977–83.
4. Sigrist NE, Doherr MG, Spreng DE. Clinical findings and diagnostic value of post-traumatic thoracic radiographs in dogs and cats with blunt trauma. J Vet Emerg Crit Care (San Antonio) 2004;14(4):259–68.
5. Schild H, Strunk H, Weber W, et al. Pulmonary contusion: CT vs plain radiogram. J Comput Assist Tomogr 1989;13(3):417–20.
6. Hyacinthe A, Broux C, Francony G, et al. Diagnostic accuracy of ultrasonography in the acute assessment of common thoracic lesions after trauma. Chest 2012; 141(5):1177–83.
7. Dicker SA, Lisciandro GR, Newell SM, et al. Diagnosis of pulmonary contusions with point-of-care lung ultrasonography and thoracic radiography compared to thoracic computed tomography in dogs with motor vehicle trauma: 29 cases (2017-2018). J Vet Emerg Crit Care (San Antonio) 2020;30(6):638–46.
8. Armenise A, Boysen RS, Rudloff E, et al. Veterinary-focused assessment with sonography for trauma-airway, breathing, circulation, disability and exposure: a prospective observational study in 64 canine trauma patients. J Small Anim Pract 2019;60:173–82.
9. Soldati G, Testa A, Silva FR, et al. Chest ultrasonography in lung contusion. Chest 2006;130(2):533–8.
10. Croce MA, Fabian TC, Davis KA, et al. Early and late acute respiratory distress syndrome: two distinct clinical entities. J Trauma 1999;46(3):361–8.
11. Volpicelli G, Mussa A, Garofalo G, et al. Bedside lung ultrasound in the assessment of alveolar-interstitial syndrome. Am J Emerg Med 2006;24(6):689–96.
12. Lichtenstein DA, Meziere GA. Relevance of lung ultrasound in the diagnosis of acute respiratory failure: the BLUE protocol. Chest 2008;134(1):117–25.
13. Volpicelli G, Elbarbary M, Blaivas M, et al. International evidence-based recommendations for point-of-care lung ultrasound. Intensive Care Med 2012;38(4): 577–91.
14. Ball CG, Ranson KM, Rodriguez-Galvez M, et al. Sonographic depiction of post-traumatic alveolar-interstitial disease: the handheld diagnosis of a pulmonary contusion. J Trauma 2009;66(3):962.
15. Lisciandro GR, Fosgate GT, Fulton RM. Frequency and number of ultrasound lung rockets (B-lines) using a regionally based lung ultrasound examination named Vet BLUE (Veterinary Bedside Lung Ultrasound Exam) in dogs with radiographically normal lung findings. Vet Radiol Ultrasound 2014;55(3):315–22.

16. Jambrik Z, Monti S, Coppola V, et al. The usefulness of ultrasound lung comets as a nonradiologist sign of extravascular lung water. Am J Cardiol 2004;93(10): 1265–70.

17. Vezzosi T, Mannucci T, Pistoresi A, et al. Assessment of lung ultrasound B-lines in dogs with different stages of chronic valvular heart disease. J Vet Intern Med 2017;31(3):700–4.

18. Lisciandro GR, Fulton RM, Fosgate GT, et al. Frequency and number of B-lines using a regionally based lung ultrasound examination in cats with radiographically normal lungs compared to cats with left-sided congestive heart failure. J Vet Emerg Crit Care (San Antonio) 2017;27(5):499–505.

19. Lisciandro GR. The Vet BLUE lung scan. In: Lisciandro GR, editor. Focused ultrasound techniques for the small animal practitioner. Ames (IA): Wiley-Blackwell; 2014. p. 166–88.

20. Ward JL, Lisciandro GR, Keene BW, et al. Accuracy of point-of-care lung ultrasonography for the diagnosis of cardiogenic pulmonary edema in dogs and cats with acute dyspnea. J Am Vet Med Assoc 2017;250(6):666–75.

21. Ward JL, Lisciandro GR, DeFranceso TD. Distribution of alveolar-interstitial syndrome in dogs and cats with respiratory distress as assessed by lung ultrasound versus thoracic radiographs. J Vet Emerg Crit Care (San Antonio) 2018;28(5): 415–28.

22. Rademacher N, Pariaut R, Pate J, et al. Transthoracic lung ultrasound in normal dogs and dogs with cardiogenic pulmonary edema: a pilot study. Vet Radiol Ultrasound 2014;55(4):447–52.

23. Francisco MJ, Rahal A, Vieira FA, et al. Advances in lung ultrasound. Einstein (Sao Paulo) 2016;14(3):443–8.

24. Lisciandro GR, Lagutchik MS, Mann KA, et al. Evaluation of a Thoracic Focused Assessment with Sonography for Trauma (TFAST) protocol to detect pneumothorax and concurrent thoracic injury in 145 traumatized dogs. J Vet Emerg Crit Care (San Antonio) 2008;18(3):258–69.

25. Walters AM, O'Brien MA, Selmic LE, et al. Evaluation of the agreement between focused assessment with sonography for trauma (AFAST/TFAST) and computed tomography in dogs and cats with recent trauma. J Vet Emerg Crit Care (San Antonio) 2018;28(5):429–35.

26. Lisciandro GR. Evaluation of initial and serial Combination Focused Assessment with Sonography for Trauma (CFAST) examination of the thorax (TFAST) and abdomen (AFAST) with the application of an abdominal fluid scoring system in 49 traumatized cats [Abstract]. J Vet Emerg Crit Care (San Antonio) 2012; 22(2):S11.

27. Lisciandro GR, Fosgate GT. Use of Vet BLUE protocol for the detection of lung atelectasis and sonographic gallbladder wall evaluation for anaphylaxis and volume overload in 63 dogs undergoing general anesthesia. Abstract. J Vet Emerg Crit Care (San Antonio) 2018;28:S15–6.

28. Neri L, Storti E, Lichtenstein D. Toward an ultrasound curriculum for critical care medicine. Crit Care Med 2007;35(5 Suppl):S290–304.

29. Harris GL, Brodbelt D, Church D, et al. Epidemiology, clinical management, and outcomes of dogs involved in road traffic accidents in the United Kingdom (2009-2014). J Vet Emerg Crit Care 2018;28(2):140–8.

30. Staffieri F, Driessen B, Monte VD, et al. Effects of positive end-expiratory pressure on anesthesia-induced atelectasis and gas exchange in anesthetized and mechanically ventilated sheep. Am J Vet Res 2010;71(8):867–74.

31. Monte VD, Bufalari A, Grasso S, et al. Respiratory effects of low versus high tidal volume with or without positive end-expiratory pressure in anesthetized dogs with healthy lungs. Am J Vet Res 2018;79(5):496–504.
32. Lisciandro GR, Romero LA, Bridgeman CH. Pilot study: Vet BLUE profiles pre- and post-anesthesia in 31 dogs undergoing surgical sterilization. Abstract. J Vet Emerg Crit Care 2015;25:S8–9.
33. Boysen SR, Lisciandro GR. The use of ultrasound in the emergency room (AFAST and TFAST). Vet Clin North Am Small Anim Pract 2013;43(4):773–97.
34. Exadaktylos AK, Sclabas G, Schmid SW, et al. Do we really need routine computed tomographic scanning in the primary evaluation of blunt chest trauma in patients with "normal" chest radiograph? J Trauma 2001;51(6):1173–6.
35. Yeguiayan J-M, Yap A, Freysz M, et al. Impact of whole-body computed tomography on mortality and surgical management of severe blunt trauma. Crit Care 2012;16(3):R101.
36. Drobatz K. Heat Stroke. In: Silverstein DC, Hopper K, editors. Small animal critical care medicine. 2nd edition. St Louis (MO): Elsevier; 2015. p. 798.

Lung Ultrasonography for Pneumothorax in Dogs and Cats

Søren R. Boysen, DVM, DACVECC

KEYWORDS

- Pneumothorax • Lung sliding • Glide sign • Lung point • Pleura
- Lung ultrasonography • Curtain sign

KEY POINTS

- The most sensitive sites for air to accumulate should be assessed to avoid missing the presence of pneumothorax, and a thorough understanding of how to interpret normal and pneumothorax-associated findings is required to arrive at an accurate diagnosis.
- Although ultrasonography is more sensitive and specific than radiographs for diagnosis of pneumothorax in human medicine, the reported accuracy in veterinary medicine is variable and likely depends on the criteria used to assess pneumothorax.
- Pneumothorax is essentially ruled out if lung sliding, a lung pulse, and/or B lines/lung consolidations are present at the sites where air is most likely to accumulate within the pleural space.
- Detecting a lung point, reverse lung sliding, asynchronous signs, and double curtain signs can help confirm pneumothorax in small animals when the diagnosis is uncertain.
- Training and experience play a role in the accuracy of lung ultrasonography for the diagnosis of pneumothorax.

 Video content accompanies this article at http://www.vetsmall.theclinics.com.

INTRODUCTION

Research in human medicine shows lung ultrasonography (LUS) has clear advantages compared with other imaging modalities for the diagnosis of pneumothorax (PTX), including speed, repeatability, real-time point-of-care scanning and interpretation, absence of radiation exposure, and lower cost compared with computed tomography (CT).[1–3] Furthermore, meta-analysis of adult and neonate studies comparing LUS and thoracic radiographs with CT show LUS outperforms radiographs for the diagnosis of PTX, with a pooled sensitivity (Se) and specificity (Sp) of 75% to 91%, 97% to 99% and 40% to 82%, 96% to 100%, respectively.[3–7] Although the Se and Sp of LUS

Veterinary Emergency and Critical Care, Department of Veterinary Clinical and Diagnostic Sciences, University of Calgary, 11877 85 Street NW, Calgary, AB T3R 1J3, USA
E-mail address: srboysen@ucalgary.ca

Vet Clin Small Anim 51 (2021) 1153–1167
https://doi.org/10.1016/j.cvsm.2021.07.003
0195-5616/21/© 2021 Elsevier Inc. All rights reserved.

are high, the accuracy varies with operator experience and the LUS criteria used to rule in or rule out the diagnosis.[1,3,5,6] The PTX LUS criteria used in human studies include B-mode findings of lung sliding, B lines, lung pulse, lung point, double lung point, pseudo–curtain sign, and mirrored ribs (neonates only), and M-mode ultrasonography findings of the barcode and seashore signs.[3,5,6,8–11] Each of these specific criteria are described in detail later. Using multiple criteria is recommended, particularly when LUS is performed by novice sonographers, because research shows combining the results of multiple LUS PTX criteria outperforms any single criterion.[1,3,5]

In contrast with human medicine, evidence-based recommendations and the accuracy of LUS to diagnose PTX in veterinary medicine are limited, being derived from 6 published studies with small patient populations; 4 clinical studies, 1 case series, and an experimental study of induced PTX in dogs.[12–17] All 4 clinical studies report only the absence of lung sliding for the diagnosis of PTX, and the true Se and Sp are hindered by a failure to compare findings with accepted reference standards, and/or by the inclusion of only small case numbers.[12–15] A case series published in dogs describes the unique identification of abnormal curtain signs as well as the lung point in addition to the absence of lung sliding to diagnose PTX; however, comparison of these findings with a reference standard was not reported and the case series included only 6 dogs.[16] A well-controlled experimental study that induced small-volume PTX (2–10 mL/kg of air) in dogs under anesthesia (n = 9) described the novel finding of the reverse sliding sign as well as lung sliding, lung pulse, lung point, and the barcode sign compared with CT; however, translation of these findings to patients with naturally occurring and larger-volume PTX in the clinical setting has not been performed.[17] This latter study does suggest LUS is more Se (89% vs 67%) and equally Sp (89%) to radiographs compared with CT when all LUS criteria are combined to diagnose PTX in dogs.[17] There is even less information available regarding LUS to diagnose PTX in cats, being restricted to 2 small clinical studies that were combined with findings from dogs, neither of which reports any cats with confirmed PTX.[12,15] A comparison of LUS criteria reported in human medicine versus cats and dogs is discussed later, which highlights some of the major unanswered research questions that remain to be investigated in veterinary medicine.

TRADITIONAL LUNG ULTRASONOGRAPHY CRITERIA TO DIAGNOSE PNEUMOTHORAX
B-mode Findings

Lung sliding
Lung sliding, also referred to as the glide sign in veterinary medicine, is the most widely applied criterion to diagnose PTX in humans and veterinary patients.[3–5,12–15] The principle of lung sliding is based on 2 key concepts: (1) when the 2 pleura (parietal and visceral) are in their normal anatomic locations, the space that separates them is not sonographically visible, meaning the 2 pleura are indistinguishable from each other and appear as a single white line (the pleural line); and (2) lung sliding is a dynamic finding and therefore only valid when the patient breathes, causing the lung to slide along the thoracic wall with the respiratory cycle. The sliding of the lung along the thoracic wall causes the pleural line (composed of the parietal and visceral pleura) to shimmer. Therefore, the presence of lung sliding (shimmering) with the respiratory cycle confirms the lungs are in contact with the thoracic wall, ruling out the presence of PTX (and other pleural space disorders) at that probe location (Video 1).

Lung sliding in humans. Overall, the absence of lung sliding is very Se for the diagnosis of PTX in people, with reported values as high as 100%.[3–5] However, much lower sensitivities have also been reported (47%–59%), which is likely explained by insufficient lung regions and/or the most sensitive sites for accumulation of air in the pleural space not being assessed, particularly when small-volume pneumothoraces are present.[3,18–20] Placing the probe below the region of free pleural air in patients with small-volume PTX detects the presence of lung sliding and leads the operator to erroneously rule out PTX for that hemithorax.[3,18] This point stresses the importance of scanning the most sensitive sites for air to accumulate and performing serial examinations to detect expanding pneumothoraces that might have initially been missed. Alternatively, it has been suggested that the presence of partial lung sliding associated with the lung point may be mistaken for true lung sliding, leading operators to mistakenly rule out PTX when the lung point actually confirms its presence (lung point is discussed later).[19] It is therefore essential to ensure the correct sites is scanned, sufficient lung regions are scanned, and the operator is comfortable with the sonographic difference between lung sliding and the lung point.

With PTX, the visceral pleura is separated from the parietal pleura by air, which renders it invisible to ultrasonography. In this situation, the pleural line is comprised of only the parietal pleura; however, it appears identical to a pleural line comprised of both pleura: it is the dynamic presence of lung sliding with the respiratory cycle that makes it possible to determine that the 2 pleura are in contact. The absence of lung sliding has a Sp of 88% to 98% for the diagnosis of PTX in people, indicating other disorders can result in a loss of lung sliding. For example, bullous emphysema, pleural adherences, single lung lobe intubation (unilateral loss of sliding only), acute respiratory distress syndrome (ARDS), subcutaneous emphysema, massive atelectasis, asthma, and previous pleurodesis have all been reported to result in the loss of lung sliding.[21–24] In critically ill humans, lung sliding is reportedly impaired in 21% to 40% of patients with ARDS or extensive pneumonia and the Sp decreases from 91% in the general population to 78% in intensive care unit patients and 60% in patients with ARDS.[21,24] Therefore, lung sliding is absent when the probe is situated over a PTX but can also be absent with disorders other than PTX. If lung sliding is absent and a diagnosis of PTX is suspected but not confirmed based on other history, clinical findings, and imaging modalities, additional LUS findings that rule in PTX should be sought, provided the patient is sufficiently stable to permit a search for these findings. However, with appropriate history and clinical findings, thoracocentesis should be performed if the patient is unstable and a loss of lung sliding is noted.[19]

The study population has also been shown to affect the Se and Sp of absent lung sliding, with the Sp being higher and the Se lower in patients with trauma compared with non–trauma-related pneumothoraces.[3,25] This finding is likely caused by populations with traumatic PTX are younger and have fewer confounding disorders such as pleural adhesions, and comprehensive evaluations for absent lung sliding are less likely in patients with trauma because of these patients being immobilized and receiving other emergency interventions that interfere with scanning.[3,5,18,26] Similarly, the Se and Sp are reportedly higher in neonates, likely because confounding lung disorders are less likely and larger areas of lung can be more rapidly evaluated.[6,10]

Small animals. Lung sliding has been assessed in 4 clinical small animal veterinary studies, a single case report, and 1 experimental study. However, because of lack of a reference standard (CT) in the 2 larger clinical canine studies (n = 32[13] and n = 29[14]) and the inclusion of mixed patient populations (cats and dogs) combined with small sample sizes in the 2 remaining clinical studies (n = 3 and 6),[12,15] the true Se and Sp of absent lung sliding to diagnose PTX in small animal patients remains unknown. In an experimental study using anesthetized dogs (n = 9) with induced PTX using infused volumes of 2, 5, and 10 mL/kg of room air through a surgically placed thoracostomy tube, the Se of absent lung sliding for detection of PTX was 11%, 56%, 67%, respectively, with an Sp of 89% regardless of the volume of air infused.[17] This study suggests the absence of lung sliding may be less sensitive in dogs than in humans, particularly with small-volume PTX, but becomes more evident as the volume of PTX increases. However, the impact of thoracostomy tubes and anesthesia on detection of lung sliding was not discussed. A small case series in dogs (n = 6) found absence of lung sliding to be equivocal in 2 cases of confirmed PTX, which also suggests further research is required to determine the accuracy of absent lung sliding to diagnose PTX.[16] Furthermore, to the authors knowledge, the incidence of absent lung sliding in critically ill small animal patients without PTX has not be determined, although rapid shallow breathing and/or panting are reported to make assessment of lung sliding more challenging.[13] Further research in small animals is needed to determine the accuracy of absent lung sliding to diagnose PTX, and whether other confounding conditions in critically ill spontaneously breathing and positive pressure–ventilated patients can cause a loss of lung sliding unrelated to PTX, as noted in humans.

B lines

B lines, occasionally referred to as lung rockets, comet-tail artifacts, and ring-down artifact, are defined by the following 5 criteria: (1) they are unfading vertical white (hyperechoic) lines that (2) originate at the lung surface, (3) move in synchrony with lung sliding (swing to and fro with the respiratory cycle), (4) extend to the far field, and (5) obscure A lines if present. The first 3 criteria are considered obligatory by most investigators, whereas the last 2 criteria are most often, but not always, present.[21,27] Because B lines arise from the lung surface, if they also originate from the pleural line, it indicates the lung surface must be in contact with the thoracic wall (Video 2). Most human studies describe the absence of B lines and lung sliding when considering the diagnosis of PTX,[3,5] which is unfortunately not the case in veterinary medicine. The 4 clinical small animal studies published to date used only the absence of lung sliding in the materials and methods, and/or failed to record the presence or absence of B lines in the results to support a diagnosis of PTX.[12–15] The presence or absence of B lines was reported in a case series of 6 dogs, although their ability to rule out PTX was not discussed.[16] For consistency and standardization between studies, the presence or absence of B lines for assessment of PTX in small animals should be specifically stated and reported along with the absence of lung siding and other LUS findings: the diagnosis of PTX necessitates that lung sliding, lung pulse, and B lines be absent, because the finding of even a single B line rules out PTX at the probe location.[3,13,21] However, because the application of LUS for assessing PTX is focused to sites where air is most likely to accumulate, and B lines only occur at sporadic locations in healthy individuals, and in low numbers, most healthy patients, as well as patients with PTX, lack B lines at the most sensitive sites for evaluation of PTX (their absence does not confirm PTX).[21,28–30] However, the incidence of B lines is higher in patients with trauma because underlying pulmonary contusions are often present, which is advantageous to both rule out PTX and identify the lung point (discussed later in relation to lung point).[14,16] In summary, similar to lung sliding, the presence of B lines rules out PTX at the probe location; however, the absence of B lines does not confirm the diagnosis, and other LUS findings should be considered along with history and clinical findings.

Lung pulse

Although not widely assessed in human or veterinary literature, the lung pulse, defined as the rhythmic movement of the visceral pleura in opposition to the parietal in synchrony with the cardiac rhythm, has been used to assess patients for PTX (Video 3).[1,3,6,10,17,21] In essence, the lung pulse can be considered a mini–lung slide that occurs independent of true lung sliding. Similar to lung sliding and B lines, the presence of a lung pulse rules out PTX when visible at the probe location, and supports a diagnosis of PTX when it is absent. It has been used in the diagnosis of atelectasis and single lung lobe intubation where lung sliding is absent over the nonintubated lung because of lack of air flow through the lung lobes, but the lung pulse is still visible.[21] The limitation of the lung pulse is that it is more difficult to identify at lung regions more distal from the heart, which is where uncontained pleural air tends to accumulate, and it is not present in well aerated lung where lung sliding becomes dominant and the lung is resistant to cardiac vibrations.[31] Therefore, similar to lung sliding with the respiratory cycle, the absence of the lung pulse is Se but not Sp for PTX. The lung pulse has not been clinically assessed in small animals. An experimental study in anesthetized dogs showed that the overall Se and Sp for the absence of a lung pulse in small-volume to moderate-volume PTX (2–10 mL/kg) was identical to the Se and Sp for the absence of lung sliding (44.4% and 88.8%, respectively).[17] The lung pulse requires further clinical research in small animal patients.

Lung point

The lung point is defined as the site within the thorax where the visceral pleura of the lung recontacts the parietal pleura of the thoracic wall in patients with PTX.[13,21,31] It is sonographically identified as a clear demarcation or sudden appearance of lung sliding that is seen at the transition from PTX to lung along the lateral thoracic wall.[21,31] The PTX side of a lung point always appears as an absence of lung sliding, absence of a lung pulse, and absence of B lines, with or without the identification of A lines (A lines can be made to appear or disappear depending on the angle of insonation between the ultrasound beams and the pleural line). In contrast, the lung side of a lung point varies in appearance depending on the underlying state of lung; it may appear as lung sliding and/or a lung pulse with or without visible A lines (eg, when spontaneous PTX is the cause; **Fig. 1**A, Video 4), or lung sliding with B lines and/or lung consolidation (eg, when pulmonary contusions or other lung disorders are present; see **Fig. 1**B, Video 5).[16] When a region of lung with an absence of lung sliding, lung pulse, and B lines is identified in patients with appropriate history and clinical findings, the probe should gradually be moved toward the hilus of the lung until fleeting, sudden inspiratory visualization of either lung sliding or B lines/consolidation is seen in an area where the absence of these signs was previously visualized.[32]

Although the Sp reported for the lung point in humans with PTX is very high (94%–100%), the Se is variable (15%–100%) and generally considered low to moderate.[3,6,10,33] A review of the human literature shows the lung point is often not identified, or is excluded from LUS studies.[3,5,34] Several studies suggest the focused nature of LUS to diagnose PTX, lack of training to correctly differentiate the lung point from lung sliding or the curtain sign, and the time and difficulty many operators experience in trying to identify the lung point preclude its routine use, particularly in patients with trauma.[3,19,34] Furthermore, evidence suggests less experienced sonographers have particular difficulty in identifying the lung point to confirm the diagnosis of PTX, with

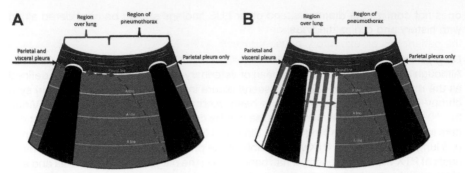

Fig. 1. The lung point with the probe situated half over a region of lung in contact with the chest wall and half over a region of PTX. Lung siding is visible where the lung is in contact with the chest wall (*red dotted line with arrow heads*), and is absent where the lung pulls away from the chest wall (*red dotted line without arrow heads*). (*A*) In this example, A lines are visible throughout the image because the lung that contacts the chest wall has no visible lung disorder at the lung surface, which appears similar to the image created below the region of PTX. The appearance of this lung point is often seen in patients with spontaneous PTX. (*B*) In this example, multiple B lines are visible where the lung contacts the chest wall (*left side*), and only A lines are visible to the right of the image where the probe is situated over a region of PTX. The appearance of this lung point is often seen in patients with trauma-induced PTX where visible lung has increased B lines and/or regions of consolidation caused by the presence of pulmonary contusions. (Images produced by Dr. Søren Boysen with permission.)

only 15% of scanners able to locate it in 1 study.[1] In patients with massive PTX, the lung does not recontact the thoracic wall and a lung point is not present.[32] In addition, although considered pathognomonic for the diagnosis of PTX by some investigators, several studies have reported a lung point or pseudo–lung point associated with several conditions unrelated to PTX, including pleural thickening and adhesion, subpleural cysts, asthma, bullous emphysema, and even in patients with healthy lungs.[22,35–38]

The accuracy of the lung point to confirm PTX in naturally occurring PTX in small animals is unknown. A small canine case series identified the lung point in 5 of 6 cases of confirmed PTX but failed to identify it in 1 dog despite multiple attempts to localize it.[16] In an experimental study using anesthetized dogs, the lung point had an Sp of 100% and an Se of 20% and 40% with PTX volumes from 2 to 10 mL/kg, respectively.[17] Although the Se of identifying the lung point increased with the volume of PTX, it remained low. It has been suggested that the lung point may be less sensitive in dogs than it is in humans, although much larger studies with larger-volume pneumothoraces are required to confirm or refute this hypothesis.[16,17] To the author's knowledge, the lung point has not been identified in cats, and more LUS research on PTX in general is required in this species.

M-mode Findings

Barcode and seashore sign

The use of M mode, which detects motion over time, can be used to detect the motion of lung sliding.[17,27,31] When the M-mode cursor is situated over the pleural line, 2 different patterns are displayed on the screen: The motionless portion of the thorax above the pleural line creates horizontal lines and the sliding below the pleural line creates a granular pattern, likened to a sandlike pattern found at the beach (Video

6).[17,27,31] The resultant picture is one that resembles waves crashing onto the sand and is therefore called the seashore sign, which can be identified in normal lung. If the patient has an expiratory pause between respirations, then the seashore sign is temporarily lost and appears as a barcode sign (Video 7). With PTX, M mode only shows 1 pattern of parallel horizontal lines above and below the pleural line, exemplifying the lack of lung sliding at the level of the pleural line. This pattern resembles a barcode or stratosphere sign.[17,27,31] The use of M mode has been suggested in people when the detection of lung sliding may be subtle using B mode alone. When both the seashore and barcode sign are visible within the same window during the active phases of respiration, it is consistent with the B-mode finding of the lung point.[27] Individual Se and Sp of M mode for detection of PTX is rarely reported because it is generally considered in conjunction with B mode to confirm the presence or absence of lung siding (eg, lung sliding is reported regardless of which mode of ultrasonography is used to detect it).[3,5,34] To the author's knowledge, M mode has not been clinically reported in dogs or cats for the detection of PTX, although it was reported in the experimental canine study by Hwang and colleagues,[17] where it was used in conjunction with B mode to determine the overall presence of lung sliding.

Combined Lung Ultrasonography Criteria

Most human studies use a combination of absent lung sliding, absent B lines/consolidations, and absent lung pulse with or without the presence of a lung point to diagnose PTX.[3,5,34,39] However, the Se and Sp of combining criteria versus individual assessment of criteria are not well defined. A recent Cochrane Review concluded that future human studies should explicitly report individual LUS findings (absence of lung sliding, absence of B lines or comet-tail artifact, presence of lung point, and absence of lung pulse) to enable assessment of the accuracy of these individual findings and their combinations.[7] Similar research recommendations would be reasonable for small animal patients as well.

NOVEL LUNG ULTRASONOGRAPHY CRITERIA TO DIAGNOSE PNEUMOTHORAX
Double Lung Point

Another LUS criterion used to diagnose PTX in human medicine is the double lung point, which is considered very rare and has not been reported in any veterinary clinical or experimental studies. The double lung point is described as the absence of lung sliding and B lines between 2 lung points.[8] It has been hypothesized that a double lung point can be detected secondary to traumatic PTX when pulmonary contusions cause pleural adhesions that trap air from rising to the most gravity-independent areas.[8,11] With the double lung point, both edges of trapped pleural air can be scanned and visualized as 2 lung points alternating on the 2 opposite sides of the probe, moving in opposite directions. One lung point appears at 1 end of the probe during inspiration, whereas the other lung point appears at the opposite end of the probe during expiration. When the air layer is small, both lung points may be visible in the same sonographic window, but, if the air layer is large, the probe will need to be moved from 1 lung point to the other. An essential feature of the double lung point is that the 2 lung points appear in opposite directions to the orientation of the probe and move in opposite directions to each other during the respiratory cycle.[11] The double lung point has not been studied in veterinary medicine, although patient positioning (lateral vs dorsal position) may influence results.

Mirrored Ribs

Mirrored ribs have been reported in human neonates with confirmed PTX and are defined as the occurrence of at least 1 rib and associated intercostal muscles appearing below the pleural line in B mode (mirroring of the rib and intercostal muscles below the pleural line) without any shadowing by the pleura or B lines.[10] It is hypothesized that mirrored ribs are caused by a long path reverberation artifact caused by repeated reflections of ultrasound beams between the transducer, the pleura, and the internal part of nonossified ribs.[10] The finding of mirrored ribs is no longer visible when the ribs become ossified, limiting their utility to neonates. The fact that mirrored ribs are a static marker is considered an advantage compared with dynamic markers such as lung sliding because still images can be used to make the diagnosis, and mirrored ribs are visible regardless of respiratory frequency or depth of respirations.[10] To the author's knowledge, mirrored ribs have not been reported in neonatal veterinary patients, although the findings of mirrored ribs in neonatal dogs and cats may have similar applications to what is reported in human medicine.

Reverse Sliding Sign

The reverse sliding sign is a unique LUS finding for diagnosis of PTX that has been reported in an experimental study in dogs under anesthesia.[17] It is defined as movement of A lines in the opposite direction to classic lung sliding during inspiration.[17] Given that A lines are an artifact created by a soft tissue–air interface, sliding is probably a misnomer, because there is no real sliding of tissues across each other at the level of A lines. Therefore, the reverse sliding sign refers to the apparent direction of movement of A lines and should not be confused for true lung sliding, which is the actual sliding of the lung surface across the thoracic wall at the level of the pleural line. The reverse sliding sign was more sensitive (85%) than all other LUS criteria assessed (absence of lung sliding, absence of lung pulse, and lung point) for detection of small-volume PTX (2–10 mL/kg) in dogs, and had a specificity of 100% compared with CT.[17] However, given the study only involved a uniform population of healthy dogs with thoracostomy tube–induced pneumothoraces under anesthesia, it is unknown whether the Se and Sp will be the same in awake spontaneously breathing dogs with larger-volume naturally occurring pneumothoraces, and patients without thoracostomy tubes or undergoing anesthesia. It is also unknown whether the reverse sliding sign can be seen with other respiratory disorders (eg, diaphragmatic paralysis) or conditions that result in a paradoxic respiratory pattern. Further research is required to answer these questions.

Curtain signs

Abnormal curtain signs, including asynchronous and double curtain signs, have been described in a clinical case series of dogs with confirmed spontaneous and trauma-induced PTX.[16] These dogs were considered to have only mild to moderate degrees of PTX, and extrapolation of these findings to larger-volume PTX is unknown. Interestingly, dogs with PTX of mild to moderate volume had all 3 types of curtains signs (normal, double, and asynchronous) present over each hemithorax, with normal curtain signs visible in the ventral third of the thorax.[16] The Se and Sp of abnormal curtain signs was not determined and only 6 dogs were included in the study, which limits the value of these findings. Much larger studies comparing abnormal curtain signs with a reference standard and other LUS criteria for diagnosis of PTX, as well as larger-volume PTX and patients in respiratory distress without evidence of PTX, are recommended to further evaluate the value of asynchronous and double curtain signs in both dogs and cats. The description of normal, asynchronous, and double curtain signs is provided in detail later; however, the theoretic pathophysiology of how abnormal curtain signs are created in dogs with PTX is explained elsewhere.[16] Although a pseudo–curtain sign has been described in human medicine with large or complete pneumothoraces extending to the lung base, which has a very similar appearance to normal curtain signs, they have not yet been described in veterinary patients. A pseudo–curtain sign appears similar to a normal curtain sign except lung sliding and B lines are absent with the pseudo–curtain sign and lung sliding, plus/minus B lines are visible with a normal curtain sign.[9]

Normal Curtain Signs

An air curtain is defined as a vertical edge artifact created when air overlies soft tissue structures, or less commonly pleural effusion, within the thorax.[9] It is visible when both air and the sonographically visible structures it overlies are identified in the same ultrasonography window.[9] Because they are created by air that overlies sonographically visible structures, curtain signs can be identified in healthy patients with air-filled lungs (lung curtains), and in patients with air or gas in the pleural space (PTX-induced curtains).[9,16] In healthy patients, lung curtains are located at the caudal lung border where air-filled lung overlies the diaphragm and soft tissue structures of the abdomen at the costophrenic recess, which represents the abdominal curtain sign (**Figs. 2 and 3**, Video 8),[9,16] and the ventral lung border where air-filled lung overlies the soft tissues of heart at the cardiac notch, referred to as a cardiac curtain sign (Video 9). When created by air-filled lung of healthy patients, the abdominal curtain sign shows distinct characteristics: it is dynamic and shifts in a cranial (expiratory) and caudal (inspiratory) direction as a result of the respiratory contraction and expansion of the lungs; regardless of the phase of the respiratory cycle, the lateral aspect of the diaphragm (and underlying abdominal soft tissue structures) is always covered by a lung curtain.[9] Therefore, during inspiration, as the lung expands into the costophrenic recess, the lung curtain appears to move caudally, covering more of the intra-abdominal

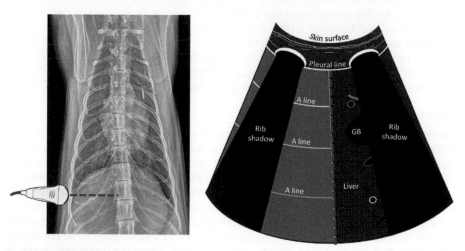

Fig. 2. Thoracic radiograph of a cat showing the probe location to identify the abdominal curtain sign, and the corresponding schematic image of the abdominal curtain sign. The dotted red line represents the point where the probe is situated half over lungs and half over visible soft tissue structures of the abdomen. GB, gall bladder. (Image produced by Dr. Søren Boysen with permission.)

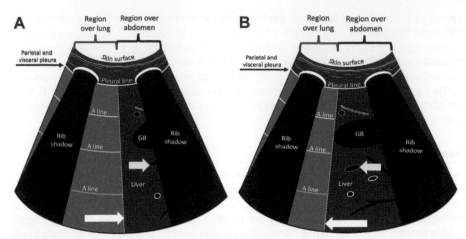

Fig. 3. The normal movement on ultrasonography of the abdominal curtain sign (*white arrow*) and abdominal contents (*yellow arrow*) in synch with each other during inspiration (*A*) and expiration (*B*). (Images produced by Dr. Søren Boysen with permission.)

structures. However, the movement of the lung curtain is caused by lung expansion and therefore is not perfectly synchronous to the movement of the intra-abdominal structures that are seen as a result of diaphragmatic activity.[9] As a result of these distinct features, there are several criteria that can be distinguished in healthy patients with a normal abdominal curtain sign: (1) there should only ever be 1 curtain sign visible at the caudal lung border, (2) which should always be visible throughout respiratory cycle (although it may become lost if it slides under a rib shadow), (3) and although it may move slightly out of synch with the abdominal content and diaphragmatic activity, both the curtain sign and visible abdominal soft tissue structures should move in the same direction during the respiratory cycle (Video 8). To avoid confusing rib shadows for the curtain sign, the author recommends assessing the curtain sign when it is centered between 2 ribs, or located just caudal to the more cranial rib, at the end of expiration. Gas-filled structures of the abdomen (eg, stomach and intestines) can give the impression of a curtain sign, but they can be differentiated from true curtain signs by the fact they are separated from the body wall by a layer of intestinal wall, or fail to create a vertical air edge artifact.[16]

Asynchronous Curtain Sign

The asynchronous curtain sign has only been described in veterinary medicine and is defined as movement of the vertical air edge artifact (PTX-induced curtain) in the opposite direction to the abdominal contents.[16] More precisely, it is the cranial movement of a PTX-induced curtain sign with concomitant caudal movement of abdominal contents during the inspiratory phase of the respiratory cycle, with caudal movement of a PTX-induced curtain sign and cranial movement of the abdominal contents during the expiratory phase of the respiratory cycle (**Fig. 4**, Video 10).[16] Therefore, it is not only the direction of movement of the curtain sign and visible abdominal structures that is important but also their direction of movement during the respiratory cycle.[16] Although not proven, in theory an asynchronous curtain sign is unlikely to occur in the absence of PTX or other pleural space disorders because the mechanics of respiration, the normal interaction of the lung, thoracic wall, diaphragm, and costophrenic recess, implies the lung would have to contract in size while the thorax expands on

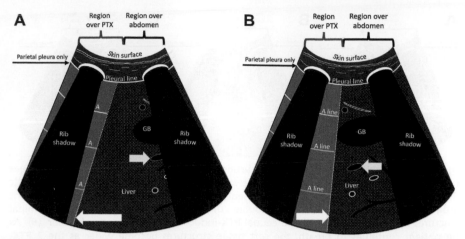

Fig. 4. The asynchronous curtain sign on ultrasonography that has been reported in dogs with PTX. During inspiration (A) the vertical edge artifact of a PTX-induced curtain sign (*white arrow*) moves cranial and in the opposite direction to the abdominal contents, which move caudally (*yellow arrow*). During expiration (B) the PTX-induced curtain sign and the abdominal contents move toward each other. A, A lines. (Images produced by Dr. Søren Boysen with permission.)

inspiration, while at the same time the diaphragm would have to contract caudally with the abdominal contents, suggesting a space would need to be created between normal air-filled lung and the costophrenic recess, which seems improbable.[40] Further research is required to determine the Se and Sp of the asynchronous curtain sign or whether other disorders can create similar findings to the asynchronous curtain sign in the absence of PTX. The asynchronous curtain sign should not be confused for paradoxic cranial movement of the diaphragm, which can occur with respiratory fatigue and diaphragmatic paresis/paralysis, particularly in proximity to the central tendon.[41,42] With paradoxic diaphragmatic movement, the central diaphragm can be drawn cranially with increased negative pleural pressure (which sonographically can appear as abdominal contents moving cranially on inspiration).[41,42] This process occurs as a result of thoracic expansion during inspiration, which increases negative pleural pressure drawing the diaphragm and abdominal contents cranially, whereas the lung slides caudally along the thoracic wall as it expands into the costophrenic recess in people. This situation creates the appearance of the lung curtain and abdominal contents moving toward each other on inspiration and away from each other on expiration, the opposite of what is expected with asynchronous curtains signs associated with PTX. Although the pathophysiologic mechanisms are similar, the asynchronous curtain sign should also not be confused for the reverse sliding sign because asynchronous curtain signs consider the direction of movement of the vertical edge air artifact in relation to the movement of visible underlying soft tissue structures and phase of respiration, whereas the reverse sliding sign only describes assessment of the direction of movement of A lines, which may or may not have a different Se and Sp for diagnosis of PTX.[16,17]

Double Curtain Sign

The double curtain sign is defined as 2 parallel vertical abdominal edge artifacts (PTX-induced curtain signs) visible in the same sonographic window, or within close

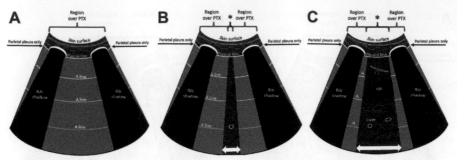

Fig. 5. The appearance of the double curtain sign on ultrasonography as it changes throughout the respiratory cycle. During the expiratory pause, between breaths, the classic PTX findings of absent lung sliding and presence of A lines may be seen (*A*). As the patient inspires, the sudden appearance of a double curtain sign, seen as soft tissue abdominal structures bordered by a cranial and caudal PTX-induced curtain sign, may be seen (*B*). As the patient continues to breath, the soft tissue structures become wider as the 2 PTX-induced curtain signs diverge away from each other (*C*). During expiration, the process is reversed and the 2 PTX-induced curtain signs converge toward each other until the soft tissue structures disappear when the lateral diaphragm pulls away from the thoracic wall. The asterisk "*" represents a region where the probe is situated over the diaphragm and associated underlying soft tissue structures at the costophrenic recess. (Images produced by Dr. Søren Boysen with permission.)

proximity to each other over the same hemithorax (Video 11).[16] Their appearance can vary and they are sometimes identified as the sudden inspiratory visualization of abdominal soft tissue structures within an area that previously contained only A lines and an absence of lung sliding (**Fig. 5**, Video 11). Alternatively, the double curtain sign may be visible throughout the respiratory cycle, appearing as abdominal soft tissue structures that are bound cranially and caudally by vertical air edge artifacts, which diverge away from each other on inspiration and converge toward each other on expiration (Video 12). In addition, it is possible for both visible edge artifacts of the double curtain sign to slide caudally on inspiration in combination with the findings described earlier (Video 13). The double curtain sign should not be confused with the reverse lung sliding sign as described earlier and should also not be confused for cardiac curtain signs, which are visible where air-filled ventral lung borders overly the cardiac structures. In theory, a double curtain sign should only exist with PTX because there can only be 1 true caudal abdominal vertical edge (lung) artifact in healthy patients.[9,16] However, mimics such as the lung point, cardiac curtain signs, subcutaneous emphysema, diaphragmatic hernias, and gas-filled intestines visible below the diaphragm should be ruled out. Similar to asynchronous curtain signs, a lot more research is needed to determine the Se, Sp, and value of double curtain signs in diagnosing PTX in small animal veterinary patients.

SUMMARY

Evidence in the human literature suggests LUS is highly accurate at diagnosing PTX, outperforming thoracic radiography, particularly when performed by experienced sonographers and when multiple LUS criteria are considered. Although LUS shows tremendous promise for the diagnosis of PTX in small animals, study results are conflicting, likely because of species differences, lack of methodology standardization between studies regarding reference standards and LUS criteria used to diagnose PTX, limited training opportunities and expertise, and inclusion of only small study populations. Further research will likely provide insight into the true accuracy of LUS and the various LUS criteria to diagnose PTX in small animal patients.

DISCLOSURE

The author receives honorariums and travel expenses for presentation of emergency and critical care topics, including point of care ultrasound, from continuing education approved events hosted by ultrasound companies and conferences around the world, and does receive remuneration from online educational companies for delivery of veterinary emergency and critical care topics, including point of care ultrasound. The author also makes available free open access veterinary point of care ultrasound educational through the University of Calgary, Faculty of Veterinary Medicine website, but otherwise declares no commercial conflicts of interest and has no funding sources to declare for this article.

SUPPLEMENTARY DATA

Supplementary data to this article can be found online at https://doi.org/10.1016/j.cvsm.2021.07.003.

REFERENCES

1. Ramos Hernández C, Núñez Delgado M, Botana Rial M, et al. Validity of lung ultrasound to rule out iatrogenic pneumothorax performed by pulmonologists without experience in this procedure. Revista Clinica Espanola 2021 May; 221(5):258–63.
2. Kiley S, Tighe P, Hajibrahim O, et al. Retrospective computed tomography mapping of intrapleural air may demonstrate optimal window for ultrasound diagnosis of pneumothorax. J Intensive Care Med 2014;29(6):342–7.
3. Staub LJ, Biscaro RRM, Kaszubowski E, et al. Chest ultrasonography for the emergency diagnosis of traumatic pneumothorax and haemothorax: a systematic review and meta-analysis. Injury 2018;49(3):457–66.
4. Alrajab S, Youssef AM, Akkus NI, et al. Pleural ultrasonography versus chest radiography for the diagnosis of pneumothorax: review of the literature and meta-analysis. Crit Care 2013;17(5):R208.
5. Dahmarde H, Parooie F, Salarzaei M. Accuracy of ultrasound in diagnosis of pneumothorax: a comparison between neonates and adults-a systematic review and meta-analysis. Can Respir J 2019;2019:5271982.
6. Fei Q, Lin Y, Yuan TM. Lung ultrasound, a better choice for neonatal pneumothorax: a systematic review and meta-analysis. Ultrasound Med Biol 2021; 47(3):359–69.
7. Chan KK, Joo DA, McRae AD, et al. Chest ultrasonography versus supine chest radiography for diagnosis of pneumothorax in trauma patients in the emergency department. Cochrane Database Syst Rev 2020;7(7):CD013031.
8. Aspler A, Pivetta E, Stone MB. Double-lung point sign in traumatic pneumothorax. Am J Emerg Med 2014;32(7):819.e1–2.
9. Lee FCY. The curtain sign in lung ultrasound. J Med Ultrasound 2017;25(2): 101–4.
10. Küng E, Aichhorn L, Berger A, et al. Mirrored ribs: a sign for pneumothorax in neonates. Pediatr Crit Care Med 2020;21(10):e944–7.

11. Volpicelli G, Audino B. The double lung point: an unusual sonographic sign of juvenile spontaneous pneumothorax. Am J Emerg Med 2011;29(3):355.e1–2.

12. Walters AM, O'Brien MA, Selmic LE, et al. Evaluation of the agreement between focused assessment with sonography for trauma (AFAST/TFAST) and computed tomography in dogs and cats with recent trauma. J Vet Emerg Crit Care (San Antonio) 2018;28(5):429–35.

13. Lisciandro GR, Lagutchik MS, Mann KA, et al. Evaluation of a thoracic focused assessment with sonography for trauma (TFAST) protocol to detect pneumothorax and concurrent thoracic injury in 145 traumatized dogs. J Vet Emerg Crit Care 2008;18:258.

14. Armenise A, Boysen RS, Rudloff E, et al. Veterinary-focused assessment with sonography for trauma-airway, breathing, circulation, disability and exposure: a prospective observational study in 64 canine trauma patients. J Small Anim Pract 2019;60(3):173–82.

15. Cole L, Pivetta M, Humm K. Diagnostic accuracy of a lung ultrasound protocol (Vet BLUE) for detection of pleural fluid, pneumothorax and lung pathology in dogs and cats. J Small Anim Pract 2021;62(3):178–86.

16. Boysen S, McMurray J, Gommeren K. Abnormal curtain signs identified with a novel lung ultrasound protocol in six dogs with pneumothorax. Front Vet Sci 2019;6:291.

17. Hwang TS, Yoon YM, Jung DI, et al. Usefulness of transthoracic lung ultrasound for the diagnosis of mild pneumothorax. J Vet Sci 2018;19(5):660–6.

18. Retief J, Chopra M. Pitfalls in the ultrasonographic diagnosis of pneumothorax. J Intensive Care Soc 2017;18(2):143–5.

19. Kirkpatrick AW, Sirois M, Laupland KB, et al. Hand-held thoracic sonography for detecting post-traumatic pneumothoraces: the Extended Focused Assessment with Sonography for Trauma (EFAST). J Trauma 2004;57(2):288–95.

20. Brook OR, Beck-Razi N, Abadi S, et al. Sonographic detection of pneumothorax by radiology residents as part of extended focused assessment with sonography for trauma. J Ultrasound Med 2009;28(6):749–55.

21. Lichtenstein D. Lung ultrasound in the critically ill. Curr Opin Crit Care 2014;20(3):315–22.

22. Del Colle A, Carpagnano GE, Feragalli B, et al. Transthoracic ultrasound sign in severe asthmatic patients: a lack of "gliding sign" mimic pneumothorax. BJR Case Rep 2019;5(4):20190030.

23. Raimondi F, Rodriguez Fanjul J, Aversa S, et al. Lung ultrasound for diagnosing pneumothorax in the critically Ill neonate. J Pediatr 2016;175:74–8.e1.

24. Martinez AN, Quinn C, Mihm F, et al. 1127: lung ultrasound: the fine line between diagnosing and ruling out pneumothorax. Crit Care Med 2018;46(1):547.

25. Ebrahimi A, Yousefifard M, Mohammad Kazemi H, et al. Diagnostic accuracy of chest ultrasonography versus chest radiography for identification of pneumothorax: a systematic review and meta-analysis. Tanaffos 2014;13(4):29–40.

26. Lichtenstein DA, Mézière GA. Relevance of lung ultrasound in the diagnosis of acute respiratory failure: the BLUE Protocol. Chest 2008;134(1):117–25.

27. Lichtenstein D, van Hooland S, Elbers P, et al. Ten good reasons to practice ultrasound in critical care. Anaesthesiol Intensive Ther 2014;46(5):323–35.

28. Lisciandro GR, Fosgate GT, Fulton RM. Frequency and number of ultrasound lung rockets (B-lines) using a regionally based lung ultrasound examination named vet BLUE (veterinary bedside lung ultrasound exam) in dogs with radiographically normal lung findings. Vet Radiol Ultrasound 2014;55(3):315–22.

29. Lisciandro GR, Fulton RM, Fosgate GT, et al. Frequency and number of B-lines using a regionally based lung ultrasound examination in cats with radiographically normal lungs compared to cats with left-sided congestive heart failure. J Vet Emerg Crit Care (San Antonio) 2017;27(5):499–505.

30. Rademacher N, Pariaut R, Pate J, et al. Transthoracic lung ultrasound in normal dogs and dogs with cardiogenic pulmonary edema: a pilot study. Vet Radiol Ultrasound 2014;55(4):447–52.

31. Husain LF, Hagopian L, Wayman D, et al. Sonographic diagnosis of pneumothorax. J Emerg Trauma Shock 2012;5(1):76–81.

32. Lichtenstein DA. Ultrasound in the management of thoracic disease. Crit Care Med 2007;35(5 Suppl):S250–61.

33. Lichtenstein D, Mezière G, Biderman P, et al. The "lung point": an ultrasound sign specific to pneumothorax. Intensive Care Med 2000;26(10):1434–40.

34. Ding W, Shen Y, Yang J, et al. Diagnosis of pneumothorax by radiography and ultrasonography: a meta-analysis. Chest 2011;140(4):859–66.

35. Aziz SG, Patel BB, Ie SR, et al. The lung point sign, not pathognomonic of a pneumothorax. Ultrasound Q 2016;32(3):277–9.

36. Lanks CW. A subpleural cyst mimicking pneumothorax. J Ultrasound Med 2019; 38(8):2233–5.

37. Steenvoorden TS, Hilderink B, Elbers PWG, et al. Lung point in the absence of pneumothorax. Intensive Care Med 2018;44(8):1329–30.

38. Zhang Z, Chen L. A physiological sign that mimics lung point in critical care ultrasonography. Crit Care 2015;19(1):155.

39. Lichtenstein DA, Mezière G, Lascols N, et al. Ultrasound diagnosis of occult pneumothorax. Crit Care Med 2005;33(6):1231–8.

40. Macklem PT. Respiratory muscle dysfunction. Hosp Pract (Off Ed 1986;21(3): 83–90, 95-6.

41. Qian Z, Yang M, Li L, et al. Ultrasound assessment of diaphragmatic dysfunction as a predictor of weaning outcome from mechanical ventilation: a systematic review and meta-analysis. BMJ Open 2018;8(9):e021189.

42. Kim WY, Suh HJ, Hong SB, et al. Diaphragm dysfunction assessed by ultrasonography: influence on weaning from mechanical ventilation. Crit Care Med 2011; 39(12):2627–30.

Section II: Non-pulmonary Thoracic and Cardiac Ultrasound

TFAST Accurate Diagnosis of Pleural and Pericardial Effusion, Caudal Vena Cava in Dogs and Cats

Gregory R. Lisciandro, DVM, DABVP DACVECC

KEYWORDS

- TFAST • Pericardial effusion • Pleural effusion • Volume status • Echocardiography

KEY POINTS

- TFAST is a standardized focused assessment with sonography examination of the thorax.
- TFAST and its tenets allow for an accurate diagnosis of pleural effusion and pericardial effusion.
- TFAST and its diaphragmatico-hepatic view allow for the assessment of patient volume status of which information may be integrated with TFAST echocardiography views.
- TFAST and its target organ approach serve as a screening test for obvious soft tissue abnormalities of the heart that often are missed or only suspected based on physical examination, laboratory test results, and radiography.
- TFAST may be used for the diagnosis and semiquantification of pneumothorax and its TFAST thirds rule used for tracking pneumothorax.
- TFAST and its fundamental echocardiography views serve as a screening test for volume status assessment, abnormalities in cardiac contractility, and left-sided and right-sided heart conditions through chamber size assessment.

 Video content accompanies this article at http://www.vetsmall.theclinics.com.

INTRODUCTION

In 2004, the first translational study of focused assessment with sonography for trauma (FAST) from humans to small animals documented that minimally trained nonradiologist veterinarians could proficiently recognize ascites and that hemoperitoneum was far more common than previously reported.[1] Moreover, pleural effusion (PE) and pericardial effusion (PCE) could be detected via the subxiphoid view by looking cranial to the diaphragm.[1,2] Thoracic FAST (TFAST) was developed at the same time as abdominal FAST (AFAST) in 2005. TFAST was used to move past the

Hill Country Veterinary Specialists and FASTVet.com, Spicewood, TX, USA
E-mail address: FastSavesLives@gmail.com

Vet Clin Small Anim 51 (2021) 1169–1182
https://doi.org/10.1016/j.cvsm.2021.07.004

AFAST-TFAST diaphragmatico-hepatic (DH) view for more intrathoracic information, including pneumothorax, PE and PCE, and echocardiography. AFAST and TFAST were combined and called combination FAST prior to the development of veterinary brief lung ultrasound examination (Vet BLUE), a more comprehensive lung ultrasound screening test over the bilaterally applied TFAST chest tube site (CTS) views.[3] It was quickly recognized that by including both cavities, a better patient assessment was achieved, similar to the use of extended FAST in people.[4]

Since 2010, when all 3 formats were combined, the ultrasound examination was named Global FAST, a unique imaging screening test of both body cavities.[5–10] Global FAST is used as an extension of the physical examination, providing an unbiased set of 15 data imaging points with exact clarity of both the abdomen and thorax, including heart (TFAST echocardiography) and lung (Vet BLUE).[5–10] Although TFAST may be used as a standalone ultrasound examination, through the standardized approach of Global FAST, sonographers avoid common imaging mistakes, such as satisfaction of search error and confirmation bias error, through selective point-of-care ultrasound (POCUS) imaging.[8] As an example, decreased volume status may be detected during focused echocardiography at the left ventricular (LV) short-axis mushroom view and the patient fluid resuscitated. However, the question of "Where is the volume loss (leak in the tank)?" never was addressed. As a result, the hemoabdomen is missed and it has to be wondered when the intra-abdominal hemorrhage, the cause of echo-cardiographic volume depletion, will be detected?—hopefully before the patient succumbs to their life-threatening condition. Global FAST automatically searches for causes of volume loss within the abdominal cavity and retroperitoneal space, missed or only partially screened for using TFAST.[5,6]

TFAST OVERVIEW
Thoracic Focused Assessment with Sonography for Trauma Standardized Methodology—Names, Views, Order, and Probe Maneuvering

TFAST is designed according to the principle that air rises and fluid falls into gravity-dependent regions called pouches.[2,11,12] Thus, the CTS view is used for pneumo-thorax, and the pericardial site (PCS) views and DH view for PE, PCE, and cardiac evaluation, including TFAST echocardiography views (**Fig. 1**).[2,11,12,13,14] TFAST is performed without shaving the patient and preferred in standing for its low impact and safety for the patient.[2,13,14,15,16] Standing (and sternal) also are truer to the law over other positioning that air rises to the chest tube site view and fluid falls into the gravity dependent TFAST pouches.[11,15,16]

TFAST AND ITS USE FOR PLEURAL EFFUSION AND PERICARDIAL EFFUSION

There are fundamental tenets to accurately diagnose PCE that is contained and rounded within the pericardial sac and PE that is uncontained and unrestrained within the pleural cavity that are imperative for the noncardiologist sonographer to learn, un-derstand, and follow (**Table 1**).[2,15,16] The reason for the importance of following these rules is that, unlike the abdominal cavity, which is forgiving (low risk) when performing abdominocentesis, the thorax has 1 major fluid-filled organ that may be mistaken for free fluid, and that is the patient's heart. Mistaking a heart chamber for PCE or PE can lead to a potentially catastrophic error in patient care, performing centesis on a pa-tient's heart (Video 1).

From experience, TFAST data collection and a clinical study published several years ago, these TFAST tenets have been developed for an accurate diagnosis of PCE and PE:

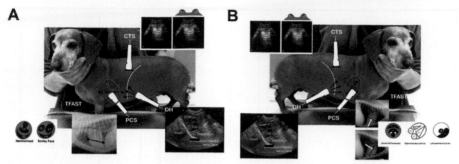

Fig. 1. The TFAST protocol is shown from the left side in A) and the right side in B). TFAST includes bilaterally applied chest tube site (CTS) views for pneumothorax, the pericardial site (PCS) views for PE and PCE and echocardiography, and the DH view for PE, PCE, volume status, lung pathology along the pulmonary-diaphragmatic interface, ascites, and soft tissue abnormalities of the gallbladder and liver. GB, gallbladder; LA, left atrium; LV, left ventricle; RA, right atrium; RV, right ventricle. (© 2021 Gregory R. Lisciandro.)

1. Image the heart toward its muscular apex where chambers are difficult to confuse for PCE at the diaphragmatico-hepatic view, the racetrack sign, and from the right pericardial site (PCS) view, the bull's eye sign; and PE as anechoic (black) triangulations (**Fig. 2**) (Videos 2–7).[2,15,16]
2. Image first caudally into the cardiac-diaphragmatic pouch and then cranially into the cardiac-cervical pouch away from heart chambers by using the TFAST slide for the curtain sign of PE (**Fig. 3**) (Video 8).[16]
3. Use only the long-axis 4-chamber view from the right pericardial site view, where all 4 chambers may be identified and fluid clearly determined to be outside the heart and contained within the pericardial sac for PCE or outside the pericardial sac for PE (**Fig. 4**) (Video 9).[2,15,16]
4. Use only the short-axis hammerhead view from the left pericardial site view, where both ventricles may be identified and fluid clearly determined to be outside the heart and contained within the pericardial sac for PCE or outside the pericardial sac for PE (see **Fig. 4**) (Video 10).[16]
5. Always image the heart in its entirety using the bright white (hyperechoic) pericardium as a landmark in the far field (**Fig. 5**).[2,15,16]
6. Avoid using right pericardial site short-axis views for the diagnosis of both PE and PCE because it is too easy to mistake the crescent-shaped right ventricle (RV) for either (see **Fig. 5**) (see Video 1).[2,15,16]
7. If all 4-chambers of the mammalian heart can be identified clearly, and there is clearly fluid outside these 4 chambers, then default to PE if it is not clearly PCE because PCE is much easier to diagnose (see **Fig. 4**) (Video 11).[16]

Pitfalls

The RV on short axis probably is the most important structure to not confuse with PCE and PE. The RV is crescent-shaped and has echogenic papillary muscles and chordae tendineae along this scanning plane. Moreover, the RV can image quite variably by the noncardiologist sonographer, with the RV appearing falsely enlarged and its normal structures mistaken for masses, thrombi, fibrin, lung (papillary muscles), and heartworms (chordae tendineae). Its crescent-shape mimics PCE and PE.

Table 1
TFAST tenets for accurately detecting pleural and pericardial effusion and cardiac tamponade

Pericardial Effusion

Imaging Strategies	TFAST-AFAST Diaphragmatico-hepatic View	TFAST Right and Left Pericardial Site Views	Thoracic Radiography	Gold Standard
(1) Image toward the muscular apex of the heart, where no heart chambers that can be mistaken for free fluid	• Racetrack sign	• Bull's eye sign on short axis	• Unreliable test for PCE and cardiac tamponade	• Ultrasound and computed tomography
(2) Identify ALL 4 cardiac chambers		• TFAST right PCS view—long-axis 4-chamber view		
(3) Identify BOTH ventricles		• TFAST left PCS view—short-axis hammerhead view		
(4) Image the heart in its entirety using the hyperechoic pericardium in the far field as a landmark				

Pleural Effusion

Imaging Strategies	TFAST-AFAST Diaphragmatico-hepatic View	TFAST Right and Left Pericardial Site Views	Thoracic Radiography	Gold Standard
(1) Image the heart in its entirety using the hyperechoic pericardium in the far field as a landmark	• Anechoic triangulations—no racetrack sign	• TFAST right and left PCS—anechoic triangulations	Good test	Debatable between ultrasound, computed tomography, and thoracoscopy

(2) TFAST slide
moving caudal
and cranial to
the heart avoiding
confounding
heart chambers

- Curtain sign of PE
- TFAST slide caudally into the cardiac-diaphragmatic pouch
- TFAST slide cranially into the cardiac-cervical pouch

© 2021 Gregory R. Lisciandro.

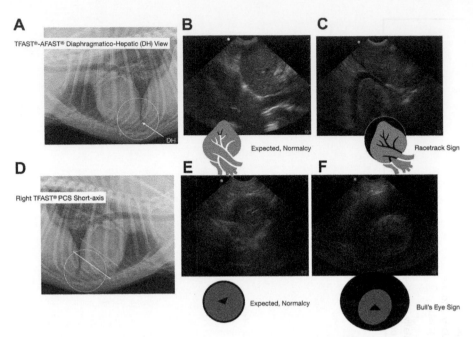

Fig. 2. Showing the rounding of PCE at the DH view and the TFAST right pericardial site view, referred to as the racetrack sign (*A–C*) and bull's eye sign (*D–F*), respectively, with correlative thoracic radiography and the expected TFAST appearance and that with PCE. (© 2021 Gregory R. Lisciandro.)

Methods to Avoid Pitfalls

- Primarily assess RV chamber size at the right pericardial site view on the long-axis 4-chamber view because the scanning plane is more reliable using the author's white dot method vs assessing right ventricular size at right pericardial site short-axis view (**Fig. 6**) (see Video 2).
- Respect the danger zone on right pericardial site short-axis and avoid diagnosing PCE and PE solely on this view. The axiom in human POCUS is "1 view is no view." In other words, the abnormality must be seen on 2 different views (see **Fig. 5**) (see Video 1).[16]
- Memorize the TFAST echocardiography chart and double-check its short-axis levels by fanning a level ventral and a level dorsal to where the sonographer is thought to be located on the cardiac (short-axis) ladder (**Fig. 7**).[16]
- Learn to fan on the short-axis and long-axis lines, the author's clockface methodology, to image the heart most consistently and learn its expected appearance (see **Fig. 7**).[16]
- Keep the screen direction of the patient's head to the left and the patient's tail to the right of the screen like all other imaging (this is in contrast to traditional echocardiography, in which the orientation was reversed, for some odd reason). This not only will help spatially orient as to the anatomy and which direction is cranial and caudal but also will help center the heart on the screen identical to how it would be done with any other structure (ie, gallbladder, kidney, urinary bladder, and so forth)

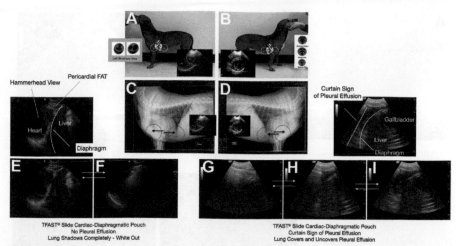

Fig. 3. Shows the TFAST slide on overlays of a dog in (*A*) and (*B*) and then with its correlative standing radiographs in (*C*) and (*D*) from the left and right side, respectively. The TFAST slide is a newer strategy again avoiding mistaking heart chambers for PE or PCE that involves sliding caudally and cranially in the cardiac-diaphragmatic pouch and the cardiac-cervical pouch (*arrows and circles*). The confounding structure is the pericardial fat that often is a darker (anechoic to hypoechoic) triangulation located in between the muscular apex often heart and the diaphragm (*E*), that shadows out (*F*) when sweeping the probe dorsally. In contrast, the presence of PE creates the curtain sign (*G–I*). Knowing how much different the heart looks dependent on the left pericardial site view (hammerhead and smiley face) and the right pericardial site view (mushroom view) also helps prevent mistaking heart chambers for PE (and PCE). (© 2021 Gregory R. Lisciandro.)

- Everyone looks at the screen. This includes the sonographer, restrainer, and patient, because it is safer in case the patient is showing aggression, turns to bite or scratch, or is decompensating. Also, the sightline to the screen should be comfortable for the sonographer (avoid looking over a shoulder) and allows the sonographer to physically see the external location and scanning plane of the probe.[17]
- Part the fur with alcohol so that the probe is as directly as possible on skin to avoid air trapping, which reduces image quality and use lots of acoustic coupling gel (author preference is alcohol-based hand sanitizer gel).
- Use the nonprobe hand on the standing patient's sternum as a V-trough to stabilize the patient or under the patient to help reduce probe pressure on the intercostal spaces when patients are in right lateral recumbency.[17]
- Follow the TFAST tenets for the accurate diagnosis of PCE and PE and avoid the trap of, "it just looks like PCE or PE."

TFAST AND THE CAUDAL VENA CAVA FOR VOLUME STATUS
Volume Status

Characterizing the caudal vena cava (CVC) in its sagittal plane as it courses through the diaphragm (and its associated hepatic veins) estimates patient volume status by its respirophasic height change as follows: fluid responsive (bounce), a change of 35% to 50%; fluid intolerant (FAT), little change (<10%), and an increased maximum height; and fluid starved/hypovolemic (flat), little change (<10%) and a decreased

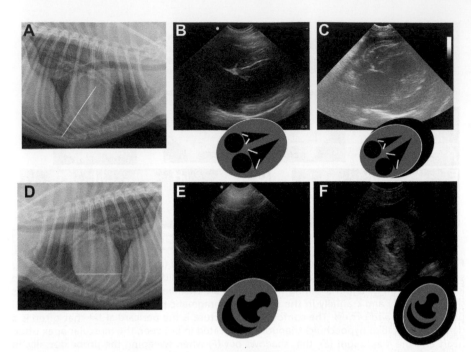

Fig. 4. The accurate diagnosis of PCE relies on imaging the heart globally, identifying the heart chambers, and seeing clearly that fluid is outside the heart and rounded within the pericardial sac. The pericardial sac attaches at 1 atrium courses around the muscular apex of the heart, and attaches at the other atrium. There are 2 major echocardiography views that satisfy these criteria. They are from the right pericardial site view the long-axis 4 chamber view [A-C] and from the left pericardial site view the hammerhead view [D-F], respectively. (© 2021 Gregory R. Lisciandro.)

maximum height (see **Fig. 7**) (see Video 11; Videos 12, 13).[9,10,12,15–20] Hepatic venous distension (tree trunk sign) likely is 100% specific for severely increased right-sided filling pressures in dogs and cats positioned in lateral, standing, or sternal[21–23]; and its finding, referred to as the tree trunk sign, plus a FAT CVC easily is recognized by properly trained nonradiologist veterinarians (see Videos 13; Video14).[15,18,19] Absolute measurements of the maximum height also have been created; however, dynamic CVC characterization as a rule trumps maximum height measurements unless there is hepatic venous distension (**Table 2**).[6,9,10,16]

TFAST FUNDAMENTAL ECHOCARDIOGRAPHY VIEWS

TFAST echocardiography views are from the right PCS view and include the LV short-axis mushroom view for volume status and contractility, the LV short-axis left atrial (LA) to aortic (Ao) view for left-sided problems (increased LA filling pressures), the long-axis 4-chamber view for right-sided problems (increased RV filling pressures), and the long-axis LV outflow tract (LVOT) and Ao valves (**Fig. 8**).[5,6,12,14–16] The eyeball method in properly trained noncardiologists has been shown effective as a screening test in people.[24] These views also serve as a screening test for cardiac-related soft tissue abnormalities because the radiographic cardiac silhouette is unreliable.[25,26] Importantly, when the sonographer is unable to obtain its echocardiography views, the absence of

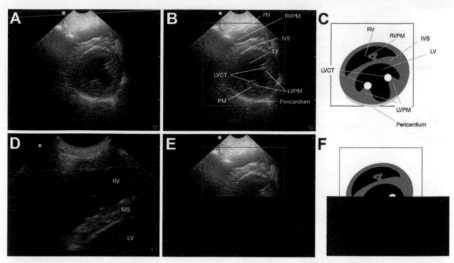

Fig. 5. The anatomy of the heart is important to understand as well as the importance of having enough depth to see the bright hyperechoic pericardium the far field. This alone prevents many imaging interpretations mistakes. Note, (A, B) there is enough depth to iden-tify the heart and its respective chambers; however, (D, E) depth is too shallow, and mistakes easily are made. The correlative cartoons (C) and (F) help show the anatomy. IVS, interven-tricular septum; LVCT, LV chordae tendineae; PLPM, LV papillary muscle; PM, papillary mus-cle; RVPM, RV papillary muscle. (© 2021 Gregory R. Lisciandro.)

wet lung during Vet BLUE rules out clinically relevant left-sided congestive heart failure and absence of a fluid-intolerant CVC rules out clinically relevant right-sided conges-tive heart failure.[12,21,22,27–32] These Global FAST fallback views allow an approach that often is easier (and faster) than echocardiography in the unstable patient (see **Fig. 7**).[5,6,9,10,14]

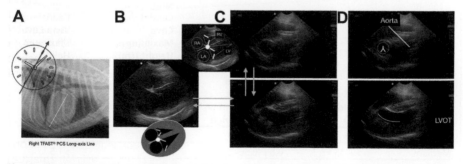

Fig. 6. The long-axis lines of the heart for the 4-chamber view are best performed by fan-ning on the long-axis line using the clockface (1-o'clock position) shown in the standing dog (same concept for cats). The white dot (hyperechoic base of the interatrial septum) is an identifiable landmark during fanning to locate the proper plane for the long-axis 4-chamber view. By fanning slightly cranially, the LVOT is added as a fourth TFAST echocardi-ography view and can screen for soft tissue abnormalities associated in that region. LA, left atrium; LV, left ventricle; LVOT, left ventricular outflow tract; RA, right atrium; RV, right ventricle. (© 2021 Gregory R. Lisciandro.)

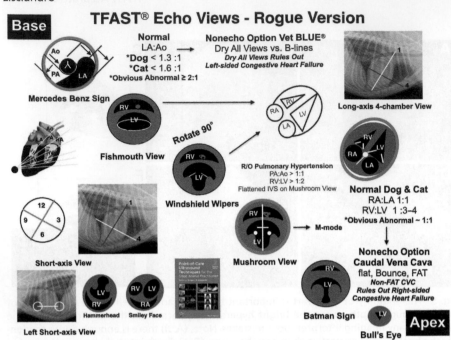

Fig. 7. The TFAST echocardiography chart that shows the different levels of the heart, those most important for left-sided and right-sided enlargement, and volume and contractility. Moreover, the appearance of the heart is remarkably different from the left versus right sides, and the fallback views can be used to support the presence of left-sided and right-sided failure while also serving as important information when TFAST echocardiography views cannot be acquired. IVS, interventricular septum; PA, pulmonary artery. (© 2021 Gregory R. Lisciandro.)

Table 2
Reference values for the maximum height of the caudal vena cava measured in longitudinal at the subxiphoid[a] view in 126 healthy dogs grouped into 3 body weight classes

Size	Body Weight (kg)	Expected Caudal Vena Cava Height Measurement (cm) and Range	Suggested Caudal Vena Cava Maximum Height (cm) for a Flat or Hypovolemic, Fluid-starved Caudal Vena Cava	Suggested Caudal Vena Cava Maximum Height (cm) for a FAT (High Central Venous Pressure)
Small/toy[b]	<9 kg	0.55 (0.40–0.70)	<0.25	>1.0
Medium	>9–15 kg	0.85 (0.50–1.10)	<0.35	>1.5
Large/giant	>15 kg	0.95 (0.80–1.20)	<0.50	>1.5

[a] The subxiphoid view is analogous to the FAST DH view and the CVC imaged in its longitudinal plane.
[b] Suggested starting point for felines while awaiting current research findings.
   Data from the study by Darnis et al. (2018) and measurements created with permission by Lisciandro GR and Vientós-Plotts AI. These values are unproved but give some guidelines for veterinary clinicians to combine with the eyeball method—bounce, FAT, and flat. © 2021 Gregory R. Lisciandro.

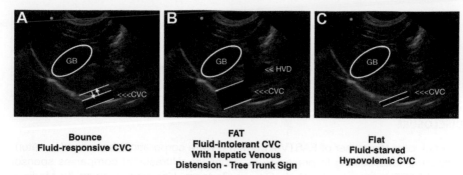

Bounce
Fluid-responsive CVC

FAT
Fluid-intolerant CVC
With Hepatic Venous
Distension - Tree Trunk Sign

Flat
Fluid-starved
Hypovolemic CVC

Fig. 8. The CVC and its associated hepatic veins are characterized by the eyeball method for its dynamic change (its distensibility) during cardiac and respiratory cycles as having a [*A*] bounce, being fluid responsive; [*B*] being FAT, distended with the tree trunk sign of hepatic venous distension; or [*C*] flat, being fluid starved or a hypovolemic CVC. CVC, caudal vena cava; HVD, hepatic venous distension; GB, gallbladder. (© 2021 Gregory R. Lisciandro.)

Recognizing Cardiac Abnormalities

The radiographic cardiac silhouette is an unreliable screening test for many cardiac-related conditions that likely are under-reported regarding prevalence because without complete echocardiography (or computed tomography), the condition would be missed.[24,25] These conditions include intracardiac and extracardiac masses, intracardiac thrombi and echogenic smoke, dilated cardiomyopathy, pulmonary hypertension, and intracardiac heartworms and caval syndrome, all of which can be suspected using the TFAST approach. The caveats are that TFAST serves as a screening test, that artifacts and cardiac anatomy can mimic pathology, and that not finding these conditions does not definitively rule them out (more advanced imaging is necessary). There is tremendous value, however, in using this approach over, or in combination with, physical examination and radiography and the patient's clinical profile.

SUMMARY

TFAST is low-impact, cost-effective, real-time information and rapid, radiation-sparing, point-of-care imaging that allows a veterinarian to see a problem list and thus better direct resuscitation and treatment and streamline the diagnostic plan. TFAST should be considered a screening test used for detecting free fluid and soft tissue abnormalities; however, its use has clear advantages over physical examination, laboratory test results, and radiography for most conditions. Global FAST and its 15 views provide an unbiased set of data imaging points that prevent the common imaging mistakes of satisfaction of search and confirmation bias errors through TFAST alone or selective POCUS imaging. Global FAST should be used as an extension of the physical examination on a daily basis for nearly all patients in the clinical setting and preempt add-on POCUS examinations.

CLINICS CARE POINTS

- The use of the TFAST tenets for the accurate diagnosis of pericardial and pleural effusion avoiding mistaking heart chambers for either.
- The use of characterization of the caudal vena cava and its associated hepatic veins are an effective means to assess patient volume status.

- TFAST echocardiography may be used to asses volume status and contractility, left- and right-sided problems through left atrial and right ventricular size, respectively.
- The TFAST thirds rule may be used to semi quantitate degree of pneumothorax for decision making while also serving as a tracking tool for static, resolving and worsening by lung point location.

DISCLOSURE

The author is the owner of FASTVet.com, a private corporation that provides veterinary ultrasound training to practicing veterinarians. Ultrasound companies sponsor Global FAST courses and include Oncura Partners, Universal Imaging, EI Medical, and Sound; and EI Medical and the Veterinary Medical Network have licensed Global FAST education materials. His spouse, Stephanie Lisciandro, is a veterinarian and Medical Director at Oncura Partners, Fort Worth, Texas. The author has no funding sources to declare for this article.

SUPPLEMENTARY DATA

Supplementary data to this article can be found online at https://doi.org/10.1016/j.cvsm.2021.07.004

REFERENCES

1. Boysen SR, Rozanski EA, Tidwell AS, et al. Evaluation of a focused assessment with sonography for trauma protocol to detect free abdominal fluid in dogs involved in motor vehicle accidents. J Am Vet Med Assoc 2004;225(8):1198–204.
2. Lisciandro GR. The use of the diaphragmatico-hepatic (DH) views of the abdominal and thoracic focused assessment with sonography for triage (AFAST/TFAST) examinations for the detection of pericardial effusion in 24 dogs (2011-2012). J Vet Emerg Crit Care 2016;26(1):125–31.
3. Lisciandro GR. Evaluation of initial and serial combination focused assessment with sonography for trauma (CFAST) examination of the thorax (TFAST) and abdomen (AFAST) with the application of an abdominal fluid scoring system in 49 traumatized cats. Abstract. J Vet Emerg Crit Care 2012;22(S2):S11.
4. Kirkpatrick AW, Sirois M, Laupland KB, et al. Hand-held thoracic sonography for detecting post-traumatic pneumothoraces: the extended focused assessment with sonography for trauma (EFAST). J Trauma 2004;57:288–95.
5. Lisciandro GR, Armenise AA. Chapter 16: focused or COAST3 - Cardiopulmonary Resuscitation (CPR), Global FAST (GFAST3), and the FAST-ABCDE exam. In: Lisciandro GR, editor. Focused ultrasound for the small animal practitioner. Ames, IA: Wiley Blackwell; 2014. p. 269–85.
6. Lisciandro GR, Lisciandro GR. Chapter 36: POCUS: Global FAST-patient monitoring and staging. In: Point-of-care ultrasound techniques for the small animal practitioner. 2nd edition. Ames IA: Wiley Blackwell; 2021. p. 685–728.
7. Hnatusko AL, Gicking JC, Lisciandro GR. Anaphylaxis-related hemoperitoneum in 11 dogs. J Vet Emerg Crit Care 2021;31(1):80–5.
8. Lisciandro GR, Gambino JM, Lisciandro SC. Case series of 13 dogs and 1 cat with ultrasonographically-detected gallbladder wall edema associated with cardiac disease. J Vet Intern Med 2021. https://doi.org/10.1111/jvim.16117.
9. Lisciandro GR. Cageside ultrasonography in the emergency room and the intensive care unit. Vet Clin North Am 2020;50(6):1445–67.

10. Lisciandro GR. Chapter 3: point-of-care ultrasound. In: Mattoon JS, Sellon R, Berry CR, editors. Small animal diagnostic ultrasound. 4th edition. St. Louis MO: Elsevier; 2020. p. 76–104.

11. Lisciandro GR, Lagutchik MS, Mann KA, et al. Evaluation of a thoracic focused assessment with sonography for trauma (TFAST) protocol to detect pneumothorax and concurrent thoracic injury in 145 traumatized dogs. J Vet Emerg Crit Care 2008;18(3):258–69.

12. Lisciandro GR. Abdominal and thoracic focused assessment with sonography for trauma, triage and monitoring in small animals. J Vet Emerg Crit Care 2011;21(2): 104–22.

13. McMurray J, Boysen S, Chalhoub S. Focused assessment with sonography in nontraumatized dogs and cats in the emergency and critical care setting. J Vet Emerg Crit Care 2016;26(1):64–73.

14. Boysen SR, Lisciandro GR. The use of ultrasound in the emergency room (AFAST and TFAST). Vet Clin North Am Small Anim Pract 2013;43(4):773–97.

15. Lisciandro GR, Lisciandro GR. Chapter 9: the thoracic FAST3 (TFAST3) exam. In: Focused ultrasound techniques for the small animal practitioner. Ames IA: Wiley Blackwell; 2014. p. 140–65.

16. Lisciandro GR, Lisciandro GR. Chapter 17: POCUS: TFAST-introduction and image acquisition. In: Point-of-care ultrasound Techniques for the small animal practitioner. 2nd edition. Ames IA: Wiley Blackwell; 2021. p. 297–336.

17. Lisciandro GR, Lisciandro GR. Chapter 5: POCUS: top ultrasound mistakes during global FAST. In: Point-of-care ultrasound Techniques for the small animal practitioner. 2nd edition. Ames IA: Wiley Blackwell; 2021. p. 39–54.

18. Ferrada P, Attand RJ, Whelan J, et al. Qualitative assessment of the inferior vena cava: useful tool for the evaluation of volume status in criticall ill patients. Am Surg 2012;78(4):468–70.

19. Ferrada P, Vanguri P, Anand RJ, et al. Flat inferior vena cava: indicator of poor prognosis in trauma and acute care surgery patients. Am Surg 2012;78(12): 1396–8.

20. Darnis E, Boysen S, Merveille AC, et al. Establishment of references values of the caudal vena cava by fast-ultrasonography through different views in healthy dogs. J Vet Intern Med 2018;32(4):1308–18.

21. Chou Y, Ward JL, Barron LZ, et al. Focused ultrasound of the caudal vena cava in dogs with cavitary effusions or congestive heart failure: a prospective observational study. PLOS ONE; 2021.

22. Himelman RB, Kircher B, Rockey DC, et al. Inferior vena cava plethora with blunted respiratory response: a sensitive echocardiographic sign of cardiac tamponade. J Am Coll Cardiol 1988;12(6):1470–7.

23. Tchernodrinski S, Arntfield R. Chapter 18: inferior vena cava. In: Point-of-care ultrasound. Soni NJ, Arntfield R, and Kory P. Elsevier: 2015; Philadelphia: pp. 135–141.

24. Ferrada P, Evans D, Wolfe L, et al. Findings of a randomized controlled trial using limited transthoracic echocardiogram (LTTE) as a hemodynamic monitoring tool in the trauma bay. J Trauma Acute Care Surg 2014;76(1):31–7.

25. Côté E, Schwarz LA, Sithole F. Thoracic radiographic findings for dogs with cardiac tamponade attributable to pericardial effusion. J Am Vet Med Assoc 2013 5; 243(2):232–5.

26. Guglielmini C, Diana A, Santarelli G, et al. Accuracy of radiographic vertebral heart score and sphericity index in the detection of pericardial effusion in dogs. J Am Vet Med Assoc 2012;241(8):1048–55.

27. Lisciandro GR, Fosgate GT, Fulton RM. Frequency of ultrasound lung rockets using a regionally-based lung ultrasound examination named veterinary bedside lung ultrasound exam (Vet BLUE) in 98 dogs with normal thoracic radiographic lung findings. Vet Radiol Ultrasound 2014;55(3):315–22.

28. Lisciandro GR, Fulton RM, Fosgate GT, et al. Frequency of B-lines using a regionally-based lung ultrasound examination (the Vet BLUE protocol) in 49 cats with normal thoracic radiographical lung findings. J Vet Emerg Crit Care 2017;27(3):267–77.

29. Lisciandro GR, Ward JL, DeFrancesco TC, et al. Absence of B-lines on Lung Ultrasound (Vet BLUE protocol) to rule out left-sided congestive heart failure in 368 cats and dogs. Abstract. J Vet Emerg Crit Care 2016;26(S1):S8.

30. Ward JL, Lisciandro GR, Keene BW, et al. Accuracy of point-of-care lung ultrasonography for the diagnosis of cardiogenic pulmonary edema in dogs and cats with acute dyspnea. J Am Vet Med Assoc 2017;250:666–75.

31. Rademacher N, Pariaut R, Pate J, et al. Transthoracic lung ultrasound in normal dogs and dogs with cardiogenic pulmonary edema: a pilot study. Vet Radiol Ultrasound 2014;55(4):447–52.

32. Vezzosi T, Mannucci A, Pistoresi F, et al. Assessment of lung ultrasound B-lines in dogs with different stages of chronic valvular heart disease. J Vet Intern Med 2017;31(3):700–4.

Focused Cardiac Ultrasonography in Cats

Kerry Loughran, DVM

KEYWORDS

- Echocardiography • Focused cardiac ultrasonography • Feline cardiomyopathy
- Heart failure • Feline aortic thromboembolism • Pleural effusion
- Pericardial effusion • Respiratory distress

KEY POINTS

Focused cardiac ultrasonography (FCU) can: be conducted by any veterinarian with appropriate training

- identify feline heart disease through the recognition of left ventricular hypertrophy, left atrial enlargement, and cavitary effusion;
- differentiate congestive heart failure (CHF) from noncardiac causes of feline dyspnea;
- screen for occult heart disease in asymptomatic cats; and
- be integrated with other diagnostics for clinical decision making regarding cats that would benefit most from referral for complete echocardiography by a veterinary cardiologist.

  Video content accompanies this article at http://www.vetsmall.theclinics.com.

INTRODUCTION

Heart disease is a common cause of morbidity and mortality in cats.[1–4] Focused cardiac ultrasonography (FCU) can identify ultrasonographic signs supportive of heart disease including left ventricular hypertrophy, left atrial enlargement, and cavitary effusion in symptomatic and asymptomatic cats (**Table 1**). In the emergency and critical care setting, FCU can improve the differentiation of congestive heart failure (CHF) from noncardiac causes of feline respiratory distress.[5,6] In primary care clinics, FCU can screen for occult heart disease in asymptomatic cats with the potential to prevent those at risk from developing cardiac complications.[7]

Echocardiography performed by a veterinary cardiologist is the gold standard of feline cardiac imaging. However, many cats may never receive an echocardiographic evaluation due to limited availability and accessibility.[8] In addition, complete echocardiography is not always possible in critical cats requiring real-time assessment and

---

Department of Clinical Sciences and Advanced Medicine, School of Veterinary Medicine, University of Pennsylvania, 3900 Delancey Street, Philadelphia, PA 19104
E-mail address: kerryl@upenn.edu

Vet Clin Small Anim 51 (2021) 1183–1202
https://doi.org/10.1016/j.cvsm.2021.07.002
0195-5616/21/© 2021 Elsevier Inc. All rights reserved.

Table 1
Prospective study results for focused cardiac ultrasonography in cats

Study/Year	Cat Population	Clinical Question	FCU Performed by	Results
Ward et al,[5] 2018	51 dyspneic cats	Is the dyspnea due to CHF?	Emergency clinicians	• FCU left atrial enlargement: 97.0% sensitive and 100% specific for CHF • Presence of pericardial effusion: 60.6% sensitive and 100% specific for CHF • Vet Blue lung scan with >1 site strongly positive for B-lines: 78.8% sensitive and 83.3% specific for CHF
Janson et al,[6] 2020	41 dyspneic cats	Is the dyspnea due to CHF?	Emergency clinicians	• FCU improved diagnostic accuracy of CHF from 73% after physical examination to 92% after FCU • The LA/Ao measured by FCU was significantly correlated with LA/Ao measured by echocardiography • The POC-BNP did not significantly change the diagnostic accuracy after FCU
Loughran et al,[7] 2019	343 apparently healthy cats	Does the cat have occult heart disease?	Nonspecialist practitioners	• In cats with mild, moderate, and marked occult heart disease, the proportion of cats having a correct diagnosis of heart disease after FCU was 45.6%, 93.1%, and 100%, respectively. • There was significant agreement between the cardiologist and the nonspecialist practitioner regarding the presence of left atrial enlargement and left ventricular hypertrophy

Abbreviations: CHF, congestive heart failure; FCU, focused cardiac ultrasonography; LA/Ao, left atrium to aorta ratio; POC-BNP, point-of-care N-terminal pro-B-type natriuretic peptide assay.

treatment. FCU can easily be learned and performed by emergency clinicians, primary care veterinarians, radiologists, internists, and other noncardiologist personnel.[9,10] When used in conjunction with other diagnostics such as physical examination, thoracic radiography, blood biomarkers, electrocardiography (ECG), Global FAST, and other point-of-care ultrasonographic examinations, feline FCU carries the potential to improve clinical decision making.[4–7]

This article reviews the definition, advantages, clinical indications, limitations, training recommendations, and a protocol for FCU in cats.

DEFINITION

FCU is defined by the American Society of Echocardiography as "a focused examination of the cardiovascular system performed by an [appropriately trained clinician, typically not a cardiologist] by using ultrasound as an adjunct to the physical examination to recognize specific ultrasonic signs that represent a narrow list of potential diagnoses in specific clinical settings."[10] FCU is now also recognized by the American College of Veterinary Internal Medicine as a useful diagnostic tool for identifying cardiomyopathy in cats.[4] FCU is generally used to address a specific binary clinical question of yes (present) or no (absent)[9] (ie, is this cat likely dyspneic because of CHF?). FCU is often one part of an integrative point-of-care ultrasonographic approach, that is, Global FAST, which would include evaluation of the pleural and abdominal cavities to look for effusions and obvious soft tissue abnormalities and the lung to look for cardiogenic pulmonary edema and other lung conditions. Fast enough to perform during a routine primary care wellness appointment and during a rapid emergency triage assessment, abnormalities on FCU can help clinicians make immediate treatment choices, such as whether to start diuretics for CHF. Moreover, FCU can guide decision making regarding referral for complete echocardiography by a veterinary cardiologist.[4] Distinct from complete echocardiography, FCU is a screening test that lacks detailed information on heart morphology and function and may fail to detect all cardiac abnormalities.[4,7,9–11]

ADVANTAGES

Cardiomyopathies are a heterogeneous group of myocardial disorders with variable causes and phenotypes.[4] There are 5 recognized phenotypes in cats including hypertrophic cardiomyopathy (HCM), restrictive cardiomyopathy (RCM), dilated cardiomyopathy (DCM), nonspecific cardiomyopathy, and arrhythmogenic right ventricular cardiomyopathy (**Table 2**). The prevalence of HCM is high (approximately 15% in the general cat population), whereas the other phenotypes are quite uncommon.[2,4,12–14] Regardless of the phenotype, the clinical disease course and certain pathologic features such as left atrial enlargement are similar.

Identifying cats with heart disease can be challenging. The diagnostic tools available including physical examination,[1,5–7,12,13,15] ECG,[7,16,17] thoracic radiography,[1,15,16,18–21] genetic testing,[22,23] and biomarker measurement[5,24–27] all have limitations. Although FCU is not meant to replace other diagnostics, it has several advantages. FCU is performed rapidly, point-of-care with portable equipment, and typically with minimal restraint without exposing the patient or staff to radiation. Moreover, ultrasonography is superior at detecting small volumes of pleural effusion (PE) and pericardial effusion (PCE) compared with radiography.[28] FCU can be performed in combination with other point-of-care ultrasonographic examinations including thoracic/abdominal focused assessment with sonography for trauma, triage, and tracking (TFAST/AFAST) and veterinary bedside lung ultrasound exam (Vet BLUE) to maximize the clinical real-time

Table 2
Classic findings for cardiomyopathy phenotypes adapted from the ACVIM consensus statement guidelines for the classification, diagnosis, and management of cardiomyopathies in cats[4]

Cardiomyopathy Phenotype	Findings
Hypertrophic cardiomyopathy	Diffuse or regional increased left ventricular wall thickness
Restrictive cardiomyopathy	Normal left ventricular dimensions with atrial enlargement
Dilated cardiomyopathy	Normal or reduced left ventricular wall thickness, left ventricular chamber dilation, systolic dysfunction, atrial enlargement
Arrhythmogenic right ventricular cardiomyopathy	Right atrial and right ventricular dilation ± left atrial and left ventricular enlargement
Nonspecific cardiomyopathy	Myocardial abnormalities that do not fit into one category

Abbreviation: ACVIM, American College of Veterinary Internal Medicine.

information gained, especially for symptomatic cats. For example, B-line lung artifacts on Vet BLUE lung ultrasonography are commonly due to alveolar-interstitial edema and can support the diagnosis of fulminant CHF.[29–32]

CLINICAL INDICATIONS

1. Any cat exhibiting clinical signs attributable to heart disease including dyspnea, collapse, and/or limb dragging.
2. Any cat in need of or currently receiving medical treatment that could result in cardiac complications such as steroid administration, parenteral fluid administration, sedation, and/or general anesthesia.
3. Any cat as part of a routine wellness examination to screen for occult cardiomyopathy.

LIMITATIONS

1. Overlap exists between the ultrasonographic appearance of mild cardiomyopathy and normal cardiac morphology, especially in older cats.[33,34] Fortunately, mild disease is often less clinically relevant and the consequences of underdiagnosing mild disease are typically not catastrophic for the cat. In addition, FCU can be performed serially, especially in equivocal or mildly diseased cats to monitor for progression toward more severe disease such as the development of left atrial enlargement.
2. FCU is not always successful. In a recent study of 343 asymptomatic cats, 8% were too fractious to complete FCU without sedation and an additional 8% produced unsatisfactory, nondiagnostic images because of increased body condition, inadequate restraint, or other physical factors.[7]
3. Cardiomyopathy phenotypes are variable and can be associated with different underlying causes such as hyperthyroidism and hypertension, which must be ruled out before idiopathic cardiomyopathy can be definitively diagnosed.[4]
4. Volume status can alter cardiac morphology. For example, dehydration or diuresis can lead to a small left ventricular chamber size and secondary increased wall thickness, known as "pseudohypertrophy," which can be confused with HCM.[35] Volume overload with intravenous fluid administration, long-acting steroids, and anemia can lead to increased chamber sizes, including left atrial size, and thereby lead to abnormal FCU measurements despite no underlying cardiomyopathy.[35–37]

TRAINING RECOMMENDATIONS

Guidelines outlining the appropriate quantity and type of training required for FCU proficiency are lacking.[9,10,38] Studies in humans, dogs, and cats suggest that FCU improves the accuracy of clinical diagnosis regardless of the degree of training or experience.[9,39–42] A published feline FCU training protocol included a short didactic lesson, a live FCU demonstration by a cardiologist, and an online instructional video (Video 3),[8] with variable amounts of supervised and unsupervised practice.[7] This protocol successfully trained veterinarians to acquire the short-axis left atrium to aorta (LA/Ao) view and left ventricular short-axis "mushroom" view, and to subjectively evaluate key cardiac features such as the left atrial size, left ventricular wall thickness, left ventricular contractile function, and the presence or absence of cavitary effusions.[7]

PROTOCOL
Equipment

FCU requires an ultrasound machine with 2D (B-mode) capabilities, a phased-array or curvilinear probe (transducer) with a small footprint, and 70% isopropyl alcohol and/or water-soluble acoustic coupling gel. Owing to the small feline thoracic size and narrow intercostal spaces, high-frequency sector probes (7–12 mHz) are best. Additional helpful equipment includes a cut-out scanning table for obtaining images in lateral recumbency, an e-collar or muzzle for uncooperative cats, and electric clippers for long-haired cats.

Optimal 2D images are obtained by choosing ultrasound settings with a high frame rate and aligning the probe perpendicular to the structures of interest.[43] The cardiac setting that provides a high-contrast image is ideal for evaluating the heart chambers and motion and is recommended if available on the ultrasound machine.[44] An adequate depth of field (usually 4–6 cm in cats) should be ensured to fit the entire heart on the screen. The risk of inadequate depth (too shallow) is that the heart chambers could be misidentified or mistaken for PCE or PE.

A summary of FCU findings should always be recorded in the cat's medical record, ideally on a standardized goal-directed template that aligns with the order of image acquisition and the clinical questions being addressed.[31,38] Whenever possible, FCU images (still or cine) should be stored for review and medical record keeping, especially when real-time assessment is difficult due to patient stability or temperament. Stored images are also invaluable for serial FCU comparison to monitor for progression of disease and response to therapy.

Cat Positioning and Preparation

FCU may be performed in right lateral recumbency, sternal, standing, or on the operator's lap. Imaging the gravity-dependent side in lateral recumbency is ideal because gravity draws the heart toward the probe and against the thoracic wall, displacing air interference from lung and optimizing the acoustic window.[43] However, standing and sternal are generally safer than lateral restraint. Flow-by oxygen can be administered during FCU to respiratory compromised cats.

Shaving a small rectangle on the thorax where the heart's apical beat is palpated can enhance image quality. Alternatively, the hair can be parted after being wetted with isopropyl alcohol. Acoustic coupling gel may then be applied to optimize coupling of the transducer with the exposed skin. Placing the probe on a wetted mat of hair will not provide a good FCU image because of the air trapping, so parting or shaving the hair is crucial. Of note, isopropyl alcohol increases the risk of a fire hazard if electrical defibrillation is needed, and therefore only gel should be used in cats at risk for ventricular fibrillation or cardiopulmonary arrest.[44]

Most cats can be restrained unsedated for FCU. Some cats may require 2 restrainers, whereas others may be too unstable, painful, or fractious to tolerate FCU. If uncooperative, light, safe sedation protocols that will not markedly alter FCU results include the following:

1. Butorphanol and midazolam (0.3 mg/kg of each intramuscularly [IM] or intravenously [IV])
2. Butorphanol (0.3 mg/kg IM or IV) and alfaxalone (0.5 mg/kg IM or titrated to effect 0.25-1 mg/kg IV)

Ultrasound Views

FCU consists of right parasternal short- and long-axis views, left-sided views, and the subcostal view (**Fig. 1**). Obtaining all views is not necessary to answer many clinical questions, and the LA/Ao view often provides the most valuable information because it is independent of ventricular remodeling that may be difficult to interpret.[5-7] If only the LA/Ao view can be obtained, FCU remains a useful diagnostic tool.

FCU views are described in the following discussion in the order for which there is the most evidence to support their use and the author's recommended order for obtaining them. For each FCU view, the probe position, visible cardiac structures, primary purpose, abnormalities to look for, and important points are highlighted. Criteria for characterizing cardiomyopathy and normal values are provided (see **Table 2**; **Table 3**). Normal values vary based on ideal body weight with measurements on the high end of the reference range expected for larger cats and measurements on the low end of the reference range expected for smaller cats.[45,46]

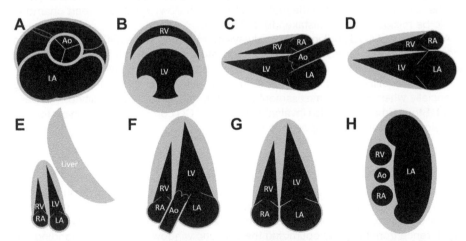

Fig. 1. Two-dimensional schematic representations of heart. Structures visualized from the right parasternal window: (*A*) the short-axis LA/Ao view, (*B*) the short-axis "mushroom" view, (*C*) the long-axis right parasternal outflow tract view, and (*D*) the long-axis right parasternal inflow view. Structures visualized from the (*E*) subcostal view. Structures visualized from the left apical window: (*F*) apical left ventricular outflow view and (*G*) apical inflow view. Structures visualized from the (*H*) left cranial window. Note that orientation for these images has the patient's head to the right and caudal to the left of the image. The ultrasound indicator dot on the screen would be to the right of the image. LA, left atrium; Ao, aorta; LV, left ventricle; RA, right atrium; RV, right ventricle.

Table 3
Normal feline cardiac ultrasonographic values in cats obtained from references cited using mean ± 2 SDs and rounded to the nearest half millimeter or percent

Parameter	Ideal View	Normal Values
Ao	La/Ao	6–12.5 mm[53]
LA	La/Ao	8–15 mm[53]
La/Ao (diameter)	La/Ao	0.8–1.6[53]
La/Ao (area)	La/Ao	2.1–2.8[35]
LVIDd	Mushroom	12–18.5 mm[53]
LVIDs	Mushroom	4–11 mm[53]
IVSd	Mushroom	3-6 mm[53]
LVFWd	Mushroom	3–5.5 mm[53]
IVSd or LVFWd/LVIDd	Mushroom	24%–38%[53]
LVFS	Mushroom	31%–75%[53]
LAD	Inflow	11–18 mm[45]
LAFS	Inflow	16%–36%[57]
RVIDd:LVIDd	Inflow	LVIDd >2RVIDd[65]
RAD:LAD (diameter)	Inflow	RAD < LAD[53,65]

Abbreviations: Ao, aorta; IVSd, interventricular septum thickness at end diastole; LA, left atrium; LAD, left atrial dimension; LAFS, left atrial fractional shortening; LVFS, left ventricular fractional shortening; LVFWd, left ventricular free wall thickness at end diastole; LVIDd, left ventricular internal dimension at end diastole; LVIDs, left ventricular internal dimension at end systole; RAD, right atrial dimension; RVIDd, right ventricular internal dimension at end diastole.

Right Parasternal Short-Axis Heart Base ("Mercedes-Benz" Left Atrium to Aorta View)

Probe position A
The probe is positioned parasternally on the right side of the thorax, most often one intercostal space cranial to the apical heart beat with the probe marker directed cranially toward the cat's elbow. The scan plane goes through the right side of the heart in the near field, the aorta in the center, and the left atrium in the far field (see **Fig. 1**A). The aorta should be round, and ideally the 3 cusps of the aortic valve should form a Y shape, referred to as the Mercedes-Benz sign, during diastole when the valves are closed. The aortic valves may be less conspicuous if a microconvex probe is used.

Primary purpose
The primary purpose of obtaining the LA/Ao view is to evaluate the size of the left atrium (**Fig. 2**, Video 1A). Left atrial size can be evaluated relative to aortic size, which minimizes the influence of patient size variability, or as a nonnormalized dimension (see **Table 3**). Left atrial area relative to aortic area can be either estimated subjectively (ie, eyeballing how many "aortas" fit inside the left atrium) or measured using a linear method of dividing the left atrial diameter by the aortic diameter (see **Fig. 2**). Performing both the area and linear methods is a good way to double check whether the left atrium is enlarged.

Detecting disease
An enlarged left atrium indicates increased left atrial pressure and is typically present in all left-sided heart diseases before and during left-sided congestive heart failure (L-CHF).[18] Although early or mild left-sided heart disease may exist before left atrial

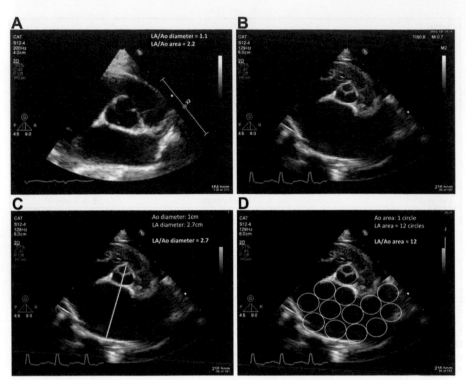

Fig. 2. LA/Ao view of (*A*) a cat with a normal heart and (*B–D*) a cat with a severely enlarged left atrium. Left atrial size is measured by diameter (*C*) and estimated by area relative to the aorta (*D*). LA, left atrium; Ao, aorta.

enlargement, moderate to severe left-sided heart disease of any type is typically accompanied by an enlarged left atrium.[47] An LA/Ao diameter ratio greater than 2.0 is highly suggestive of L-CHF in cats exhibiting clinical signs.[48] If the left atrium is normal in size, the presence of L-CHF is highly unlikely.[5,6,18,48] Moreover, a normal-sized left atrium seen in combination with dry lung on all views of Vet BLUE lung ultra-sonography provides strong evidence that L-CHF is not present.[5]

Hydration status can influence cardiac chamber dimensions. Increased left atrial size is a hallmark of fluid overload.[35–37] Serial FCU should be considered during administration of parenteral fluids (and may be combined with Vet BLUE and TFAST) to screen for developing L-CHF from volume overload and is a recommended application of FCU in human medicine.[9]

Challenges of measuring the feline left atrium include: (1) an angle of interrogation that incorporates a pulmonary vein that prevents visualization of the left atrial wall and thus the operator may need to extrapolate the margins of the left atrium for measurement; and (2) if the scan plane is directed too far dorsally in the basilar direction, the right pulmonary artery can obscure the view of the left atrium.

The left atrium can also be evaluated in any of its views for spontaneous echogenic contrast, which appears as a swirling of blood referred to as left atrial "smoke" (**Fig. 3**A, Video 1B). The presence of spontaneous echogenic contrast suggests that aggregates of cellular material are forming due to blood stasis (Virchow triad) and may lead to the development of an intracardiac thrombus, most commonly seen

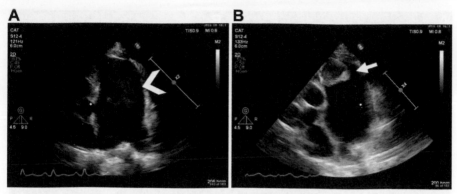

Fig. 3. Left cranial view of (*A*) a cat with left atrial spontaneous echogenic contrast (chevron) and (*B*) a cat with a thrombus in the left auricle (*arrow*).

wedged in the left auricle (see **Fig. 3**B).[49–52] As a result, aortic or arterial thromboemboli (ATE) become a possible sequela.

Important points
Evaluating left atrial size is clinically useful in symptomatic[5,6] and asymptomatic[7] cats. Left atrial size measurement with FCU is strongly correlated with left atrial size measured by echocardiography.[6,7] Diuretic therapy should be considered for any cat with an enlarged left atrium and clinical signs of L-CHF. Further supportive evidence may be gained by performing lung ultrasonography such as Vet BLUE because in the absence of B-lines, cardiogenic pulmonary edema is unlikely.[29,30] Prophylactic treatment with clopidogrel should be considered in any cat with an enlarged left atrium, left atrial spontaneous echogenic contrast, and/or an observed intracardiac thrombus to prevent ATE (barring any contraindications).[4]

Right Parasternal Short-Axis Ventricular Level ("Mushroom" View)

Probe position B
Moving from the LA/Ao view to the "mushroom" view requires fanning apically from the same external point on the thoracic wall. The scan plane is directed through the right ventricle, which appears as a half-moon crescent in the near field, and the left ventricle in the far field at the level where the mitral valve chordae tendineae attach to the papillary muscles (see **Fig. 1**B). The left ventricle is the structure of interest, but the right ventricle can also be evaluated. This level along the short axis is called the "mushroom" view because the cavity of the left ventricle looks like a mushroom.

Primary purpose
The primary purpose of the "mushroom" view is evaluation of left ventricular chamber size, contractility, and wall thickness (**Fig. 4**, Video 2A). This view is especially important for categorizing types of cardiomyopathy (see **Table 2**). Wall thickness is measured at end diastole when the heart is full. Fractional shortening (FS) is calculated by freezing a loop to measure the left ventricular internal dimension at end diastole when it is most full (LVIDd) and at end systole when it is most empty (LVIDs). FS is calculated as (LVIDd-LVIDs)/LVIDd.

Detecting disease
An HCM phenotype is characterized by left ventricular concentric hypertrophy recognized via FCU as (1) increased septal or left ventricular wall thickness measured at end

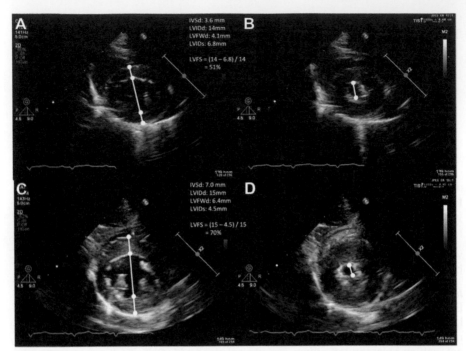

Fig. 4. Right parasternal left ventricular "mushroom" view. The left ventricle of a normal cat in (A) diastole and (B) systole; and the left ventricle of a cat with hypertrophic cardiomyopathy in diastole (C) and systole (D). The left ventricular measurements and fractional shortening calculation [(LVIDd – LVIDs)/LVIDd] are displayed. IVSd, interventricular septum thickness at end-diastole; LVIDd, left ventricular internal dimension at end diastole; LVFWd, left ventricular free wall thickness at end diastole, LVIDs, left ventricular internal dimension at end systole.

diastole (see **Table 3**), (2) enlarged papillary muscles, and/or (3) left ventricular cavity obliteration at the end of systole (see **Fig. 4**, Video 2B).[53–55] Objectively measuring wall thickness is superior to estimating or eyeballing whether concentric hypertrophy of the left ventricle is present because rapid feline heart rates and patient movement can cause the left ventricle to subjectively appear thick even when measurements are normal. The sonographer must learn to use the freeze function and roll the cine ball through frames to capture the correct view of interest.

Although HCM is by far the most common cardiomyopathy phenotype, it is important for the sonographer to be aware of phenotype variability (see **Table 2**). For example, cats with RCM exhibit normal left ventricular wall thickness and contractility. However, if the left atrium is enlarged, heart disease could be present. Challenges in evaluating the left ventricle include (1) determining whether any observed asymmetry of the left ventricle is due to probe positioning versus true myocardial asymmetry, of which the latter can be a sign of disease, and (2) determining if the scan plane is too far apical, which could lead to the incorrect diagnosis of left ventricular hypertrophy.[31,54]

The right side of the heart can also be evaluated from the "mushroom" view. Flattening of the interventricular septum, an enlarged right ventricular chamber, and/or increased right ventricular wall thickness suggests right ventricular volume or pressure overload (see **Table 3**). The accuracy and utility of evaluation of the right side of the heart with FCU in cats has not been reported, and therefore, referral for complete echocardiography is best if right-sided heart abnormalities are suspected. However, evidence in human medicine supports that evaluation of the size of the right side of the heart with FCU is clinically helpful.[9,10]

Important points
Despite the imaging challenges, evaluation of the left ventricular wall thickness using FCU is significantly correlated with echocardiographic measurements in cats.[7] Increased wall thickness could indicate HCM. Decreased contractility could indicate DCM or end-stage HCM. Normal wall thickness combined with left atrial enlargement could indicate RCM (see **Table 2**). If features of cardiomyopathy are present, caution with treatments that could be contraindicated in cats with heart disease and referral for evaluation by a veterinary cardiologist is appropriate.

Right Parasternal Long-Axis 5-Chamber (Outflow) View and 4-Chamber (Inflow) View

Probe positions C and D
The probe is rotated 90° to change from the short-axis views to the long-axis views. For the outflow view, the probe marker points toward the cat's shoulder. The scanning plane is directed through the right ventricle and right atrium in the near field and the left atrium and left ventricle in the far field with the aorta between the left and right atrium (see **Fig. 1**C). For the inflow view, the probe marker points dorsally toward the cat's neck. Compared with the outflow view, the aorta is no longer visible and the left atrium and right atrium are adjacent with the interatrial septum between them (see **Fig. 1**D).

Primary purpose
The long-axis inflow and outflow views can be used to look for left ventricular hypertrophy, decreased left ventricular contractility, and right-sided heart enlargement (see **Table 3**). Care should be taken not to include papillary muscle in any of the measurements to avoid a false-positive diagnosis of left ventricular hypertrophy. Left atrial size and function can also be assessed.

Detecting disease
The outflow view is especially valuable to evaluate the interventricular septum. Some cats with HCM exhibit focal thickening of the basilar septum, and this can contribute to a left ventricular outflow tract obstruction (**Fig. 5**).

The inflow view provides a useful image of the left and right atria (see **Fig. 5**; **Fig. 6**). In dyspneic cats, a cutoff value for left atrial size of 1.65 cm has a sensitivity and specificity of 87% for diagnosing CHF.[56] Minimum and maximum left atrial diameter measurements abbreviated as LADmin and LADmax, respectively, can also be used to calculate left atrial FS as (LADmax-LADmin)/LADmax, which decreases progressively with more advanced disease (see **Table 3**).[47,57,58]

Important points
The right parasternal long-axis views provide information about chamber sizes, wall thickness, and contractility. Although these views are used less frequently and their clinical utility as part of FCU has not been specifically studied, cardiac information provided is similar to the short-axis views. In some cases, long-axis images may be easier to ascertain and can serve to double-check one's FCU assessment.

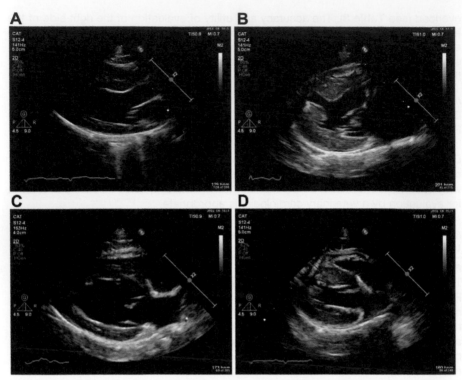

Fig. 5. Right parasternal long-axis outflow view in (*A*) a normal cat and (*B*) a cat with hypertrophic cardiomyopathy and pronounced upper septal thickening. Right parasternal inflow view in (*C*) a normal cat and (*D*) a cat with severe left ventricular concentric hypertrophy from idiopathic hypertrophic cardiomyopathy.

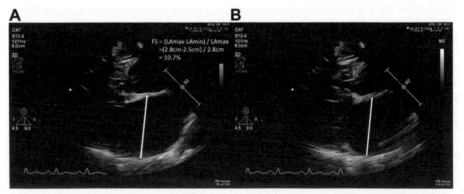

Fig. 6. Right parasternal long-axis inflow view in a cat with severe left atrial enlargement measured when the atrium is the biggest (*A*) and when the atrium is the smallest (*B*). The left atrial fractional shortening calculation [(LADmax-LADmin)/LADmax] is displayed. LAD, left atrial dimension.

Subcostal View (Diaphragmaticohepatic View)

Probe position E

The probe is positioned caudal to the xiphoid in a longitudinal plane with footprint facing cranially and the marker pointing caudodorsally toward the spine. The scan plane is directed through the liver in the near field, the diaphragm in the middle of the field of view, and the heart in the far field (see **Fig. 1E**). In AFAST and TFAST protocols, this same view is analogous to their diaphragmaticohepatic (DH) view.

Primary purpose

The subcostal view evaluates for pleural, pericardial, and abdominal effusion as well as venous congestion (eg, distended caudal vena cava and hepatic veins).

Detecting disease

In cats, the presence of PCE is highly specific for diagnosing L-CHF.[5] The amount typically ranges from scant to mild without evidence of tamponade (collapse of the right-sided heart chambers), but there can occasionally be larger volumes in severe or chronic cases of feline CHF. In one study, 75% of cats with any degree of PCE had the final diagnosis of CHF.[59] In another study, any degree of feline PCE was 100% specific for heart failure.[5] Other far less common causes of feline PCE include feline infectious peritonitis and neoplasia such as lymphoma. PCE most commonly appears as an anechoic space around the heart, rimmed by the hyperechoic pericardium creating a circular appearance (**Fig. 7**).

PE is a common consequence of feline L-CHF and right-sided congestive heart failure (R-CHF), unlike in dogs. In FCU views, PE appears as an anechoic space surrounding the heart and lungs (see **Fig. 7**). Importantly, the diaphragm often creates a mirror image of the gallbladder into the thorax, which can be mistaken for PE if the sonographer is not aware of this potential artifact. However, mirror image artifact requires a strong air-soft tissue interface and rules out PE in that scanning plane.

Distinguishing PE from PCE can be challenging. The machine must be set to display enough depth to see the heart in its entirety, using the landmark of the hyperechoic pericardium in the far field, so that heart chambers are identified and not mistaken for PE or PCE. If the pericardium is hard to identify, one should turn the gain down and look in the far field for the hyperechoic pericardium, which as a rule is the brightest structure in the thoracic cavity. Other general principles are that PCE is rounded being contained within the pericardial sac. In contrast, PE is uncontained, and thus more triangulated in appearance within the pleural cavity (see **Fig. 7**). However, PE may be symmetric, unilateral, compartmentalized, and have varied degrees of echogenicity depending on its cause.

Of note, PE and PCE often exist simultaneously in feline CHF. In these cases, the pericardium is sandwiched between 2 anechoic spaces with the PCE on one side and the PE on the other. Although a scant amount of PE and PCE is physiologic, it is not typically appreciable on FCU.

Abdominal effusion can occur with feline R-CHF or biventricular CHF but is not present with isolated L-CHF and is overall less commonly associated with heart disease in cats than dogs.[60] If there is R-CHF or biventricular CHF, the hepatic veins and caudal vena cava are typically visibly distended and the hepatic parenchyma may appear subjectively hypoechoic.[31]

Importantly, all FCU views can be used to detect PE and PCE. As a general rule, suspect effusion should always be documented at more than one FCU view with enough depth to see the heart in its entirety to prevent false-positives[54,61] (see **Fig. 7**).

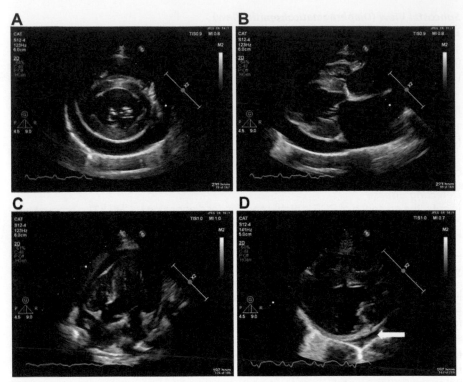

Fig. 7. Pericardial effusion visualized from the (*A*) short-axis left ventricular "mushroom" view, (*B*) right parasternal long-axis inflow view, and (*C*) left ventricular long-axis outflow view in cats with cardiomyopathy. Pleural effusion (*arrow*) visualized from the (*D*) left ventricular "mushroom" view in a cat with cardiomyopathy.

Important points

The subcostal view, which is part of the AFAST and TFAST protocols, is most helpful and efficient as a single view (and advantageous for circumventing the air interference of transthoracic views) to look for evidence of L-CHF and R-CHF including PE, PCE, ascites, and distension of the caudal vena cava and hepatic veins. In cats with L-CHF, PE and PCE are common either alone or in combination with cardiogenic pulmonary edema. Ascites along with distension of the caudal vena cava and hepatic veins may be present if there is R-CHF or biventricular CHF.

Left Apical and Left Cranial Views

Probe positions F, G, and H

For the left apical views, the probe is positioned at the parasternal aspect of the left side of the thorax, near the apical beat with the marker aimed caudodorsally toward the cat's lumbar spine. The scan plane is directed to go through the cardiac apex in the near field with the cardiac base in the far field. The probe is rotated slightly clockwise and fanned to be more perpendicular with the thorax to go from the left ventricular outflow view (see **Fig. 1**F) to the 4-chamber left apical view without the aorta (see **Fig. 1**G). For the left cranial view, the probe is moved cranially into the axillary region and the marker points cranially. The probe should be fanned so that it is almost parallel with the thorax. The structure of interest in the left cranial view is the left atrium (see **Fig. 1**H).

Primary purpose and detecting disease

The left apical views provide a subjective impression of chamber sizes, wall thickness, and contractility using similar criteria as described for the right-sided inflow and outflow views. The left cranial view offers the best image to see spontaneous echogenic contrast and/or intracardiac thrombi by advantageously providing a clearer view of the left auricle (see **Fig. 3**).

Important points

The left-sided apical and cranial views can be performed only when necessary and feasible. These views are likely unnecessary for most cats if good right-sided views are acquired. However, in some cats, especially those with severe pulmonary parenchymal disease in which air-filled lung obscures right parasternal FCU views, obtaining these left-sided views can be helpful. In complete echocardiography, the left-sided views are important for Doppler measurements of mitral inflow velocity and left ventricular outflow velocity and assessment of valvular insufficiencies, which are not part of FCU.

Combining Focused Cardiac Ultrasonography with Other Point-of-Care Ultrasound Scans

Integrating point-of-care ultrasound information, that is, AFAST, TFAST, and Vet BLUE, can be helpful especially when FCU is too risky or the cat is too uncooperative for restraint because these other examinations are generally lower impact (less restraint) for the patient. For example, the absence of PE combined with dry lung in all Vet BLUE views usually rules out L-CHF and places feline asthma at the top of the differential list in cats with non-trauma-induced respiratory distress. On the other hand, nondistended caudal vena cava and hepatic veins rule out any clinically relevant R-CHF at the AFAST-TFAST DH view. Evaluating lung via Vet BLUE and evaluating the caudal vena cava and hepatic veins via the AFAST-TFAST DH views are referred to as the Global FAST non-echo fallback views when FCU is not possible and are explained in more detail.

Another clinically helpful manner in which to take advantage of the Global FAST non-echo fallback views is to better assess FCU findings. For example, if during FCU the LA/Ao appears to be markedly enlarged ($\geq$2), then the use of Vet BLUE allows for the assessment of cardiogenic pulmonary edema and its degree through its B-line scoring system combined with its number of positive regions. Thus, in this case, dry lung on Vet BLUE supports the absence of L-CHF in the presence of likely left-sided heart disease that is nonemergent but requires follow-up. If the cat has respiratory distress then the FCU finding combined with dry lung during Vet BLUE better supports primary respiratory disease with concurrent left-sided heart disease without overt L-CHF. This strategy has been documented in cats without PE and PCE.[5,30,31] Furthermore, in cats with wet lung (B-lines), especially with an enlarged LA/Ao ($\geq$2), B-line scoring combined with numbers of positive regional Vet BLUE views helps guide appropriate heart failure and loop diuretic therapy as recently shown in dogs.[62] There are other causes of B-lines in cats including pneumonia, hemorrhage, and inflammatory conditions, and pseudo B-lines caused by nodular disease.[63]

Centesis

FCU can be used to guide pleurocentesis in cats. Therapeutic pleurocentesis is commonly performed in cats with CHF to treat respiratory distress from pressure atelectasis. By physically removing the PE, necessary diuretic therapy dose and frequency can be reduced. Point-of-care ultrasonography can not only be used to find the largest pocket of PE but also can be used to avoid the serious complication of cardiac puncture. Pericardiocentesis is not typically indicated in cases of feline PCE caused by CHF because (1) the amount of PCE is usually small; (2) the PCE should respond to diuretic therapy, which is the treatment of choice; (3) either the left or both atria are enlarged, which can increase the likelihood of life-threatening cardiac puncture; and (4) cats with severe heart disease are often receiving an antithrombotic therapy, which can increase the risk for bleeding. However, in cats with noncardiac causes of large-volume PCE, FCU can guide needle or catheter placement for drainage.

Cardiopulmonary Resuscitation

FCU should be used during cardiopulmonary resuscitation in conjunction with the ECG to look for coordinated cardiac contractions that would suggest return of spontaneous circulation and rule out the presence of pulseless electrical activity and asystole.[9,10,64]

SUMMARY

Feline FCU performed by a trained noncardiologist veterinarian is a useful diagnostic tool for identifying heart disease in both symptomatic and asymptomatic cats. Designed to be an extension of the physical examination, FCU can improve clinical decision making especially when used in conjunction with other diagnostic tests. Advantages include that it is rapid to perform, provides real-time information, requires minimal feline restraint, is radiation sparing, and has a high accuracy for detecting moderate to severe heart disease. Moreover, serial FCU examinations may be used for monitoring patients and guiding therapy.

DISCLOSURE

No commercial or financial conflicts of interest. No funding sources.

ACKNOWLEDGMENTS

The author would like to thank Erin Achilles, Sarah Benjamin, Tatiana Cooke, Anna Gelzer, Clare Gruendel, Terry Huh, Marie Keith, Marc Kraus, Éva Larouche-Lebel, Rory Loughran, Mark Oyama, Nicola Parisi, Megan Poad, John Rush, and Gabriela Villanueva for their thoughtful suggestions in the making of this article.

SUPPLEMENTARY DATA

Supplementary data related to this article can be found online at https://doi.org/10.1016/j.cvsm.2021.07.002.

REFERENCES

1. Rush JE, Freeman LM, Fenollosa NK, et al. Population and survival characteristics of cats with hypertrophic cardiomyopathy: 260 cases (1990-1999). J Am Vet Med Assoc 2002;220(2):202–7.
2. Payne J, Luis Fuentes V, Boswood A, et al. Population characteristics and survival in 127 referred cats with hypertrophic cardiomyopathy (1997 to 2005). J Small Anim Pract 2010;51(10):540–7.
3. Fox PR, Keene BW, Lamb K, et al. Long-term incidence and risk of noncardiovascular and all-cause mortality in apparently healthy cats and cats with preclinical hypertrophic cardiomyopathy. J Vet Intern Med 2019;33(6):2572–86.

4. Luis Fuentes V, Abbott J, Chetboul V, et al. ACVIM consensus statement guidelines for the classification, diagnosis, and management of cardiomyopathies in cats. J Vet Intern Med 2020;34(3):1062–77.

5. Ward JL, Lisciandro GR, Ware WA, et al. Evaluation of point-of-care thoracic ultrasound and NT-proBNP for the diagnosis of congestive heart failure in cats with respiratory distress. J Vet Intern Med 2018;32(5):1530–40.

6. Janson CO, Hezzell MJ, Oyama MA, et al. Focused cardiac ultrasound and point-of-care NT-proBNP assay in the emergency room for differentiation of cardiac and noncardiac causes of respiratory distress in cats. J Vet Emerg Crit Care 2020; 30(4):376–83.

7. Loughran KA, Rush JE, Rozanski EA, et al. The use of focused cardiac ultrasound to screen for occult heart disease in asymptomatic cats. J Vet Intern Med 2019; 33(5):1892–901.

8. Association AVM. Reports and statistics. Secondary Reports and statistics. 2019. Available at: https://www.avma.org/resources-tools/reports-statistics. Accessed January 1, 2021.

9. Via G, Hussain A, Wells M, et al. International evidence-based recommendations for focused cardiac ultrasound. J Am Soc Echocardiogr 2014;27(7):683 e1–83 e33.

10. Spencer KT, Kimura BJ, Korcarz CE, et al. Focused cardiac ultrasound: recommendations from the American Society of Echocardiography. J Am Soc Echocardiogr 2013;26(6):567–81.

11. Rush J. Two Minute screening Echocardiogram for cats. North Grafton (MA): Youtube; 2018.

12. Paige CF, Abbott JA, Elvinger F, et al. Prevalence of cardiomyopathy in apparently healthy cats. J Am Vet Med Assoc 2009;234(11):1398–403.

13. Wagner T, Fuentes VL, Payne JR, et al. Comparison of auscultatory and echocardiographic findings in healthy adult cats. J Vet Cardiol 2010;12(3):171–82.

14. Ferasin L, Sturgess CP, Cannon MJ, et al. Feline idiopathic cardiomyopathy: a retrospective study of 106 cats (1994-2001). J Feline Med Surg 2003;5(3):151–9.

15. Payne JR, Brodbelt DC, Luis Fuentes V. Cardiomyopathy prevalence in 780 apparently healthy cats in rehoming centres (the CatScan study). J Vet Cardiol 2015;17(Suppl 1):S244–57.

16. Schober KE, Maerz I, Ludewig E, et al. Diagnostic accuracy of electrocardiography and thoracic radiography in the assessment of left atrial size in cats: comparison with transthoracic 2-dimensional echocardiography. J Vet Intern Med 2007;21(4):709–18.

17. Moise NS, Dietze AE, Mezza LE, et al. Echocardiography, electrocardiography, and radiography of cats with dilatation cardiomyopathy, hypertrophic cardiomyopathy, and hyperthyroidism. Am J Vet Res 1986;47(7):1476–86.

18. Schober KE, Wetli E, Drost WT. Radiographic and echocardiographic assessment of left atrial size in 100 cats with acute left-sided congestive heart failure. Vet Radiol Ultrasound 2014;55(4):359–67.

19. Litster AL, Buchanan JW. Radiographic and echocardiographic measurement of the heart in obese cats. Vet Radiol Ultrasound 2000;41(4):320–5.

20. Carlisle CH, Thrall DE. A comparison of normal feline thoracic radiographs made in dorsal versus ventral recumbency. Vet Radiol 1982;23(1):3–9.

21. Toal RL, Losonsky JM, Coulter DB, et al. Influence of cardiac cycle on the radiographic appearance of the feline heart. Vet Radiol 1985;26(2):63–9.

22. Wess G, Schinner C, Weber K, et al. Association of A31P and A74T polymorphisms in the myosin binding protein C3 gene and hypertrophic cardiomyopathy in Maine Coon and other breed cats. J Vet Intern Med 2010;24(3):527–32.

23. Granstrom S, Godiksen MT, Christiansen M, et al. Genotype-phenotype correlation between the cardiac myosin binding protein C mutation A31P and hypertrophic cardiomyopathy in a cohort of Maine Coon cats: a longitudinal study. J Vet Cardiol 2015;17(Suppl 1):S268–81.

24. Connolly DJ, Magalhaes RJ, Syme HM, et al. Circulating natriuretic peptides in cats with heart disease. J Vet Intern Med 2008;22(1):96–105.

25. Fox PR, Rush JE, Reynolds CA, et al. Multicenter evaluation of plasma N-terminal probrain natriuretic peptide (NT-pro BNP) as a biochemical screening test for asymptomatic (occult) cardiomyopathy in cats. J Vet Intern Med 2011;25(5):1010–6.

26. Machen MC, Oyama MA, Gordon SG, et al. Multi-centered investigation of a point-of-care NT-proBNP ELISA assay to detect moderate to severe occult (pre-clinical) feline heart disease in cats referred for cardiac evaluation. J Vet Cardiol 2014;16(4):245–55.

27. Lalor SM, Connolly DJ, Elliott J, et al. Plasma concentrations of natriuretic peptides in normal cats and normotensive and hypertensive cats with chronic kidney disease. J Vet Cardiol 2009;11(Suppl 1):S71–9.

28. Soni NJ, Franco R, Velez MI, et al. Ultrasound in the diagnosis and management of pleural effusions. J Hosp Med 2015;10(12):811–6.

29. Ward JL, Lisciandro GR, DeFrancesco TC. Distribution of alveolar-interstitial syndrome in dogs and cats with respiratory distress as assessed by lung ultrasound versus thoracic radiographs. J Vet Emerg Crit Care (San Antonio) 2018;28(5):415–28.

30. Ward JL, Lisciandro GR, Keene BW, et al. Accuracy of point-of-care lung ultrasonography for the diagnosis of cardiogenic pulmonary edema in dogs and cats with acute dyspnea. J Am Vet Med Assoc 2017;250(6):666–75.

31. Lisciandro GR. Cageside Ultrasonography in the Emergency Room and Intensive Care Unit. Vet Clin North Am Small Anim Pract 2020;50(6):1445–67.

32. Lisciandro GR, Fulton RM, Fosgate GT, et al. Frequency and number of B-lines using a regionally based lung ultrasound examination in cats with radiographically normal lungs compared to cats with left-sided congestive heart failure. J Vet Emerg Crit Care (San Antonio) 2017;27(5):499–505.

33. Haggstrom J, Luis Fuentes V, Wess G. Screening for hypertrophic cardiomyopathy in cats. J Vet Cardiol 2015;17(Suppl 1):S134–49.

34. Fox PR. Hypertrophic cardiomyopathy. Clinical and pathologic correlates. J Vet Cardiol 2003;5(2):39–45.

35. Campbell FE, Kittleson MD. The effect of hydration status on the echocardiographic measurements of normal cats. J Vet Intern Med 2007;21(5):1008–15.

36. Wilson HE, Jasani S, Wagner TB, et al. Signs of left heart volume overload in severely anaemic cats. J Feline Med Surg 2010;12(12):904–9.

37. Smith SA, Tobias AH, Fine DM, et al. Corticosteroid-associated congestive heart failure in 12 cats. Intern J Appl Res Vet Med 2004;2(3):159–70.

38. Adamson R, Morris AE, Woan JS, et al. Development of a Focused Cardiac Ultrasound Image Acquisition Assessment Tool. ATS Scholar 2020;1(3):260–77.

39. Panoulas VF, Daigeler AL, Malaweera AS, et al. Pocket-size hand-held cardiac ultrasound as an adjunct to clinical examination in the hands of medical students and junior doctors. Eur Heart J Cardiovasc Imaging 2013;14(4):323–30.

40. Kobal SL, Trento L, Baharami S, et al. Comparison of effectiveness of hand-carried ultrasound to bedside cardiovascular physical examination. Am J Cardiol 2005;96(7):1002–6.

41. Hezzell MJ, Ostroski C, Oyama MA, et al. Investigation of focused cardiac ultrasound in the emergency room for differentiation of respiratory and cardiac causes of respiratory distress in dogs. J Vet Emerg Crit Care 2020;30(2):159–64.

42. Tse YC, Rush JE, Cunningham SM, et al. Evaluation of a training course in focused echocardiography for noncardiology house officers. J Vet Emerg Crit Care (San Antonio) 2013;23(3):268–73.

43. Côté E, MacDonald KA, Meurs KM, Sleeper MM. Echocardiography. Feline Cardiology, 2011:51-67.

44. DeFrancesco T. Focused or COAST3—ECHO (Heart). Focused Ultrasound Techniques for the Small Animal Practitioner, 2014:189-205.

45. Schober K, Savino S, Yildiz V. Reference intervals and allometric scaling of two-dimensional echocardiographic measurements in 150 healthy cats. J Vet Med Sci 2017;79(11):1764–71.

46. Häggström J, Andersson ÅO, Falk T, et al. Effect of Body Weight on Echocardiographic Measurements in 19,866 Pure-Bred Cats with or without Heart Disease. J Vet Intern Med 2016;30(5):1601–11.

47. Abbott JA, MacLean HN. Two-Dimensional Echocardiographic Assessment of the Feline Left Atrium. J Vet Intern Med 2006;20(1).111–9.

48. Patata V, Caivano D, Porciello F, et al. Pulmonary vein to pulmonary artery ratio in healthy and cardiomyopathic cats. J Vet Cardiol 2020;27:23–33.

49. Vititoe KP, Fries RC, Joslyn S, et al. Detection of intra-cardiac thrombi and congestive heart failure in cats using computed tomographic angiography. Vet Radiol Ultrasound 2018;59(4):412–22.

50. Schober KE, Maerz I. Assessment of left atrial appendage flow velocity and its relation to spontaneous echocardiographic contrast in 89 cats with myocardial disease. J Vet Intern Med 2006;20(1):120–30.

51. Côté E, MacDonald KA, Meurs KM, Sleeper MM. Arterial Thromboembolism. Feline Cardiology, 2011:303-322.

52. Hogan DF, Brainard BM. Cardiogenic embolism in the cat. J Vet Cardiol 2015;17: S202–14.

53. Adin DB, Diley-Poston L. Papillary muscle measurements in cats with normal echocardiograms and cats with concentric left ventricular hypertrophy. J Vet Intern Med 2007;21(4):737–41.

54. Boon JA. Veterinary echocardiography. Ames (IA): John Wiley & Sons; 2011.

55. Côté E, MacDonald KA, Meurs KM, Sleeper MM. Hypertrophic Cardiomyopathy. Feline Cardiology, 2011:101-175.

56. Smith S, Dukes-McEwan J. Clinical signs and left atrial size in cats with cardiovascular disease in general practice. J Small Anim Pract 2012;53(1):27–33.

57. Linney CJ, Dukes-McEwan J, Stephenson HM, et al. Left atrial size, atrial function and left ventricular diastolic function in cats with hypertrophic cardiomyopathy. J Small Anim Pract 2014;55(4):198–206.

58. Kochie SL, Schober KE, Rhinehart J, et al. Effects of pimobendan on left atrial transport function in cats. J Vet Intern Med 2021;35(1):10–21.

59. Hall DJ, Shofer F, Meier CK, et al. Pericardial effusion in cats: a retrospective study of clinical findings and outcome in 146 cats. J Vet Intern Med 2007; 21(5):1002–7.

60. Côté E, MacDonald KA, Meurs KM, Sleeper MM. Pleural Effusion. Feline Cardiology, 2011:19-23.

61. Lisciandro G. The Thoracic FAST3 (TFAST3) Exam. Focused Ultrasound Techniques for the Small Animal Practitioner, 2014:140-165.
62. Murphy SD, Ward JL, Viall AK, et al. Utility of point-of-care lung ultrasound for monitoring cardiogenic pulmonary edema in dogs. J Vet Intern Med 2021; 35(1):68–77.
63. Lisciandro GR, Lisciandro SC. POCUS: Vet BLUE – Clinical Integration. Point-of-Care Ultrasound Tech Small Anim Pract 2021;459–507.
64. Breitkreutz R, Price S, Steiger HV, et al. Focused echocardiographic evaluation in life support and peri-resuscitation of emergency patients: a prospective trial. Resuscitation 2010;81(11):1527–33.
65. Visser LC, Sloan CQ, Stern JA. Echocardiographic Assessment of Right Ventricular Size and Function in Cats With Hypertrophic Cardiomyopathy. J Vet Intern Med 2017;31(3):668–77.

Focused Canine Cardiac Ultrasound

Teresa C. DeFrancesco, DVM, DACVIM (Cardiology), DACVECC[a],*,
Jessica L. Ward, DVM, DACVIM (Cardiology)[b]

KEYWORDS

- Echocardiography • Congestive heart failure • Dyspnea • Respiratory distress
- Pulmonary edema • Ascites • Pleural effusion • Pericardial effusion

KEY POINTS

- In a dog in severe respiratory distress, focused cardiac ultrasound (FCU) findings of a severely enlarged left atrium and diffuse B-lines on lung ultrasound are corroborative evidence of left-sided congestive heart failure, whereas the FCU findings of a severely enlarged and thickened right ventricle with a flattened interventricular septum are indicative of right heart pressure overload possibly related to pulmonary hypertension.
- In a dog with ascites, the FCU findings of a distended, nonfluctuating caudal vena cava, distended hepatic veins, and right heart enlargement provide corroborative evidence for right-sided congestive heart failure.
- FCU is useful in both diagnosis and treatment of pericardial effusion and cardiac tamponade. The finding of a hypoechoic to anechoic ring of fluid around the heart, right atrial collapse, and a nonfluctuating distended caudal vena cava in a dog is diagnostic for pericardial effusion with cardiac tamponade and an indication for a therapeutic pericardiocentesis.
- In a dog that presents collapsed and hypotensive, an FCU, together with other diagnostic findings, can help differentiate between common etiologies, such as pericardial effusion with cardiac tamponade, severe dilated cardiomyopathy with myocardial failure, and hypovolemia due to fluid loss.

INTRODUCTION

Focused cardiac ultrasound (FCU), or focused echocardiography, is a useful point-of-care diagnostic imaging tool typically performed in symptomatic dogs in the acute care setting. Unlike formal or complete echocardiography, FCU is a time-sensitive examination involving a select subset of targeted ultrasound views to identify severe

[a] Department of Clinical Sciences, College of Veterinary Medicine, North Carolina State University, 1052 William Moore Dr, Raleigh, NC 27607, USA; [b] Department of Veterinary Clinical Sciences, College of Veterinary Medicine, Iowa State University, 1809 S. Riverside Dr, Ames, IA 50010, USA
* Corresponding author.
E-mail address: tdefranc@ncsu.edu

Vet Clin Small Anim 51 (2021) 1203–1216
https://doi.org/10.1016/j.cvsm.2021.07.005

abnormalities in cardiac chamber size or systolic function. FCU should be performed as part of an integrated thoracic ultrasound, including interrogation of the pleural space, lungs, and caudal vena cava (CVC). Most often, the goal of FCU is to identify cardiovascular disease severe enough to cause emergent clinical signs (dyspnea, tachypnea, syncope, hypotension or cavitary effusions); FCU findings then can be used in combination with signalment, history, and physical examination to prioritize relevant differential diagnoses and guide emergency treatment.

In dogs, FCU is most helpful in the timely diagnoses of pericardial effusion and tamponade or structural heart diseases severe enough to cause left-sided congestive heart failure (L-CHF) or right-sided congestive heart failure (R-CHF). FCU also has proved useful in characterizing a hypotensive dog of uncertain etiology by identifying conditions, such as severe structural heart disease (eg, dilated cardiomyopathy [DCM]), pericardial effusion with cardiac tamponade, and extreme hypovolemia. More recently, FCU has been shown to play an important role in cardiopulmonary resuscitation by helping to identify any possible underlying causes for a nonshockable cardiac arrest (such as cardiac tamponade, critical hypovolemia, and massive pulmonary embolism) and in recognizing spontaneous cardiac activity that can be helpful in prognosis.[1] The improved diagnostic accuracy of FCU in certain conditions over the cardiac physical examination alone is the reason why point-of-care thoracic ultrasound has been coined the "visual stethoscope of the 21st century."[2]

IMAGE ACQUISITION CONSIDERATIONS
Transducer and Patient Positioning

The microconvex (curvilinear) probe is the most commonly used transducer in FCU because it is the most widely available (**Table 1**). A phased-array transducer, however, is preferred for cardiac imaging due to its ability to achieve high sampling rates (allowing for better temporal resolution in a beating heart) and smaller footprint (less rib and lung interference). Most newer compact ultrasound units have a cardiac preset that

Table 1	
General ultrasound machine and transducer settings recommended for focused cardiac ultrasound in dogs	
Setting	**Recommendations for Focused Cardiac Ultrasound**
Transducer	Microconvex (curvilinear) most commonly used; however, phased-array is preferable if available to improve temporal resolution.
Preset	Cardiac (if available); inverts image left-to-right so that atria are on right side of screen and optimizes for high contrast (vs shades of gray)
Frequency	Contingent on size of dog: higher frequencies for smaller dogs and lower frequencies for larger dogs. Choose highest frequency that allows optimal image quality.
Contact	Alcohol + ultrasound gel ($\pm$ shave hair if very thick)
Patient positioning	Sternal (often most practical, especially in respiratory distress) or right lateral from underneath (bring dog to edge of table/cage or use a custom echocardiography table with cutout)
Depth	Visualize the entire heart so that it fills at least 2/3 of the screen. This might not be possible in some large dogs if using a small ultrasound unit and high frequency probe (size of heart exceeds maximal depth).
Gain	Adjust for appropriate contrast at given depth. The lumen of the heart (blood) should be anechoic (black).

optimizes image quality to enhance temporal resolution and inverts the image left-to-right to achieve standard echocardiographic orientation used by cardiologists (with atria to the right of the screen in right parasternal views). Shaving hair typically is not necessary because good coupling can be achieved with alcohol and gel, and many dogs have thinner hair in the parasternal region. The most common patient position for FCU is the standing or sternal position, which is the most practical and safest for a dog in respiratory distress. If a patient is comfortable in lateral recumbency, then right lateral is preferred so images can be obtained from the recumbent side, with the dog positioned close to the edge of the table (or on a custom echocardiography table with a cutout) so that the heart can be imaged from underneath. In this position, gravity allows the heart to lie closer to the thoracic wall, which improves image quality especially in large dogs. The heart also can be imaged from above (the nonrecumbent hemithorax), particularly in small to medium-sized dogs or thin narrow-chested larger dogs.

Acoustic Windows and Key Cardiac Views

Two basic acoustic windows, specifically the right parasternal and subxiphoid windows, facilitate the key standard views of the heart and allow qualitative evaluation of cardiac structure and function (**Fig. 1**). The right parasternal acoustic window is located on the right hemithorax at approximately the location of the cardiac apex beat (where the heartbeat is palpated). Both short-axis and long-axis views of the heart can be obtained at this acoustic window. Because the window is small, slight movements of the transducer (rotation, sliding, fanning, and rocking) are necessary to get the standard cardiac views and to optimize the image quality. Key short-axis views are obtained of the left ventricle (LV) just below the mitral valve (mushroom view), and at the level of the heart base (left atrium [LA] to aorta [Ao], or LA:Ao view). These standard cardiac views are important to allow a qualitative evaluation of cardiac chamber size. Nonstandard cardiac views also can be helpful especially to better characterize a suspected cardiac mass or thrombus. The subxiphoid window facilitates the imaging of the CVC and the apical regions of the heart and possible pericardial or pleural effusions.

RECOGNIZING NORMAL CARDIAC ANATOMY AND FUNCTION

Examples of standard FCU views from normal dogs are shown in **Figs. 2A–5A**. Because dogs come in all sizes, the quantitative assessment of normal cardiac dimensions is dependent on body weight. Charts of normal values based on body weight can be referred to or normalized values for quantitative LV dimensions used.[3,4] The immediate goal of FCU, however, typically is a qualitative assessment of cardiac chamber and great vessel sizes. During a qualitative, or eyeball, assessment of cardiac chamber size, the operator compares the chamber sizes to each other or to the Ao (**Table 2**). Assessing the shape and curvature of the cardiac chambers also can be helpful. For example, in a parasternal long-axis view, the lumen of the LV should be 3-times to 4-times larger than the right ventricle (RV). The LV should be shaped like a bullet with parallel walls and a rounded apex. If the RV is the same size or larger than the LV in this view, this is indicative of right heart enlargement. Conversely, if the LV has a rounded shape and the interventricular septum is deviated toward the RV, this is indicative of LV volume overload (see **Fig. 3**). It is important to emphasize the importance of obtaining the standard views for these assessments of cardiac size. If the FCU image is off-angle, errors in image interpretation can occur similar to when a patient is twisted on a thoracic radiograph. The assessment of LV systolic

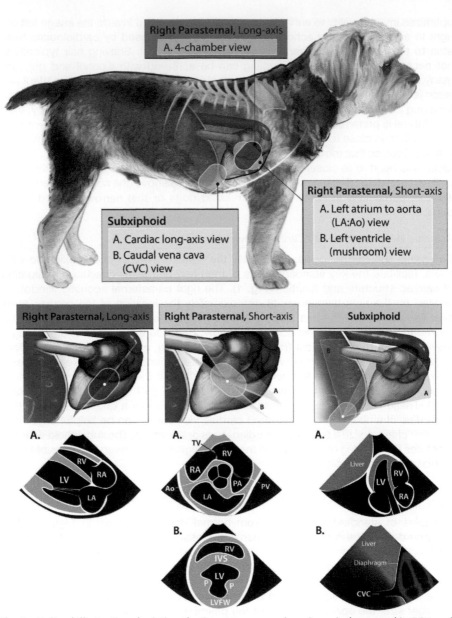

Fig. 1. Stylized illustration depicting the 2 most common imaging windows used in FCU and associated cardiac views: right parasternal long-axis (4-chamber), right parasternal short-axis (LV [mushroom] and LA:Ao views), and subxiphoid (cardiac long-axis and CVC views). Transducer orientation and corresponding schematic diagrams of FCU views are shown. IVS, interventricular septum; LVFW, LV free wall; P, papillary muscle; PA, pulmonary artery; PV, pulmonic valve. The black and white cardiac schematics labeled A and B (lower part of the figure) refer to the views from which these images are obtained. The views are labeled A and B and color coded in the upper half of the image.

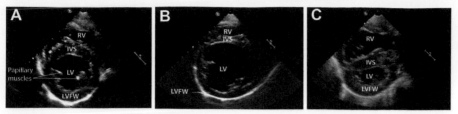

Fig. 2. Standard FCU right parasternal short-axis LV (mushroom) image of a normal dog compared with dogs with severe left and RV enlargement. (*A*) Normal dog; (*B*) dog with L-CHF and secondary to DCM, demonstrating severe LV dilation; and (*C*) dog with R-CHF secondary to severe pulmonary hypertension, demonstrating severe RV enlargement and flattening of the IVS. IVS, interventricular septum; LVFW, LV free wall.

function also usually is a qualitative assessment made in both parasternal long-axis and short-axis views. Systolic function can be assessed subjectively in the right parasternal short-axis (mushroom) view by observing the change in the size of the LV lumen from maximal diastole to maximal systole or can be quantified by calculating fractional shortening (**Box 1**). Normal fractional shortening is between 25% and 45% in most dogs.

SEVERE LEFT HEART DISEASE AND L-CHF

L-CHF in dogs manifests as pulmonary edema. The most common clinical presentation of L-CHF in dogs is acute respiratory distress (dyspnea/tachypnea); additional clinical signs can include syncope, exercise intolerance, hyporexia, and cough.[5,6] Key radiographic features of L-CHF in dogs include cardiomegaly (increased vertebral heart score), evidence of severe LA enlargement, pulmonary venous distension, and an interstitial or alveolar pulmonary pattern consistent with cardiogenic edema.[6,7]

Findings on FCU that can support a clinical diagnosis of L-CHF are analogous to the expected radiographic features and include severe LA dilation in combination with numerous B-lines on lung ultrasound (**Table 3**). Generally, dogs with L-CHF have severe LA dilation visible on right parasternal short-axis heart base views (with LA:Ao ratio usually >2:1 [see **Fig. 4**]). An uncommon exception to this rule is the setting of peracute chordae tendineae rupture, where the sudden massive worsening of mitral regurgitation causes LA pressure to rise rapidly and cause pulmonary edema before the LA has time to dilate and remodel. Combining FCU findings with identification of B-lines on lung ultrasound is important in the presumptive diagnosis of L-CHF,

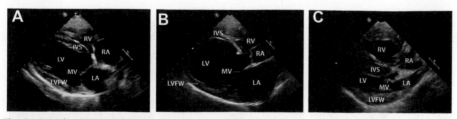

Fig. 3. Standard FCU right parasternal long-axis image of a normal dog compared with dogs with severe left and right heart disease. (*A*) Normal dog; (*B*) dog with L-CHF secondary to severe DCM, demonstrating severe LA and ventricular dilation; and (*C*) dog with R-CHF secondary to severe pulmonary hypertension, demonstrating RA and RV enlargement, RV hypertrophy, and underfilling of the left heart. IVS, interventricular septum; LVFW, LV free wall; MV, mitral valve.

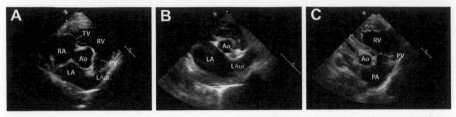

Fig. 4. Standard FCU right parasternal short-axis image at the heart base (LA:Ao view) in a normal dog compared with dogs with severe left and right heart disease. (*A*) Normal dog; (*B*) dog with L-CHF secondary to severe MMVD, demonstrating severe LA enlargement; and (*C*) dog with R-CHF secondary to severe pulmonary hypertension, demonstrating a severely enlarged main pulmonary artery. LAur, left auricle; PA, main pulmonary artery; PV, pulmonic valve; TV, tricuspid valve.

because numerous B-lines per intercostal space (termed, *strong positive sites*, on lung ultrasound) are suggestive of the presence of interstitial or alveolar fluid. Dogs with respiratory distress due to L-CHF typically have bilateral strong positive sites for B-lines, often with a diffuse distribution of infinite coalescing B-lines with lung ultrasound.[8,9]

Additional FCU findings supportive of L-CHF differ based on the underlying cardiac disease. The most common left heart diseases in dogs are myxomatous mitral valve disease (MMVD) and DCM. Advanced MMVD is most common in older small-breed dogs and is associated with a loud left apical systolic heart murmur on physical examination; echocardiographic features include a thickened mitral valve, severe mitral regurgitation, severe LA enlargement, and LV volume overload (eccentric hypertrophy) with normal to hyperdynamic LV systolic function.[6] In dogs with L-CHF secondary to MMVD, right parasternal long-axis 4-chamber FCU views reveal a thickened mitral valve with possible prolapse of a leaflet into the LA. Pericardial effusion in a dog with L-CHF and cardiogenic shock should raise suspicion for LA rupture as a complication of severe MMVD; in such cases, a crescent-shaped thrombus may be visible within the pericardial space (**Fig. 6**).

DCM is more common in middle-aged large breed dogs, although a DCM phenotype associated with consumption of boutique, exotic, and grain-free diets recently has been recognized and can affect any breed.[10,11] Tachyarrhythmias are common in DCM, but murmurs may be soft or absent; the most salient echocardiographic features are severe LV dilation with severely decreased LV systolic function.[12,13] In dogs

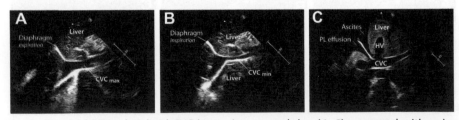

Fig. 5. Standard FCU subxiphoid CVC image in a normal dog (*A*, *B*) compared with a dog with R-CHF (*C*). (*A*) Normal dog on expiration, demonstrating maximal CVC diameter; (*B*) normal dog on inspiration, demonstrating minimum CVC diameter; and (*C*) dog with R-CHF (ascites and pleural effusion), demonstrating an enlarged CVC and hepatic veins (HV). HV, hepatic veins. PL, pleural.

Table 2
Transducer sites and cardiac views for focused cardiac ultrasound, structures evaluated at each view, and normal cardiac anatomy to recognize

Site + View	Structures Evaluated	Normal Structure and Function
Right parasternal short-axis at the level LV below the mitral valve (mushroom view)	LV size LV wall thickness LV systolic function RV size	LV size in diastole (weight-based normal values) LV wall thickness: subjective LV systolic function: subjective RV should be small crescent shape. Interventricular septum should be rounded (not flattened).
Right parasternal short-axis at the heart base (LA:Ao view)	LA size MPA size	LA:Ao should be <1.3:1 (severe LA dilation if > 2:1) MPA:Ao should be 1:1
Right parasternal long-axis 4-chamber	RA and RV size LA and LV size LV systolic function	LA and RA size should be equal with neutral interatrial septum position LV 3×–4× size and thickness of RV LV should be bullet-shaped (not round). LV systolic function: subjective
Subxiphoid cardiac long-axis	Presence of pericardial or pleural effusion	Cardiac apex should be next to liver with no evidence of pericardial or pleural effusion.
Subxiphoid sagittal CVC	CVC size CVC collapsibility Hepatic veins	CVC maximal diameter (compared with weight-based normal values) CVC_{max}:Ao <0.6 CVC collapsibility >30% Hepatic veins should not be prominent.

Abbreviations: MPA, main pulmonary artery.

with L-CHF secondary to DCM, the LV is severely dilated and spherical, and LV systolic function is markedly hypodynamic (with fractional shortening typically <20%) and normalized LV end-diastolic diameters of greater than 1.9.

FCU findings always should be integrated with patient signalment, history, and physical examination findings when considering a diagnosis of L-CHF. A small breed dog presenting for acute tachypnea with a loud left apical systolic heart murmur whose FCU reveals severe LA enlargement and multifocal B-lines can be treated confidently for L-CHF (presumed MMVD). A small breed dog without a heart murmur is highly unlikely to have L-CHF, regardless of FCU findings (unless the dog is consuming a boutique, exotic, or grain-free diet, in which cases DCM becomes a relevant differential diagnosis). A small breed dog presenting for cough with normal respiratory rate and effort and a loud left apical systolic heart murmur whose lung ultrasound shows no B-lines is highly unlikely to have L-CHF, regardless of severity of LA dilation on FCU.[14] A large breed dog with rapid atrial fibrillation, LV dilation and systolic dysfunction, and numerous multifocal B-lines is likely to have L-CHF, even if FCU cannot confirm severe LA dilation.[15]

SEVERE RIGHT HEART DISEASE AND RIGHT-SIDED CONGESTIVE HEART FAILURE

R-CHF occurs when elevated right heart filling pressures cause increased systemic venous hydrostatic pressure, resulting in development of cavitary effusions. The

---

Box 1
Formula for calculating Fractional shortening

- Fractional Shortening

$$FS = \frac{LVEDD - LVESD}{LVEDD} \times 100$$

---

most common manifestation of R-CHF in dogs is ascites; other locations of fluid accumulation (which can occur in combination) are pleural effusion, small-volume pericardial effusion (without tamponade), and rarely peripheral edema.[16,17] Additional clinical signs of R-CHF can include syncope, exercise intolerance, hyporexia, and cachexia.

Findings on FCU that can support a clinical diagnosis of R-CHF are reflective of underlying severe structural right heart disease or elevated systemic venous pressures and include right atrial (RA) dilation, RV dilation or hypertrophy, and a large indistensible (fat) CVC (see **Table 3**). Dogs with severe right heart disease typically have severe RA and RV dilation on FCU, with right parasternal long-axis views showing the RA and RV being the same size or larger than the LA and LV, respectively (see **Fig. 2**). Also, in long axis, the interatrial septum may bow toward the LA due to increased RA pressure. RV dilation also may be seen on right parasternal short-axis views, with the RV larger than the mushroom LV. Subxiphoid views of the CVC reveal CVC distension, with maximal diameter above weight-based normal (or indexed to the Ao) and decreased collapsibility of the CVC with respiratory fluctuations. A recent study found that CVC:Ao greater than 0.63 and CVC collapsibility index less than 30% were greater than 90% sensitive and specific for a diagnosis of R-CHF compared with noncardiac causes of cavitary effusion in dogs.[18]

As with L-CHF, additional FCU findings supportive of R-CHF differ based on the underlying cardiac disease. Causes of R-CHF in dogs include pulmonary arterial hypertension (PAH), congenital heart disease (pulmonic stenosis and tricuspid valve dysplasia), myxomatous (degenerative) tricuspid valve disease, or neoplasia. Additionally, although most dogs with DCM or MMVD progress to L-CHF, some may manifest with R-CHF or biventricular congestive heart failure, in particular dogs with concurrent atrial fibrillation or PAH.[6,12,17]

Dogs with severe PAH represent a specific clinical scenario with distinct recognizable FCU features (see **Table 3**). Because PAH results in RV systolic pressure overload, right parasternal long-axis and short-axis views reveal RV concentric hypertrophy (thickening) as well as enlargement, with RV wall thickness similar to or greater than the LV; the LV often appears small and volume underloaded. RV pressure overload also results in flattening of the interventricular septum on right parasternal short-axis views of the LV, giving a flattened top to the mushroom appearance of the LV (see **Fig. 3**). Severe PAH also results in main pulmonary artery enlargement, with pulmonary artery diameter larger than the Ao in right parasternal short-axis heart base views. For ultrasound systems equipped with color and spectral Doppler, systolic PA pressure can be estimated by measuring tricuspid regurgitation velocity; patients symptomatic for PAH typically have tricuspid regurgitation velocities greater than 4 m/s.[19]

Clinical and FCU suspicion for severe PAH should prompt a diagnostic investigation for the underlying cause of PAH. Diseases in dogs that can result in PAH include

Table 3
Focused cardiac ultrasound findings supportive of cardiovascular disease as the cause of emergent clinical signs in dogs

Cardivascular Disease	Compatible Clinical Signs	Supportive Focused Cardiac Ultrasound Findings	Implications for Diagnosis or Treatment
L-CHF	• Dyspnea • Tachypnea • Syncope	• Severe LA dilation • Strong positive B-line sites on lung ultrasound • ±Severe LV dilation • ± Severe LV systolic dysfunction	• DDx: MMVD, DCM • Tx: furosemide, pimobendan
R-CHF	• Cavitary effusions (ascites > pleural effusion) • Syncope	• Severe RA/RV dilation • Distended CVC with decreased collapsibility • ± RV hypertrophy • ± Interventricular septal flattening	• DDx: pulmonary hypertension, tricuspid valve dysplasia, pulmonic stenosis, myxomatous tricuspid valve disease • Tx: therapeutic centesis, furosemide, pimobendan, ±sildenafil
PAH	• Dyspnea • Tachypnea • Syncope	• RV dilation and hypertrophy • Interventricular septal flattening • Main pulmonary artery dilation • ± Distended CVC with decreased collapsibility	• DDx: heartworm disease, pulmonary thromboembolism, chronic bronchopulmonary disease • Tx: sildenafil
Pericardial effusion and tamponade	• Syncope/ collapse • ± Ascites	• Variable-volume pericardial effusion • RA/RV diastolic collapse • Distended CVC with decreased collapsibility • ± Ascites • ± Gallbladder halo sign	• DDx: cardiac neoplasia (RA/right auricle or heart base), idiopathic pericarditis • Tx: pericardiocentesis
LA rupture	• Collapse and dyspnea in dog with known MMVD	• Small-volume pericardial effusion • RA/RV diastolic collapse • Hyperechoic tubular structure in pericardium (thrombus) • LA dilation • Mitral valve thickening	• Tx: Pericardiocentesis (if severely hypotensive); medical management with pimobendan, judicious preload and afterload reduction
Volume-responsive shock	• Collapse, weakness • Hypotension	• Small LV end-diastolic dimension (volume underload) • Small CVC with collapsibility >30% • ± LV systolic obliteration (kissing LV walls) • ± Subjectively thickened LV walls (pseudohypertrophy)	• Intravenous fluid therapy

Abbreviations: DDx, differential diagnoses; Tx, treatment.

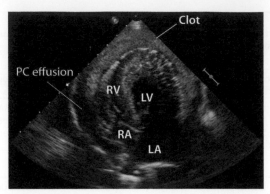

Fig. 6. Left apical cardiac ultrasound view in a dog with a LA rupture secondary to severe MMVD, demonstrating a hyperechoic tubular clot within small-volume pericardial fluid surrounding the heart. PC, pericardial.

heartworm disease, chronic bronchopulmonary disease (eg, dynamic airway disease/obstruction, chronic bronchitis, or pulmonary fibrosis), and pulmonary thromboembolic disease.[19,20] FCU cannot differentiate these underlying causes of PAH; however, in dogs with severe heartworm disease, heartworms sometimes can be seen as double-lined (railroad-track) structures within the pulmonary artery, or even within the heart (RV or RA) in cases of heartworm caval syndrome.

Note that severe left heart disease also can lead to so-called postcapillary PAH via passive backup of elevated pulmonary venous pressure across the capillary bed to cause elevated pulmonary arterial pressures.[21] FCU findings in postcapillary PAH, however, generally reflect the severe primary left heart disease, with features of L-CHF (discussed previously) predominating. Diagnosis of PAH in these cases is based on estimating systolic pulmonary artery pressures with tricuspid regurgitation velocity.

As in cases of suspected L-CHF, FCU findings always should be integrated with patient signalment, history, and physical examination findings when considering a diagnosis of R-CHF. A small breed dog presenting for acute dyspnea with a soft right-sided systolic heart murmur whose FCU shows RV enlargement and septal flattening with normal LA size should be treated for PAH, not L-CHF. Almost all dogs with R-CHF have ascites as part of their manifestation of cavitary effusion; isolated pleural effusion almost never is caused by R-CHF. Presence of a murmur or tachyarrhythmia increases clinical suspicion for R-CHF if FCU findings are equivocal. Diagnostic centesis remains critical to the emergency diagnostic work-up of cavitary effusion; hemorrhagic or septic cavitary effusion should be treated as noncardiac regardless of FCU findings.

PERICARDIAL EFFUSION AND CARDIAC TAMPONADE

FCU is one of the most useful clinical tools for a timely and accurate diagnosis of pericardial effusion and cardiac tamponade in the dog. The first step is to recognize clinical scenarios when pericardial effusion and cardiac tamponade may be present. Dogs with pericardial effusion and cardiac tamponade usually present for collapse, extreme lethargy, possible cough/retching, shortness of breath, abdominal distention, and inappetence. On physical examination, muffled heart sounds and tachycardia with weak and variable pulses (called *pulses paradoxus*) are suggestive of pericardial effusion. FCU, however, allows the visualization and characterization of the suspected pericardial effusion. In normal dogs, there is no visible pericardial effusion on an ultrasound examination. The sonographic appearance of pericardial effusion is a variable amount of (typically) anechoic fluid encircling the heart. Pericardial effusion is best observed low toward the apex of the heart, as seen via the subxiphoid or an apical transducer positon.[22] Observing the fluid from multiple views and changing a dog's position also may be helpful, because pleural effusion is more gravity dependent and displaces ventrally, whereas pericardial effusion is contained within its sac and more fixed in position. When pericardial effusion is suspected, evidence of cardiac tamponade should be looked for, which develops when the pressure in the pericardial sac exceeds that of the RV end-diastolic pressure, resulting in diminished RV diastolic filling and low cardiac output. Cardiac tamponade and increased intrapericardial pressure can develop with either large-volume or small-volume effusions depending on the time course in which the effusion develops. The FCU criteria for cardiac tamponade are diastolic collapse of the RA (and possibly RV) with a distended CVC with decreased collapsibility (**Fig. 7**). In some dogs with cardiac tamponade, the gallbladder may become thickened and edematous with a hypoechoic rim (gallbladder halo sign).[23]

FCU also can help determine the etiology of the pericardial effusion (see **Table 3**). The most common cause of pericardial effusion in older dogs is cardiac neoplasia, most commonly RA hemangiosarcoma in large-breed dogs and chemodectomas (heart base tumors) in brachycephalic dogs[24,25] (**Fig. 8**). These neoplastic masses often are quite large and may be visible when imaging the RA or heart base. Any suspected mass should be confirmed and documented in multiple views, including scanning from the left hemithorax. Other cardiac or pericardial neoplasms that are less common include mesothelioma, lymphoma, and metastatic carcinomas. If no mass is identified, benign idiopathic pericardial effusion is possible, but concern for occult neoplasia remains. After pericardiocentesis and patient stabilization, a diagnostic echocardiogram performed by a specialist and a cardiac troponin I are recommended to confirm or refute a suspected mass lesion in a dog with pericardial effusion.[26,27] Another important cause of pericardial effusion in an older small-breed dog with MMVD is an LA rupture, as discussed previously. In these cases, a hyperechoic tubular-shaped thrombus is visible surrounding the heart within (usually) small-volume pericardial effusion (see **Fig. 6**).

Finally, FCU is helpful when performing pericardiocentesis. The ultrasound can be used to guide the centesis in real time (termed, *ultrasound-guided*), or the ultrasound can be used to simply identify the optimal site for the centesis (termed, *ultrasound-assisted*). In people, ultrasound guidance has been shown to improve the safety of

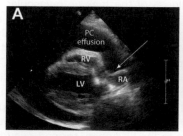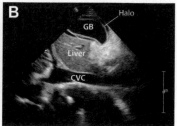

Fig. 7. FCU images demonstrating pericardial effusion and cardiac tamponade. (*A*) Right parasternal long-axis view from a dog with large-volume pericardial effusion demonstrating a collapsed RA (*arrow*) indicative of cardiac tamponade and (*B*) subxiphoid view from a dog with pericardial effusion and cardiac tamponade, demonstrating a distended CVC and edematous gallbladder wall (halo sign). GB, gallbladder; PC, pericardial.

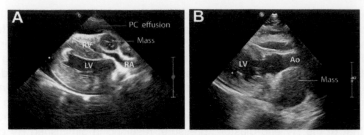

Fig. 8. Right parasternal long-axis views from dogs with pericardial effusion secondary to cardiac neoplasia. (A) Right parasternal long-axis view demonstrating small-volume pericardial effusion, evidence of RA collapse, and a mass lesion in the RA wall (highly probable hemangiosarcoma due to its location and mixed echogenicity). (B) Right parasternal long-axis image demonstrating a large round heart base mass of homogenous echogenicity adjacent to the Ao (probable chemodectoma). PC, pericardial.

pericardiocentesis.[28] If there is concern for a possible intracardiac puncture during the pericardiocentesis, a small infusion of agitated saline can be helpful to confirm placement of the needle or catheter. Bubbles appear within the cardiac chamber with an intracardiac puncture.[29]

ASSESSMENT OF VOLUME RESPONSIVENESS

Assessing of the volume status in a dog in an undifferentiated shock state is challenging. With physical examination alone, a clinician often is uncertain about the underlying cause and initial therapeutic approach in a dog presenting with collapse and hypotension. Commonly, the initial treatment of circulatory failure is often fluid resuscitation to increase stroke volume, organ perfusion, and oxygen delivery. Not all patients with circulatory collapse, however, benefit from additional fluids. If a dog is not fluid-responsive, additional intravenous fluids actually may be harmful, leading to fluid shifts into the extravascular space, leading to end-organ edema and dysfunction. FCU, together with a comprehensive focused ultrasound examination, can assess the "the pump, the tank and the pipes" in a dog with undifferentiated hypotension.[30] Evaluating the pump (the heart) using FCU can identify severe structural heart disease (eg, DCM), pericardial effusion with cardiac tamponade, sepsis-induced myocardial dysfunction, and massive pulmonary embolism leading to right heart enlargement, all conditions in which aggressive intravenous fluid resuscitation is not advised. The fullness of the tank (intravascular volume) can be assessed by FCU by evaluating the LV end-diastolic diameter and the size and collapsibility of the CVC. A dog that is fluid-responsive typically has a small, difficult-to-image CVC with greater than 30% change in diameter with respirations, whereas a dog that is not fluid-responsive has a distended (or fat) CVC with less than 25% to 30% respiratory fluctuations. A very small LV end-diastolic diameter with vigorous cardiac contractions obliterating the ventricular lumen in systole (kissing of the LV walls) is suggestive of either a distributive shock (eg, anaphylaxis) or a hypovolemic (eg, hemorrhagic) shock state. In such cases, the LV walls also may appear subjectively thickened relative to the LV lumen, termed *pseudohypertrophy*. Care should be taken, however, to be at the correct short-axis level of the heart (just below the mitral valves) because too ventral could create a false-positive result. LV systolic obliteration and a small, distensible CVC suggest a fluid-responsive shock state.

SUMMARY

FCU is a qualitative point-of-care, low-stress, and time-sensitive examination of the heart and great vessels that gives clinicians additional information to make immediate treatment decisions by rapidly diagnosing potentially life-threatening conditions and improving the management of a critically ill patient. FCU can be most helpful in the diagnosis of L-CHF, R-CHF, and pericardial effusion with cardiac tamponade and in assessing fluid responsive in undifferentiated shock states.

DISCLOSURE

The authors have no conflicts of interest to disclose.

REFERENCES

1. Gardner K, Clattenburg E, Wroe P, et al. The Cardiac Arrest Sonographic Assessment (CASA) exam - A standardized approach to the use of ultrasound in PEA. Am J Emerg Med 2018;36:729–31.

2. Gillman LM, Kirkpatrick AW. Portable bedside ultrasound: the visual stethoscope of the 21st century. Scand J Trauma Resusc Emerg Med 2012;20:18.

3. Cornell CC, Kittleson MD, Della Torre P, et al. Allometric scaling of M-mode cardiac measurements in normal adult dogs. J Vet Intern Med 2004;18:311–21.

4. Visser LC, Ciccozzi MM, Sintov DJ, et al. Echocardiographic quantitation of left heart size and function in 122 healthy dogs: a prospective study proposing reference intervals and assessing repeatability. J Vet Intern Med 2019;33:1909–20.

5. Fox PR. The history. In: Fox P, Sisson D, Moise N, editors. Textbook of canine and feline cardiology: principles and clinical practice. 2nd edition. London: Saunders; 1999. p. 41–5.

6. Keene BW, Atkins CE, Bonagura JD, et al. ACVIM consensus guidelines for the diagnosis and treatment of myxomatous mitral valve disease in dogs. J Vet Intern Med 2019;33:1127–40.

7. Diana A, Guglielmini C, Pivetta M, et al. Radiographic features of cardiogenic pulmonary edema in dogs with mitral regurgitation: 61 cases (1998-2007). J Am Vet Med Assoc 2009;235:1058–63.

8. Ward JL, Lisciandro GR, Keene BW, et al. Accuracy of point-of-care lung ultrasonography for the diagnosis of cardiogenic pulmonary edema in dogs and cats with acute dyspnea. J Am Vet Med Assoc 2017;250:666–75.

9. Ward JL, Lisciandro GR, DeFrancesco TC. Distribution of alveolar-interstitial syndrome in dogs and cats with respiratory distress as assessed by lung ultrasound versus thoracic radiographs. J Vet Emerg Crit Care 2018;28:415–28.

10. Freeman L, Stern J, Fries R, et al. Diet-associated dilated cardiomyopathy in dogs: what do we know? J AM Vet Med Assoc 2018;253:1390–4.

11. Adin D, DeFrancesco TC, Keene B, et al. Echocardiographic phenotype of canine dilated cardiomyopathy differs based on diet type. J Vet Cardiol 2019; 21:1–9.

12. Borgarelli M, Santilli RA, Chiavegato D, et al. Prognostic indicators for dogs with dilated cardiomyopathy. J Vet Intern Med 2006;20:104–10.

13. Tidholm A, Häggström J, Borgarelli M, et al. Canine idiopathic dilated cardiomyopathy. Part I: aetiology, clinical characteristics, epidemiology and pathology. Vet J 2001;162:92–107.

14. Martindale JL, Wakai A, Collins SP, et al. Diagnosing acute heart failure in the emergency department: a systematic review and meta-analysis. Acad Emerg Med 2016;23(3):223–42.
15. Friederich J, Seuß AC, Wess G. The role of atrial fibrillation as a prognostic factor in doberman pinschers with dilated cardiomyopathy and congestive heart failure. Vet J 2020;264:105535.
16. Brewster RD, Benjamin SA, Thomassen RW. Spontaneous cor pulmonale in laboratory beagles. Lab Anim Sci 1983;33:299–302.
17. Ward J, Ware W, Viall A. Association between atrial fibrillation and right-sided manifestations of congestive heart failure in dogs with degenerative mitral valve disease or dilated cardiomyopathy. J Vet Cardiol 2019;21:18–27.
18. Chou YY, Ward J, Barron L, et al. Diagnostic utility of caudal vena cava measurementsin dogs with cavitary effusions or heart failure [abstract]. J Vet Intern Med 2020;34:2846.
19. Reinero C, Visser LC, Kellihan HB, et al. ACVIM consensus statement guidelines for the diagnosis, classification, treatment, and monitoring of pulmonary hypertension in dogs. J Vet Intern Med 2020;34:549–73.
20. Kellihan HB, Stepien RL. Pulmonary hypertension in dogs: diagnosis and therapy. Vet Clin North Am Small Anim Pract 2010;40:623–41.
21. Kellihan HB, Stepien RL. Pulmonary hypertension in canine degenerative mitral valve disease. J Vet Cardiol 2012;14:149–64.
22. Lisciandro GR. The use of the diaphragmatico-hepatic (DH) views of the abdominal and thoracic focused assessment with sonography for triage (AFAST/TFAST) examinations for the detection of pericardial effusion in 24 dogs (2011-2012). J Vet Emerg Crit Care 2016;26:125–31.
23. Lisciandro GR, Gambino JM, Lisciandro SC. Thirteen dogs and a cat with ultrasonographically detected gallbladder wall edema associated with cardiac disease. J Vet Intern Med 2021;35(3):1342–6.
24. MacDonald KA, Cagney O, Magne ML. Echocardiographic and clinicopathologic characterization of pericardial effusion in dogs: 107 cases (1985–2006). J Am Vet Med Assoc 2009;235:1456–61.
25. Stafford Johnson M, Martin M, Binns S, et al. A retrospective study of clinical findings, treatment and outcome in 143 dogs with pericardial effusion. J Small Anim Pract 2004;45:546–52.
26. Shaw SP, Rozanski EA, Rush JE. Cardiac troponins I and T in dogs with pericardial effusion. J Vet Intern Med 2004;18:322–4.
27. Chun R, Kellihan HB, Henik RA, et al. Comparison of plasma cardiac troponin I concentrations among dogs with cardiac hemangiosarcoma, noncardiac hemangiosarcoma, other neoplasms, and pericardial effusion of non-hemangiosarcoma origin. J Am Vet Med Assoc 2010;237:806–11.
28. Tsang T, El-Najdawi E, Seward J, et al. Percutaneous echocardiographically guided pericardiocentesis in pediatric patients: evaluation of safety and efficacy. J Am Soc Echocardiogr 1998;11:1072–7.
29. Ainsworth C, Salehein O. Echo-guided pericardiocentesis: let the bubbles show the way. Circulation 2011;123:e210–1.
30. Perera P, Mailhot T, Riley D, et al. The RUSH exam: rapid ultrasound in SHock in the evaluation of the critically Ill. Emerg Med Clin North Am 2010;28:29–56.

Section III: Focused Ultrasound of the Abdomen

AFAST Target-Organ Approach and Fluid Scoring System in Dogs and Cats

Gregory R. Lisciandro, DVM

KEYWORDS

- Point-of-care ultrasonography • AFAST • Ascites • Fluid scoring system
- Volume status

KEY POINTS

- AFAST is a standardized ultrasonography examination of the abdomen with exact clarity to its 5 views.
- AFAST and its target-organ approach serve as a screening test for obvious soft tissue abnormalities that are often missed or only suspected based on physical examination, laboratory test results, and radiography.
- AFAST and its abdominal fluid scoring system help better characterize a positive examination using the small-volume effusion/bleeder versus large-volume effusion/bleeder concept, and also records positive and negative views.
- AFAST abdominal fluid scoring allows patients to be tracked as being static (no score change), worsening (increasing score), or resolving (decreasing score).
- AFAST may be used for additional valuable clinical information without any additional views, including characterization of the caudal vena cava and hepatic veins, urinary bladder volume measurements, pneumoperitoneum, and gastrointestinal motility.

 Video content accompanies this article at http://www.vetsmall.theclinics.com.

INTRODUCTION

In 2004, in the first translational study of focused assessment with sonography for trauma (FAST) from humans to small animals documented that minimally trained nonradiologist veterinarians could proficiently recognize ascites, and that hemoperitoneum was far more common than previously reported.[1] Moreover, pleural effusion (PE) and pericardial effusion (PCE) could be detected via the subxiphoid view by looking cranial to the diaphragm.[1,2] Since 2004, veterinary FAST has been revamped as abdominal FAST (AFAST) by naming views based on target organs, adding the umbilical view' standardizing view order and probe manipulation; developing an abdominal fluid scoring system to semiquantitate ascites over

Hill Country Veterinary Specialists and FASTVet.com, Spicewood, TX, USA
E-mail address: FastSavesLives@gmail.com

Vet Clin Small Anim 51 (2021) 1217–1231
https://doi.org/10.1016/j.cvsm.2021.07.006
0195-5616/21/© 2021 Elsevier Inc. All rights reserved.

subjective terms of trivial, mild, moderate, and severe; and incorporating other information, such as free air, estimation of urinary bladder volume, gastrointestinal motility, and characterization of the caudal vena cava (CVC) and its associated hepatic veins.[3–9]

Thorax FAST (TFAST) and Vet BLUE are additional abbreviated ultrasonography examinations of the thorax and lung, respectively.[10–12] When all 3 formats are combined, they are referred to as Global FAST, a unique imaging screening test of both body cavities.[7,13–15] Global FAST is applied as an extension of the physical examination, providing an unbiased set of 15 data imaging points with exact clarity of both the abdomen and thorax, including heart and lung.[7,13–15] Although AFAST may be used as a stand-alone ultrasonography examination, through the standardized approach of Global FAST, sonographers avoid common imaging mistakes such as satisfaction of search error and confirmation bias error through selective point-of-care ultrasonography (POCUS) imaging.[16–19] For example, gallbladder wall edema may be detected during AFAST but misinterpreted as canine anaphylaxis (or cholecystitis) when the patient has cardiac disease that is missed because Global FAST and its TFAST component was not performed.[18]

AFAST OVERVIEW
AFAST Standardized Methodology: Names, Views, Order, and Probe Maneuvering

Views are named by their target organs as follows: the diaphragmaticohepatic (DH) view (subxiphoid), the splenorenal (SR) view (left flank), the cystocolic (CC) view (caudal abdomen), the added splenointestinoumbilical (SI-U) view (level of the umbilicus, previously named the hepatorenal umbilical view), and the hepatorenal (HR5th) view (right flank) as the final fifth view.[3–5,7,14,15,20–22] The first 4 views, DH, SR, CC, and SI-U, are part of the abdominal fluid scoring system (**Fig. 1**, Videos 1–4).[3–5,7,14,15,20–22] The HR5th view is scored but not part of the total score (**Fig. 2**, Video 5). Each AFAST view is used not only for the detection of free fluid but also for obvious soft tissue abnormalities commonly missed by physical examination, laboratory testing, and radiography (**Table 1**).[3–5,7,14,15,20–22]

AFAST has been standardized from its beginning regarding its order of views, its probe maneuvers, its fluid scoring system, and recording of its findings on goal-directed templates.[3,4,21] The order follows the DH view to the SR view to the CC view to the SI-U view ending at the most gravity-dependent view, where in higher-scoring effusions abdominocentesis is likely to be performed. The HR5th view is the final AFAST view and often performed after the TFAST and Vet BLUE components of Global FAST as the most efficient manner to perform Global FAST and to dissociate the HR5th view from the total abdominal fluid score.

Probe maneuvers are standardized with a minimum of a fan, rock, and return to the starting point with scanning orientation maintained in the longitudinal plane.[3,4,21] Transverse orientation may be considered an add-on skill. Support for standardizing the probe maneuver comes from the original FAST study, which provided a table that compared scanning orientation (longitudinal vs transverse) with positive examinations. The investigators reported that 397 of 400 views matched when comparing longitudinal with transverse planes for the detection of free fluid (ascites).[1] Moreover, anatomy is generally more recognizable in longitudinal planes, and thus standardization of probe maneuvers is advantageous for beginning sonographers. It is unknown what difference, if any, is made by using both scanning planes during AFAST for obvious soft tissue abnormalities. Transverse orientation should be considered an add-on skill.

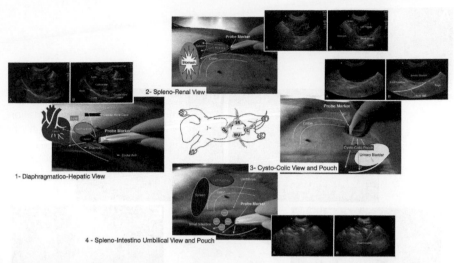

Fig. 1. The first 4 views of AFAST with their respective target organs that make up the abdominal fluid scoring system. The order is always the same, starting with a window into the abdomen and thorax of the DH view, followed by the window into the retroperitoneal space and peritoneal cavity of the SR view, followed by the CC view, and ending at the most gravity-dependent SI-U view (formerly called the hepatorenal umbilical view), where abdominocentesis is likely to be performed. There are specific pouches at the CC (CC pouch) and SI-U (umbilical pouch) views at which the probe is directed into the most gravity-dependent region where fluid would gravitate. Each view is negative for free fluid and obvious soft tissues abnormalities with unlabeled and labeled images. (© 2021 Gregory R. Lisciandro.)

Adding on the Focused Spleen

The AFAST order has evolved to include a focused spleen examination following the SI-U view through the recognition of a unique canine complication of anaphylaxis referred to as an anaphylactic-related, heparin-induced, medically treated hemoabdomen (discussed later in relation to gallbladder wall edema).[17,21,22] The positioning that is most favorable and efficient for performing AFAST followed by a focused spleen is from the left side of standing patients, and in right lateral recumbency because the spleen courses from the region of the umbilicus to the left kidney.[22] The focused spleen is performed by sliding and fanning, sliding and fanning cranially and then caudally with an overlapping methodology (**Fig. 3**, Video 6).[22] Transverse orientation may be considered an add-on skill. The focused spleen screens for any obvious soft tissue abnormalities, primarily being masses and obvious heterogenous echogenicity, referred to as a Swiss cheese or moth-eaten appearance (**Table 2**).[22,23] Rules of thumb include (1) any mass that deforms the capsule of the spleen should be considered serious until proved otherwise; and (2) findings of heterogenous echogenicity, such as Swiss-cheese bright (hyperechoic) spleen rule out lymphoma and Swiss-cheese dark (hypoechoic) spleen rule out splenic torsion, with both conditions typically having marked splenomegaly.[22,23]

AFAST AND ITS TARGET-ORGAN APPROACH
Soft Tissue Screening Test

AFAST was designed with a target-organ approach from its inception in 2005.[3] Fanning, rocking, and returning to your starting point serves as a screening test for

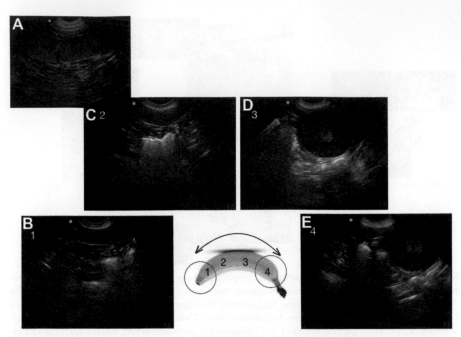

Fig. 2. The focused spleen is performed after the first 4 views of AFAST because it is usually present or close to the SI-U view. The probe is applied to the spleen by sliding and fanning, sliding and fanning until you run out of spleen both cranially and caudally as a screening test for soft tissue abnormalities. A banana is used to show how the probe is moved along imaging sections of the spleen. Here is a detected splenic mass that deforms the capsule of the spleen that looks large but is only 4 cm in maximum dimension. This small splenic mass is unlikely to be detected by physical examination or laboratory testing, and is likely to be overlooked on radiography, but is easily seen on ultrasonography. (© 2021 Gregory R. Lisciandro.)

obvious soft tissue organ abnormalities within the abdomen, including the liver, gallbladder, kidneys, spleen, urinary bladder, uterus, spleen, and small intestine. Often these abnormalities are completely missed or only suspected based on physical examination, laboratory testing, and radiographic findings (see **Table 1**). Sonographers should have the attitude that AFAST is a screening test and that its findings are suspect until confirmed by additional imaging when indicated. Moreover, soft tissue abnormalities are also screened for within the thorax at the AFAST DH view, including the heart (cardiac bump), pleural cavity, and the lung along the diaphragm (pulmonary-diaphragmatic interface).[1,2,5,7,21,24–26]

AFAST AND ITS ABDOMINAL FLUID SCORING SYSTEM
Semiquantitating Free Fluid

The use of FAST ultrasonography in people has been shown to approximate the sensitivity and specificity of the gold standard test of computed tomography.[1] In veterinary medicine, AFAST findings have been mainly been compared with plain radiography.[3] AFAST was clearly superior in not only determining whether fluid was present but also by semiquantitating its volume through fluid scoring. AFAST always carries value in its most fundamental use of refuting or confirming the presence of free fluid and in scoring its degree. Examples of ascites are shown in Videos 7–11. Ascites, often

Table 1
AFAST and its target-organ approach for soft tissue abnormalities

AFAST Soft Tissue Abnormalities	
DH view: the probe is placed immediately caudal to the xiphoid, fanned through the liver and gallbladder, rocked cranially to evaluate the heart and its cardiac bump, followed by the lung and pleural cavity, then returned to the starting point, and imaging the CVC as it traverses the diaphragm	Gallbladder wall abnormalities • Edema • Masses • Rupture Gallbladder lumen abnormalities • Sludge • Mucocele • Calculi Biliary tract distension Liver parenchymal abnormalities • Masses and cysts • Heterogenous echogenicity CVC • Distension • Thrombi • *Dirofilaria* • Masses Pleural effusion Pericardial effusion Lung abnormalities • B lines • Signs of consolidation (shred, tissue, nodule, wedge)
SR View: the probe is placed immediately caudal to the costal arch where it meets the sublumbar muscles, fanned through the left kidney, rocked cranially to evaluate the spleen, then returned to the starting point of the left kidney	Retroperitoneal abnormalities • Fluid • Masses Renal parenchyma • Renal pelvic dilatation: pyelectasia and hydronephrosis • Cysts: cortical and perinephric • Masses • Infarction Ureteral distension Splenic abnormalities Vascular (great vessels, renal vessels) • Thrombus • Masses Pneumoperitoneum
CC view: the probe is placed immediately lateral to midline over the caudal abdomen, fanned through the urinary bladder, then rocked cranially where it meets the body wall in its pouch, then returned to the starting point of the urinary bladder	Bladder wall abnormalities • Masses Bladder lumen • Sediment • Calculi • Thrombus Urogenital abnormalities
SIU views: the probe is placed at the level of the umbilicus, fanned through the small intestine and spleen making sure the scanning plane passes through the umbilical pouch, rocked cranially, and then returned to the starting point	Midabdominal masses Small intestine • Ileus and distension

(continued on next page)

Table 1 (continued)	
AFAST Soft Tissue Abnormalities	

Focused spleen: the probe is used by sliding and fanning, sliding and fanning following the spleen cranially and caudally, noting that the spleen courses from approximate midline to the left kidney making right lateral recumbency advantageous when scanning from the patient's left side when standing or sternal	Spleen parenchymal abnormalities
	• Masses and cysts
	• Infarction
	• Heterogenous echogenicity
	  ○ Dark Swiss cheese: rule out torsion
	  ○ Bright Swiss cheese: rule out lymphoma

HR5th Bonus view: the probe is placed caudal to the costal arch and sublumbar muscles, similar to the SR view or over the 10th–12th intercostal spaces, fanned through the right kidney and adjacent right liver	Retroperitoneal abnormalities • Fluid • Masses Renal parenchyma • Renal pelvic dilation: pyelectasia and hydronephrosis • Cysts: cortical and perinephric • Masses • Infarction Ureteral distension Liver abnormalities Vascular (great vessels, renal and portal vessels) • Thrombus • Masses • Shunts • Volume status

This material is reproduced and modified with permission of John Wiley & Sons, Inc., Point-of-Care Ultrasound Techniques for the Small Animal Practitioner, Wiley ©2020 and © 2021 Gregory R. Lisciandro.

caused by a serious disease, should now never be missed by clinicians with access to ultrasonography. Furthermore, performing AFAST and fluid scoring takes less time than it took to type this paragraph.

AFAST Abdominal Fluid Scoring System

The AFAST abdominal fluid scoring system is validated in either lateral recumbency, making each view gravity unequal and thus serving as an inherent depth gauge. AFAST views are scored as 0, 1/2, or 1, with 1/2 being considered a weak positive, and a 1 a strong positive (**Fig. 4**) using more than and less than the maximum fluid dimension of 5 mm for cats and 1 cm for dogs.[14,15,20] Those totaling less than 3 are considered as small-volume bleeder/effusions and those greater than or equal to 3 as large-volume bleeder/effusions.[14,15,20,22] The HR5th view is similarly scored but not part of the total abdominal fluid score.[20,22] Fluid that is safely accessible should be sampled and tested because ultrasonography cannot reliably characterize free fluid based on echogenicity.

Clinical Applications of Fluid Scoring

Patient score helps anticipate the need for blood transfusion, surgical intervention, and expected degree of hypovolemia, and thus guides fluid resuscitation and decision

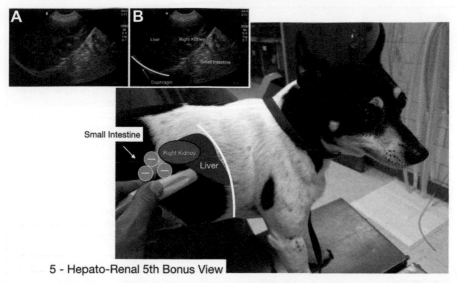

5 - Hepato-Renal 5th Bonus View

Fig. 3. Shown is the HR 5th bonus view. Its target organs are the right kidney and adjacent right liver and it is often done standing so that gas-filled small intestine falls away from the view. This view is scored but not part of the total score of the abdominal fluid scoring system. (© 2021 Gregory R. Lisciandro.)

making.[3,7] Knowing this information real time at triage and during patient rounds as an extension of the physical examination is important for case management.[27–29] For example, if trauma is suspected, fluid resuscitation will be modified in the presence of an AFAST-positive examination with the presumption that the fluid represents intra-abdominal hemorrhage until proved otherwise. The use of the AFAST fluid scoring system also provides important information regarding expected degrees of anemia in bleeding dogs and cats. For example, small-volume bleeders are not expected to become anemic because there is not enough intra-abdominal blood volume to do so.[3] Thus, if a small-volume bleeder is anemic in the acute setting, there are 4 major considerations. First, the anemia is preexisting, so compare with the initial packed cell volume. Two, the patient is bleeding somewhere else, so do a good physical examination and a Global FAST to search other cavities and spaces. Third, the anemia is from hemodilution after fluid resuscitation. In addition, the anemia could be a laboratory error. In low-scoring patients, the location of the positive views may lend support to the source of the hemorrhage or effusion; for example, sepsis. Last, the abdominal fluid scoring system provides a means to track (monitor) patients by quickly determining whether the fluid score is static (no change in score), worsening (increasing score), or resolving (decreasing score).

Expectations for Resolution of Hemoabdomen and Lavage Fluid

When bleeding has abated, and coagulation abnormalities, if present, are corrected, expect near resolution of the hemoabdomen within 48-hours as a rule of thumb in the author's experience.[21] Lavage fluid should always be completely removed because, for unknown reasons, it lasts (unlike blood) several days and thus confounds imaging interpretation (unpublished data). However, any fluid that is safely accessible may be sampled and tested.

Table 2
Rule-outs for the finding of gallbladder wall edema in dogs and cats

Condition	Expected Characterization of the CVC	Speculated Pathophysiology
[a]Canine anaphylaxis[30]	Flat, hypovolemic CVC	Massive histamine release resulting in acute marked hepatic venous congestion (increased ALT level)
[a]Pericardial effusion[18]	FAT, distended, hypervolemic CVC	Marked hepatic venous congestion from obstruction of blood flow to the right atrium
[a]Right-sided congestive heart failure[18,31] (dilated cardiomyopathy, pulmonary hypertension, tricuspid disease)	FAT, distended, hypervolemic CVC	Marked hepatic venous congestion from backflow of blood from the right atrium
Cholecystitis[32]	Variable	Direct inflammation
Pancreatitis[32]	Variable	Direct inflammation
Sepsis[33]	Variable	Direct inflammation (normal ALT level)
Acute hemorrhagic diarrhea syndrome[34]	Variable	Direct inflammation (variable ALT level)
Hypoproteinemia (third spacing)[32]	Variable	Vascular leak
Immune-mediated hemolytic anemia[21]	Variable	Likely immune mediated and volume overload
Posttransfusion[21]	Variable to FAT, hypervolemia	Likely immune mediated and volume overload

Abbreviations: ALT, alanine transaminase
 [a] Conditions that are most important to consider in the acute triage setting of acute collapse and weakness in a previously clinically normal patient.
 © 2021 Gregory R. Lisciandro.

AFAST EXTRAS
Gallbladder Wall Edema

Gallbladder wall edema (GBWE), sonographic striation of white-black-white, or white-gray-white, regardless of thickness, is a unique marker for canine anaphylaxis (AX) because the canine shock organs are liver and gastrointestinal tract (Videos 12 and 13).[30] This sonographic finding has also been referred to as the gallbladder halo sign. In the acute setting of weakness or collapse in a previously healthy dog, GBWE supports AX (anaphylactic gallbladder) and right-sided heart failure (cardiac gallbladder), most commonly caused by PCE (see the videos concerning TFAST).[18,21,31] However, when PCE is absent, TFAST echocardiography is needed. An algorithm is provided (**Fig. 5**). Other GBWE causes typically do not present with acute collapse (cholecystitis, pancreatitis, hepatitis, hypoalbuminemia, immune-mediated hemolytic anemia, acute hemorrhagic diarrhea syndrome, sepsis, and post-transfusion) (see **Table 2**).[21,22,32–34] The cardiac gallbladder also has been documented in cats and humans.[16,18]

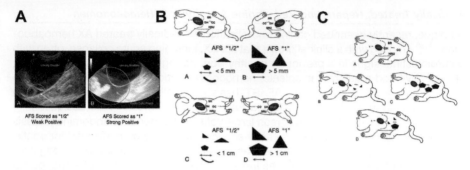

Fig. 4. The abdominal fluid scoring system has been modified with scoring now of 0 (negative), 1/2 (weak positive), and 1 (strong positive), at each respective view, called the visual method. (*A*) The cartoon shows scores of 1/2 and 1 in the CC pouch. (*B*) The measurements method may be used with less than and more than 5 mm in cats, and less than and more than 1 cm maximum dimension in dogs for scores of 1/2 and 1, respectively. (*C*) Examples of how the modification better categorizes patients. A true abdominal fluid score of 3 (1 + 1+1), contrasted with (*B*) being a score of 1 1/2 (1/2 + 1/2 + 1/2) and (*D*) of 2 (1/2 + 1/2 + 1). Now small-volume bleeder/effusion is considered less than 3 and large-volume bleeder/effusion greater than or equal to 3. (© 2021 Gregory R. Lisciandro.)

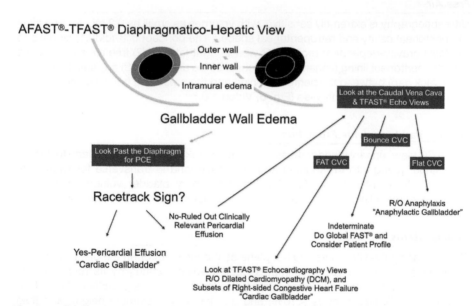

Fig. 5. A diagnostic algorithm for when gallbladder wall edema is detected at triage and differentiating an anaphylactic gallbladder from a cardiac gallbladder by first looking past the diaphragm for the racetrack sign of PCE. If present, the patient most likely has a cardiac gallbladder caused by PCE. If absent, characterize the CVC and hepatic veins. If fluid intolerant (FAT), then it is likely a cardiac gallbladder and you must do TFAST echocardiography. If flat, it is then likely an anaphylactic gallbladder. If no PCE is found and the CVC has a bounce, then the full Global FAST and clinical profile of the patient should be considered for patient assessment. A rule-out list for gallbladder wall edema is available for other causes of gallbladder wall edema in **Table 2**. (© 2021 Gregory R. Lisciandro.)

Medically Treated, Heparin-Induced, Canine Anaphylactic Hemoabdomen

A unique, recently described canine complication is medically treated AX hemoabdomen.[21,35] Any dog with a clinical profile that fits AX, including acute collapse, often with gastrointestinal signs in a previously healthy dog, sonographic GBWE, a small CVC, absent cavitated mass that is splenic, hemoconcentration, increased serum alanine transaminase level, and a positive AFAST, has a medically treated AX hemoabdomen until proved otherwise.[17,21,30,35,36] Global FAST tracking with an AFAST-assigned fluid score categorizes small-volume versus large-volume bleeder, and abdominocentesis with fluid analysis (when ascites is safely accessible) should be performed for confirmation. Glucocorticoid and histamine-2 antagonists mitigate the acquired coagulopathy.[35,36] Traditional coagulation testing (prothrombin time [PT]; activated partial thromboplastin [aPTT]) are variable, although theoretically the aPTT should be discordantly increased because of heparin from mast cell degranulation.[17,35] Surgery is not indicated and is risky, often fatal anecdotally, so veterinarians must recognize this newly described complication.[35] When bleeding has stopped, and coagulation abnormalities, if present, are corrected, expect near resolution of the hemoabdomen within 48 hours as a rule of thumb.[35] A free-of-charge webinar on this unique canine phenomenon is available at FASTVet.com (https://fastvet.com/fastvet-monthly-webinar-march-2021-canine-anaphylaxis-more-than-the-gallbladder-halo-sign-and-canine-anaphylactic-hemoabdomen-a-complication-every-veterinarian-should-know/).

Free Air

Ultrasonography is extremely sensitive, with volumes as small as 0.2 mL, for free air in the peritoneal cavity and retroperitoneal space.[8] The concept is 3-fold: (1) air rises to the least gravity-dependent region (SR view in right lateral); (2) free air is continuous with the peritoneal lining (enhanced peritoneal stripe sign); and (3) any small anechoic gap (black gap) between the peritoneal lining and the presumed free air is gastrointestinal tract until proved otherwise (**Fig. 6**, Video 14).[8,37]

Urinary Bladder Volume Estimation

At the CC view, urinary bladder measurements are taken in the sagittal plane for length (L) (without going into the trigone) and height (H), and in transverse for width (W). L × H × W (centimeters) ×0.625 estimates urinary bladder volume (milliliters)[6]. Thus, over time, clinicians have a noninvasive means to estimate urinary output.

Volume Status

Characterizing the CVC in its sagittal plane as it courses through the diaphragm (and its associated hepatic veins) estimates patient volume status by its respirophasic height change as follows: fluid responsive (bounce), a change of 35% to 50%; fluid intolerant (FAT), little change (<10%) and an increased maximum height; and fluid starved/hypovolemic (flat), little change (<10%) and a decreased maximum height.[4,7,13,21,22,31,38–40] Hepatic venous distension (tree-trunk sign) is likely 100% specific for severely increased right-sided filling pressures in dogs and cats positioned in lateral, standing, or sternal[41]; and its finding, plus a FAT CVC, is easily recognized by properly trained nonradiologist veterinarians. Absolute measurements of the maximum height have also been created; however, dynamic CVC characterization as a rule trumps maximum height measurement unless there is hepatic venous distension.[14,15,40]

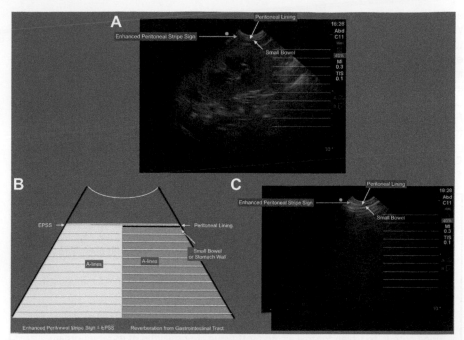

Fig. 6. The detection of free air within the peritoneal and retroperitoneal space is a simple concept. Free air must be opposed directly to the peritoneal lining or body wall without any interposing structures. The peritoneal lining and fascial plane of the body wall are a hyperechoic line to which the free air should be continuous. Both free air and air-filled gastrointestinal tract shadow or cast A lines through the far field depending on the angle on insonation. Any black (anechoic) gap between should be considered gas-filled small intestine or stomach wall as shown in (A) through (C). This same concept works when imaging lung because gastrointestinal tract, specifically the stomach, can mimic the lung surface. The effect of free air highlighting the peritoneal lining has been called the enhanced peritoneal stripe sign (EPSS). (© 2021 Gregory R. Lisciandro.)

Gastrointestinal Motility

The stomach/proximal duodenum and the jejunum may be observed for peristalsis, expecting 4 to 5 minute^{-1} and 1 to 3 minute^{-1}, respectively, if food is present in the canine gastrointestinal tract, helping detect ileus (Video 15).[9] With food absence, including intentional fasting, ileus occurs in normalcy and must be placed into clinical context.[9]

SUMMARY

AFAST and its standardized methodology are easily taught and have value in rapidly ruling in and ruling out free intra-abdominal fluid (<3 minutes). AFAST has a simple abdominal fluid scoring system that is easily learned and that proves to be clinically helpful in both bleeding and nonbleeding patients, and also serving as a tracking (monitoring) tool. AFAST also serves as a soft tissue screening test for obvious abnormalities of its target organs often missed or only suspected based on physical examination, laboratory test results, and radiography. AFAST is low-impact (minimal restraint and no shaving), cost-effective, real-time, rapid (<3 minutes), radiation-sparing, point-of-care imaging that allows veterinarians to see their problem lists and thus better direct resuscitation and treatment, and streamline the diagnostic plan. Without adding any additional views, AFAST may also be used for patient volume status by characterizing the CVC and hepatic veins, screening for pneumoperitoneum, estimating urinary bladder volume and urine output over time, and assessing gastro-intestinal motility. Global FAST and its 15 views provide an unbiased set of data imaging points that prevent the common imaging mistakes of satisfaction of search and confirmation bias errors through AFAST alone or selective POCUS imaging. Global FAST should be used as an extension of the physical examination on a daily basis for nearly all patients in the clinical setting and preempt add-on POCUS examinations.

CLINICS CARE POINTS

- FAST ultrasound is nearly the same sensitivity and specificity as the gold standard test of computed tomography in people for the detection of free fluid.
- The AFAST applied abdominal fluid scoring system semi-quantitates ascites and helps better categorize small versus large volume bleeding and effusion for decision making regarding blood transfusion and fluid resuscitation.
- The AFAST applied abdominal fluid scoring system outperforms abdominal radiography and serosal detail for the presence of fluid and its degree.
- AFAST is used to assess volume status by characterization of the caudal vena cava and hepatic via its Diaphragmatico-Hepatic view. AFAST is used to estimate urinary bladder volume and urine output, to screen for free air, and soft tissue abnormalities of its target-organs.

DISCLOSURE

The author is the owner of FASTVet.com, a private corporation that provides veterinary ultrasonography training to practicing veterinarians. Ultrasonography companies sponsor Global FAST courses and include Oncura Partners, Universal Imaging, El Medical, and Sound; and El Medical and the Veterinary Medical Network have licensed Global FAST education materials. His spouse, Stephanie Lisciandro, is a veterinarian and Medical Director at Oncura Partners, Fort Worth, Texas. The author has no funding sources to declare for this article.

SUPPLEMENTARY DATA

Supplementary data to this article can be found online at https://doi.org/10.1016/j.cvsm.2021.07.006.

REFERENCES

1. Boysen SR, Rozanski EA, Tidwell AS, et al. Evaluation of a focused assessment with sonography for trauma protocol to detect free abdominal fluid in dogs involved in motor vehicle accidents. J Am Vet Med Assoc 2004;225(8):1198–204.
2. Lisciandro GR. The use of the diaphragmatico-hepatic (DH) views of the abdominal and thoracic focused assessment with sonography for triage (AFAST/TFAST) examinations for the detection of pericardial effusion in 24 dogs (2011-2012). J Vet Emerg Crit Care 2016;26(1):125–31.
3. Lisciandro GR, Lagutchik MS, Mann KA, et al. Evaluation of an abdominal fluid scoring system determined using abdominal focused assessment with

sonography for trauma in 101 dogs with motor vehicle trauma. J Vet Emerg Crit Care 2009;19(5):426–37.

4. Lisciandro GR. Abdominal and thoracic focused assessment with sonography for trauma, triage and monitoring in small animals. J Vet Emerg Crit Care 2011;21(2): 104–22.

5. McMurray J, Boysen S, Chalhoub S. Focused assessment with sonography in nontraumatized dogs and cats in the emergency and critical care setting. J Vet Emerg Crit Care 2016;26(1):64–73.

6. Lisciandro GR, Fosgate GT. Use of AFAST Cysto-Colic view urinary bladder measurements to estimate urinary bladder volume in dogs and cats. J Vet Emerg Crit Care 2017;27(6):713–7.

7. Boysen SR, Lisciandro GR. The use of ultrasound in the emergency room (AFAST and TFAST). Vet Clin North Am Small Anim Pract 2013;43(4):773–97.

8. Kim SY, Park KT, Yeon SC, et al. Accuracy of sonographic diagnosis of pneumoperitoneum using the enhanced peritoneal stripe sign in Beagle dogs. J Vet Sci 2014;15(2):195–8.

9. Sanderson JJ, Boysen SR, McMurray JM, et al. The effect of fasting on gastrointestinal motility in healthy dogs as assessed by sonography. J Vet Emerg Crit Care 2017;27(6):645–50.

10. Lisciandro GR, Lagutchik MS, Mann KA, et al. Evaluation of a thoracic focused assessment with sonography for trauma (TFAST) protocol to detect pneumothorax and concurrent thoracic injury in 145 traumatized dogs. J Vet Emerg Crit Care 2008;18(3):258–69.

11. Lisciandro GR, Fosgate GT, Fulton RM. Frequency of ultrasound lung rockets using a regionally-based lung ultrasound examination named veterinary bedside lung ultrasound exam (Vet BLUE) in 98 dogs with normal thoracic radiographic lung findings. Vet Radiol Ultrasound 2014;55(3):315–22.

12. Lisciandro GR, Fulton RM, Fosgate GT, et al. Frequency of B-lines using a regionally-based lung ultrasound examination (the Vet BLUE protocol) in 49 cats with normal thoracic radiographical lung findings. J Vet Emerg Crit Care 2017;27(3):267–77.

13. Lisciandro GR, Armenise AA. Chapter 16: focused or COAST[3] - cardiopulmonary resuscitation (CPR), Global FAST (GFAST[3]), and the FAST-ABCDE exam. In: Lisciandro GR, editor. Focused ultrasound for the small animal practitioner. Ames, IA: Wiley Blackwell; 2014. p. 269–85.

14. Lisciandro GR. Cageside ultrasonography in the emergency room and the intensive care unit. Vet Clin North Am 2020;50(6):1445–67.

15. Lisciandro GR. Chapter 3: point-of-care ultrasound. In: Mattoon JS, Sellon R, Berry CR, editors. Small animal diagnostic ultrasound. 4th edition. St. Louis, MO: Elsevier; 2020. p. 76–104.

16. Lichtenstein DA. Gallbladder. In: Lichtenstein DA, editor. Whole body ultrasound in the critically Ill. London: Springer; 2010. p. 59–67.

17. Hnatusko AL, Gicking JC, Lisciandro GR. Anaphylaxis-related hemoperitoneum in 11 dogs. J Vet Emerg Crit Care 2021;31(1):80–5.

18. Lisciandro GR, Gambino JM, Lisciandro SC. Case series of 13 dogs and 1 cat with ultrasonographically-detected gallbladder wall edema associated with cardiac disease. J Vet Intern Med 2021. https://doi.org/10.1111/jvim.16117.

19. Lisciandro GR, Gambino JM, Lisciandro SC. The wedge sign: a possible lung ultrasound sign for pulmonary thromboembolism. J Vet Emerg Crit Care; 2021, in press.

20. Lisciandro GR, Fosgate GT, Romero LA, et al. The expected frequency and amount of free peritoneal fluid estimated using the abdominal FAST-applied abdominal fluid scores in clinically normal adult and juvenile dogs. J Vet Emerg Crit Care 2021;31(1):43–51.

21. Lisciandro GR. Chapter 2: the abdominal FAST[3] (AFAST[3]) exam. In: Lisciandro GR, editor. Focused ultrasound Techniques for the small animal practitioner. Ames, IA: Wiley Blackwell; 2014. p. 17–43.

22. Lisciandro GR. Chapter 6: POCUS: AFAST-Introduction and Image Acquisition. In: Lisciandro GR, editor. Point-of-care ultrasound techniques for the small animal practitioner. 2nd edition. Ames, IA: Wiley Blackwell; 2021. p. 57–110.

23. Lisciandro SC, Young S. Chapter 9: POCUS: spleen. In: Lisciandro GR, editor. Point-of-care ultrasound techniques for the small animal practitioner. 2nd edition. Ames IA: Wiley Blackwell; 2021. p. 173–88.

24. Lisciandro GR. Chapter 9: the thoracic FAST[3] (TFAST[3]) exam. In: Lisciandro GR, editor. Focused ultrasound techniques for the small animal practitioner. Ames, IA: Wiley Blackwell; 2014. p. 140–65.

25. Lisciandro GR. Chapter 17: POCUS: TFAST-Introduction and Image Acquisition. In: Lisciandro GR, editor. Point-of-care ultrasound Techniques for the small animal practitioner. 2nd edition. Ames, IA: Wiley Blackwell; 2021. p. 297–336.

26. Lisciandro GR, Lisciandro SC. Chapter 22: POCUS: Vet BLUE-introduction and image acquisition. In: Lisciandro GR, editor. Point-of-care ultrasound techniques for the small animal practitioner. 2nd edition. Ames, IA: Wiley Blackwell; 2021. p. 425–58.

27. Rozycki GS, Ballard RB, Feliciano DV, et al. Surgeon-performed ultrasound for the assessment of truncal injuries: lessons learned from 1540 patients. Ann Surg 1998;228(4):557–67.

28. Ollerton JE, Sugrue M, Balogh Z, et al. Prospective study to evaluate the influence of FAST on trauma patient management. J Trauma 2006;60:785–91.

29. Blackbourne LH, Soffer D, McKenney M, et al. Secondary ultrasound examination increases the sensitivity of the FAST exam in trauma. J Trauma 2004;57(5):934–8.

30. Quantz JE, Miles MS, Reed AL, et al. Elevation of alanine transaminase and gallbladder wall abnormalities as biomarkers of anaphylaxis in canine hypersensitivity patients. J Vet Emerg Crit Care 2009;19(6):536–44.

31. Nelson NC, Drost WT, Lerche P, et al. Noninvasive estimation of central venous pressure in anesthetized dogs by measurement of hepatic venous blood flow velocity and abdomen al venous diameter. Vet Rad Ultrasound 2010;51(3):313–23.

32. Nyland TG, Larson MM, Mattoon JS. Liver. In: Mattoon JS, Nyland TG, editors. Small animal diagnostic ultrasound. 3rd edition. St. Louis, MO: Elsevier Saunders; 2015. p. 332–99.

33. Walters AM, O'Brien MA, Selmic LE, et al. Comparison of clinical findings between dogs with suspected anaphylaxis and dogs with confirmed sepsis. J Am Vet Med Assoc 2017;251(6):681–8.

34. Lisciandro GR, Johnson CB, Gambino JM, et al. Prevalence of sonographically-detected gallbladder wall edema in dogs diagnosed with acute hemorrhagic diarrhea syndrome. Abstract. J Vet Emerg Crit Care 2020;S1(30):S15–6.

35. Lisciandro GR. Abdominal FAST (AFAST)-detected hemorrhagic abdominal effusion in 11 dogs with acute collapse and gallbladder wall edema (Halo Sign) with presumed anaphylaxis. Abstract. J Vet Emerg Crit Care 2016;26(S1):S8–9.

36. Lisciandro GR. Chapter 7: POCUS: AFAST-clinical integration. In: Lisciandro GR, editor. Point-of-care ultrasound techniques for the small animal practitioner. 2nd edition. Amoc, IA· Wiley Blackwell; 2021. p. 111–48.

37. Boysen SR, Gambino JM. Chapter 12: POCUS: gastrointestinal and pancreas. In: Lisciandro GR, editor. Point-of-care ultrasound Techniques for the small animal practitioner. 2nd edition. Ames, IA: Wiley Blackwell; 2021. p. 225–44.
38. Ferrada P, Attand RJ, Whelan J, et al. Qualitative assessment of the inferior vena cava: useful tool for the evaluation of volume status in critically ill patients. Am Surg 2012;78(4):468–70.
39. Darnis E, Boysen S, Merveille AC, et al. Establishment of references values of the caudal vena cava by fast-ultrasonography through different views in healthy dogs. J Vet Intern Med 2018;32(4):1308–18.
40. Lisciandro GR. Chapter 36: POCUS: global FAST-patient monitoring and staging. In: Lisciandro GR, editor. Point-of-care ultrasound Techniques for the small animal practitioner. 2nd edition. Ames, IA: Wiley Blackwell; 2021. p. 685–728.
41. Chou Y, Ward JL, Barron LZ, et al. Focused ultrasound of the caudal vena cava in dogs with cavitary effusions or congestive heart failure: a prospective observational study. PLoS One 2021;16(5):e0252544.

Focused Ultrasound Examination of Canine and Feline Emergency Urinary Tract Disorders

Laura Cole, MA, VetMB, MVetMed CertVPS, CertAVP(ECC), DACVECC, DECVECC*,
Karen Humm, MA, VetMB, MSc CertVA, DACVECC, DECVECC, FHEA, MRCVS,
Helen Dirrig, BVetMed(Hons), MVetMed(Hons), DACVR, DECVDI, MRCVS

KEYWORDS

- Urinary • Ultrasound • Emergency • Acute kidney injury • Urinary obstruction

KEY POINTS

- Small animals with urinary tract disorders can present critically ill with severe acid–base and electrolyte abnormalities.
- Point-of-care ultrasound examinations can be performed safely in the unstable animal without chemical restraint to help guide further diagnostics and therapy.
- The kidneys can be assessed in the splenorenal and hepatorenal views, and bladder in the cystocolic view, of previously described focused abdominal ultrasound protocols.
- Alongside history and physical examination findings, point-of-care ultrasound examination may expedite the diagnosis of specific causes of azotemia, including urethral and ureteral obstruction and chronic kidney disease.
- Patients with a urinary tract emergency may benefit from a complete abdominal ultrasound examination once they are clinically stable.

 Video content accompanies this article at http://www.vetsmall.theclinics.com.

INTRODUCTION

Emergency point-of-care ultrasound (POCUS) examination is an invaluable tool for the assessment and management of the emergency patient. It is being used increasingly in human medicine for the investigation of abdominal pain and urologic emergencies.[1–3] A veterinary POCUS protocol—abdominal focused assessment with sonography for trauma, triage and tracking (AFAST)—has been demonstrated to be useful in

---

Clinical Science and Services, The Royal Veterinary College, The University of London, Hawkshead Lane, Hatfield, AL9 7TA
* Corresponding author.
E-mail address: lcole3@rvc.ac.uk

Vet Clin Small Anim 51 (2021) 1233–1248
https://doi.org/10.1016/j.cvsm.2021.07.007

the assessment of unstable small animals.[4–6] Animals presenting with urinary tract emergencies can be critically ill and POCUS examination, as a noninvasive diagnostic tool, can be performed early without the need for chemical restraint in the unstable animal to help guide further diagnostics and therapy. The AFAST splenorenal and hepatorenal views allows assessment of both kidneys and the cystocolic view allows assessment of the urinary bladder. This article discusses the usefulness of POCUS examinations in the assessment and management of animals presenting with upper and lower urinary tract disorders.

UPPER AND LOWER URINARY TRACT POINT-OF-CARE ULTRASOUND TECHNIQUE

Urinary tract POCUS examinations can be performed as part of the AFAST protocol.[5] Animals can be standing, sternal, or in lateral recumbency. The ultrasound transducer should be placed in the splenorenal view (left flank caudal to the costal arch and immediately ventral to the sublumbar muscles), hepatorenal view (right flank caudal to the costal arch and immediately ventral to the sublumbar muscles), and in the cystocolic view (caudolateral abdomen cranial to the pelvis). It is recommended to fan through each kidney in both transverse and longitudinal planes (Video 1 and 2). The urinary bladder should be examined along its length in both the transverse and longitudinal planes (Video 3). Care should be taken not to apply excessive pressure with the probe in the cystocolic view because this pressure may not only distort the urinary bladder's shape, but also may prevent the detection of small volumes of fluid in the cystocolic view.

PROBE SELECTION AND MAXIMIZING IMAGE QUALITY

In larger patients with deep kidneys, a convex or microconvex probe may be most useful. These probes have a lower frequency ($\leq$5 MHz) to maximize penetration and a small footprint to allow intercostal or subcostal views, and are particularly useful for the more cranial right kidney. They may also allow easier assessment of the caudal abdominal region (bladder and urethra). In smaller dogs and cats, for all portions of the urinary tract, a higher frequency (8–12 MHz) linear probe is recommended for optimal resolution. Image depth and gain should be adjusted dynamically to maximize visualization of the structures of interest. It is very important in unshaved patients to part the hair and place the probe as directly on skin as possible.

NORMAL ULTRASOUND APPEARANCE OF THE URINARY SYSTEM

Ultrasound examination of the kidneys involves assessing the renal anatomy, echogenicity, and size. First, the outer margin should show a smooth, clearly defined hyperechoic capsule and the kidney should be symmetric and oval or kidney bean shaped. Three distinct regions should be identified: the renal cortex, the renal medulla, and the renal sinus (Fig. 1). Corticomedullary definition is seen as a clearly defined interface between the hyperechoic cortex and more hypoechoic medulla. The renal sinus is the most hyperechoic structure within the kidney, owing to the presence of fat, which surrounds the renal pelvis and vascular branches that enter the renal parenchyma. The empty renal pelvic diverticula and the interlobar and arcuate vessels are seen as regularly spaced hyperechoic structures crossing the renal parenchyma of similar echogenicity to the renal sinus. Some mild acoustic shadowing can occur distal to these vessels and the renal sinus, which should not be misinterpreted as mineralization (see Figs. 1A and B, compared with Fig. 2C). Radiographs may complement ultrasound examination in the assessment of renal mineralization.[7] When compared with

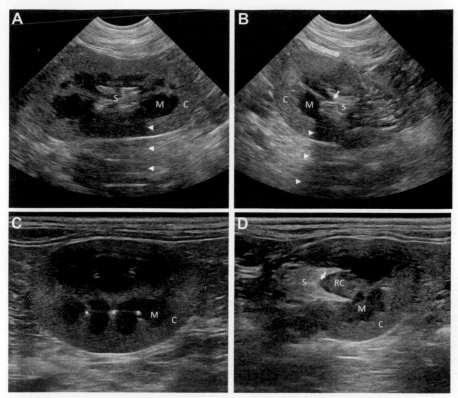

Fig. 1. Normal dog (*A, B*) and cat (*C, D*) kidney in longitudinal (*A, C*) and transverse (*B, D*) orientations. Renal cortex (*C*), renal medulla (*M*), renal sinus (*S*), renal crest (RC). The *arrow* in (*B*) and (*D*) points to the site of the renal pelvis (empty in these cases), at the tip of the renal crest. *Arrowheads* indicate the shadowing that can be identified distal to the renal sinus. *Asterisks* (*) denote the ventral sets of diverticula and interlobar vessels.

other abdominal organs, the renal cortex is usually hypoechoic to the spleen and similar to the liver. Because echogenicity will vary depending on image settings including depth and gain, comparisons between organs should always be performed without altering these settings.

To assess the renal pelvis, transverse images are preferred, using the renal crest as a landmark to identify the adjacent V-shaped structure, which may be seen using high-frequency transducers. Pelvis size is determined by measuring from the renal crest to the beginning of the ureter (**Fig. 3**B). Mild dilation with anechoic fluid can occur in patients with normal renal function, up to approximately 3 mm, but the proximal ureter is generally not identified in normalcy.[8]

When assessing renal size, long axis measurements are generally used. Renal length in normal cats ranges between 2.9 and 5.1 cm, with minor differences between the right and left kidneys and different breeds and sexes.[9–12] In dogs, the normal size ranges are very broad, and measurements depend on ratios of renal length to other structures, limiting their use in an emergency setting.[13,14] With these caveats in mind, it may be more important to assess the symmetry of a patient's left and right kidneys and take into account the size, but also other features, such as shape and architecture, when assessing for abnormalities.

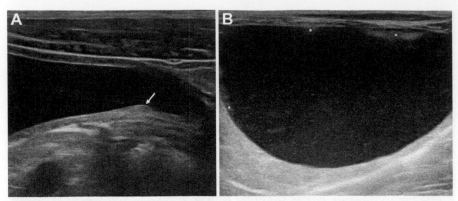

Fig. 2. (*A*) Small, smooth, luminal protrusion indicating the ureteral papilla (*arrow*) and region of the trigone in this normal male dog. (*B*) Presumed lipiduria in a cat with lipid droplets noted on an otherwise normal urinalysis. Artifacts can appear as luminal material (*).

The normal urinary bladder should have a smooth, uniform wall and anechoic contents. Wall thickness depends on bladder distension; therefore, measurements should be performed with caution, particularly in a relatively empty urinary bladder. In dogs and cats, wall thickness should not exceed 3.0 mm and 1.7 mm, respectively.[15,16] The ureteral papillae may be identified as small, smoothly marginated luminal protrusions, which can help to mark the region of the trigone at the dorsal aspect of the bladder neck (**Fig. 4**A). Urinary bladder contents are usually anechoic, but patient-related or image artefact–related factors can alter this appearance in otherwise normal animals. In particular, lipiduria in normal cats can be seen as suspended echoes within the urinary bladder (see **Fig. 4**B).[17] The proximal urethra is often identified as a tubular structure extending caudally from the bladder neck, usually empty of fluid.

POINT-OF-CARE ULTRASOUND EXAMINATION AND ACUTE KIDNEY INJURY

Acute kidney injury (AKI) is a diverse condition with multiple etiologies and variable presentation, but all causes lead to a decrease in the glomerular filtration rate, tubular dysfunction, and abnormal urine output.[18] Ultrasound findings reported in azotemic dogs and cats with AKI include variation in renal size, alterations in corticomedullary definition, increased echogenicity of the renal cortex and/or medulla, pyelectasia, and retroperitoneal fluid at the periphery of one or both kidneys (perinephric fluid) (see **Fig. 3**, Video 4).[19–21] However, most renal ultrasound findings in AKI are relatively subtle and nonspecific (**Table 1**) and many animals with AKI have a normal gross renal architecture.[20,22] Therefore, a diagnosis of AKI should not be excluded based on a normal renal ultrasound examination.

Perinephric fluid is identified at the hepatorenal and splenorenal views. Although it is associated with a variety of diseases (see **Table 1**), the presence of unilateral perinephric fluid and pyelectasia should increase the suspicion for a ureteral obstruction, whereas large volumes of perinephric fluid bilaterally may raise concern for fluid overload owing to oliguric or anuric AKI.[20,23] Perinephric fluid secondary to AKI is thought to be a transudate that forms as a result of either tubular back-leak of ultrafiltrate secondary to decreased glomerular filtration and/or as a result of increased tubular permeability, which overwhelms the normal lymphatic drainage.[24,25] Perinephric fluid can also occur secondary to urinary tract rupture and urine leakage, hemorrhage, or

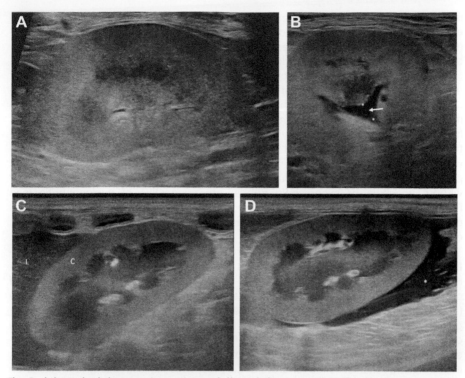

Fig. 3. (A) Marked decrease in corticomedullary definition with diffuse hyperechogenicity of the renal parenchyma, in a cat with AKI of unknown etiology. (B) Transverse image of the left kidney of a cat with AKI due to a suspected intoxication. The renal pelvis is mildly dilated with anechoic fluid (*arrow*). There is decreased corticomedullary definition. Asterisks indicate locations for measuring the renal pelvic size. (C and D) Right kidney of a young dog with confirmed leptospirosis and marked interstitial nephritis on histopathology. Note in C the marked renal cortical hyperechogenicity (C) relative to the adjacent liver parenchyma (L) and in D the anechoic perinephric fluid (*).

infection. The uroretroperitoneum or uroabdomen should be considered in an animal with perinephric fluid and a history of trauma or recent surgery, such as ovariohysterectomy. In these cases, contrast-enhanced radiographs may be useful to help confirm the presence of a rupture and urine leak. If the volume of fluid is small, then serial POCUS examinations should be performed. Urine leakage or clinically relevant hemorrhage will cause an increase in perinephric fluid over time.

Some renal ultrasound findings have been associated with particular AKI etiologies. A halo sign (increased cortical and medullary echogenicity with persistence of areas of lesser intensity at the corticomedullary junction) (**Fig. 5**A and B) has been described in patients with ethylene glycol toxicity.[26] This appearance is thought to be secondary to oxalate crystal deposition in the renal cortex, and therefore may suggest more advanced disease. However, in the original study of 15 affected dogs and cats, a halo sign was absent in 40% of patients[26] and a halo sign has also been described in patients with other causes of AKI.[20,27] A medullary rim sign, a distinct hyperechoic line in the renal medulla (see **Fig. 5**C) is reported in a range of AKI etiologies, including leptospirosis, hypercalcemic nephropathy, and feline infectious peritonitis,[21,28,29] but is also seen in a large number of animals with no renal dysfunction; therefore, its presence should not be overinterpreted.[28,29] More recent studies have differentiated a thin medullary rim sign from a thick medullary rim sign (a band sign) and found the latter to be more commonly associated with kidney disease.[29,30]

Both renal lymphoma and pyelonephritis are relatively common causes of AKI that require etiology-specific treatment alongside supportive care. Commonly reported ultrasound findings with renal lymphoma include nephromegaly, a decrease in corticomedullary definition, hypoechoic masses or subcapsular thickening, and pyelectasia (see **Fig. 5**D).[31–34] However, many animals with lymphoma have no or subtle renal ultrasound changes and abdominal lymphadenopathy is only seen in one-half of cases with primary renal lymphoma.[31–33] Renal fine-needle aspirates should, therefore, be performed if renal lymphoma is suspected. Pyelectasia and ureteral dilation, with or without anechoic or hyperechoic debris, are suggestive of pyelonephritis (see **Fig. 2**A).[10,11] A diagnosis of pyelonephritis is usually confirmed by a positive bacterial culture of urine collected by pyelocentesis, which should only be performed by an experienced practitioner.[35]

It can be difficult to differentiate AKI from chronic kidney disease (CKD) in some patients. Preexisting CKD will likely influence the animal's prognosis and therefore early recognition is beneficial. The presence of small and/or irregular kidneys and loss of corticomedullary definition on POCUS examination are nonspecific findings of CKD (see **Fig. 2**B and C) and misshapen, irregular, small kidneys in a young animal are suggestive of renal dysplasia (see **Fig. 2**D). However, alterations in renal architecture cannot be correlated directly with renal function.[36] Also, animals with more longstanding CKD may develop acute-on-chronic kidney disease secondary to infection, inflammation, renal ischemia, or ureteral disease, which is less readily identifiable on ultrasound examination.[37,38]

Table 1	
Differential diagnosis of pyelectasia and perinephric fluid in dogs and cats	
Ultrasound Finding	**Differential Diagnosis**
Pyelectasia	Intravenous fluid therapy
	Diuretic therapy
	Infection (pyelonephritis/ureteritis)
	Chronic kidney disease
	AKI (toxin, infection, ischemia, other)
	Ureteral obstruction (stone, stricture, trauma, blood clot)
	Ectopic ureters or other congenital abnormality
	Renal neoplasia (lymphoma)
	Lower urinary tract obstruction
Perinephric fluid	AKI (toxin, infection, ischemia, other)
	Ureteral obstruction
	Infection (pyelonephritis, ureteritis, renal abscess)
	Neoplasia
	Trauma (blood or urine leakage)
	Renal or ureteral rupture following severe infection or obstruction (urine leakage)
	Perinephric pseudocyst
	Lower urinary tract obstruction
	Fluid overload

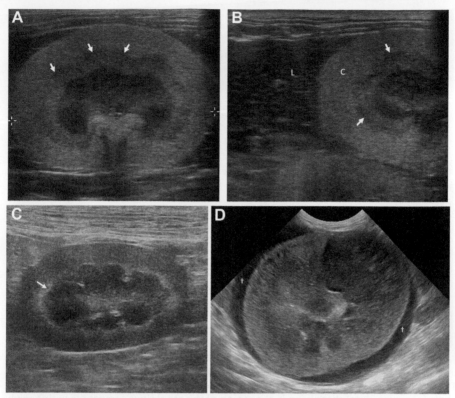

Fig. 4. (*A* and *B*) Right kidney of a cat with confirmed ethylene glycol intoxication exhibiting the halo sign (*arrows*). (*A*) longitudinal image; (*B*) note the marked hyperechogenicity of the cortex (*C*) compared with the liver parenchyma (*L*). (*C*) Longitudinal image of a hyperechoic medullary rim (*arrow*) in the left kidney of a Pug with no evidence of renal dysfunction. (*D*) Transverse image of the left kidney of a cat with confirmed renal lymphoma, showing reduced corticomedullary definition and a hypoechoic subcapsular rim (†), which showed vascularization on Doppler examination, confirming this was not fluid.

The management of AKI is largely supportive, with a particular focus on fluid balance, which requires close monitoring of urine output to guide fluid therapy. Although urethral catheterization and urine collection is the optimal method for urine output measurement, POCUS examination of the bladder can aid in the recognition of oliguria or anuria if the clinician has concerns about urethral catheterization (eg, severe thrombocytopenia, coagulopathy, or the presence of a urinary tract infection). Urinary bladder volume (in milliliters) estimation in dogs and cats can be performed using the formula: Length × Width × Height (cm) × 0.2 × π (**Fig. 6**). It should be noted that measurements are susceptible to bias at very large and small bladder volumes.[39] A 3-dimensional ultrasound method for estimation of bladder volume is used human medicine and a commercial device (BladderScan, PrimePlus) Verathon has been shown to be useful in dogs.[40,41]

To summaries, the cause of AKI cannot be determined reliably with a POCUS examination and recognizing subtle renal architectural changes requires skill and experience. Therefore, although POCUS examination can help to recognize gross abnormalities, it does not replace a more complete urinary tract ultrasound examination with a suitably trained clinician.

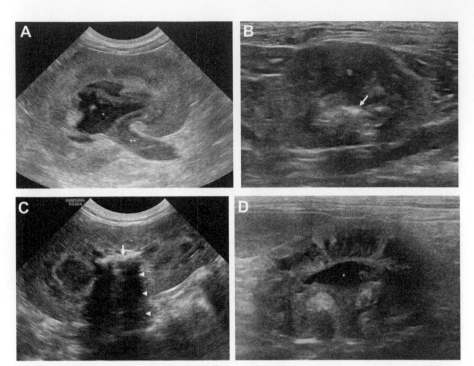

Fig. 5. (*A*) Left kidney of a dog with pyelonephritis with a dilated renal pelvis (*) and proximal ureter (**) containing echogenic debris. (*B*) Right kidney of a cat with IRIS stage 2 CKD. The renal outline is irregular, there is reduced corticomedullary definition, and a hyperechoic focus with distal shadowing in the region of the renal sinus compatible with a nephrolith (*arrow*). (*C*) Left kidney of a hypercalcemic dog with renal pelvic mineralization (*arrow*) and marked associated distal shadowing (*arrowheads*). (*D*) Left kidney of a 6-month-old dog with presumed renal dysplasia. The kidney is misshapen with no visible corticomedullary definition. There are numerous echogenic striations within the parenchyma. The renal pelvis is moderately dilated with anechoic fluid (*).

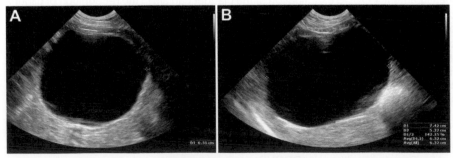

Fig. 6. (*A* and *B*) Example of urinary bladder volume estimation using bladder width (*A*) and bladder length and height (*B*) measured in centimeters yields an estimation in milliliters. In this case, bladder volume would be $7.42 \times 6.31 \times 5.22 \times 0.2 \times \pi = 153$ mL.

POINT-OF-CARE ULTRASOUND EXAMINATION AND URETERAL OBSTRUCTION

Ureteral obstruction can cause azotemia, severe electrolyte derangements, and anuria but with prompt surgical intervention (eg, placement of a subcutaneous ureteral bypass system), bilateral ureteral obstruction is associated with a good short-term prognosis when compared with oliguric or anuric AKI.[42]

POCUS findings compatible with ureteral obstruction include renal asymmetry, pyelectasia, unilateral perinephric fluid, ureteral dilation, and calculi within the ureter.[20,43] Pyelectasia of more than 13 mm has been commonly associated with ureteral obstruction.[8,43,44] However, a consensus statement has defined urolith-associated ureteral obstruction as the presence of a ureterolith, proximal ureteral dilation, and any degree of pyelectasia (**Figs. 7**A and B, Video 5).[45]

Urologic POCUS examination is used by human nephrologists and emergency clinicians for investigating acute flank pain (a symptom of ureteral obstruction) in humans. When compared with radiologists, emergency doctors are relatively proficient in identifying ureteral obstruction based on a subjective assessment of the degree of hydronephrosis.[46,47] Emergency veterinarians detected moderate to severe pyelectasia, renal asymmetry, and perinephric fluid in cats with ureteral obstruction but rarely identified ureteroliths or ureteral dilation in 1 study.[48] However, a highly skilled ultrasonographer is usually required for a complete assessment of the ureter from the kidney to the ureterovesicular junction. The most common urolith-causing ureteral obstruction in cats is the radiopaque stone calcium oxalate; therefore, radiographs may be a useful adjunct.[49]

Other causes of ureteral obstruction include strictures, ureteral trauma (including iatrogenic injury associated with abdominal surgery), and blood clots, all of which are less readily detected with ultrasound examination.[50] If the clinical suspicion for ureteral obstruction is high, but the ultrasound findings are equivocal, antegrade pyelography may be indicated. This procedure involves the injection of a water-soluble iodinated contrast agent directly into the renal pelvis under ultrasound guidance and subsequent serial radiographic assessment. Obstruction is identified by contrast abruptly terminating in the ureter (see **Fig. 7**C). In light of the possible complications associated with pyelography, including hemorrhage, sepsis, and urine leakage, this procedure should be only performed by a suitably trained clinician.

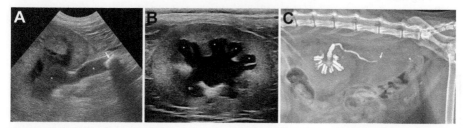

Fig. 7. (*A*) Right kidney of a dog with pyelonephritis and ureteral obstruction owing to a struvite stone (*arrow*). Note the marked shadowing distal to the stone and the dilation of the renal pelvis and proximal ureter with markedly echogenic material (*). (*B*) Longitudinal image showing hydronephrosis of the right kidney of a cat with a ureteral obstruction. The contents of the dilated renal pelvis are anechoic and there is dilation of the renal pelvic diverticula (*). (*C*) Lateral radiograph of a cat after a positive contrast left antegrade pyelography. The renal pelvis and proximal ureter are dilated with contrast. The ureteral contrast column tapers and abruptly stops just cranial to a small mineralized ureterolith (*arrow*). Note other mineralized foci overlying both kidneys, at the distal aspect of the right ureter (*arrowhead*) and within the urinary bladder.

Although severe pyelectasia (>13 mm) is strongly suggestive of ureteral obstruction, a range of pelvic dimensions have been described in cats requiring ureteral surgery and the degree of pyelectasia alone cannot be readily used to differentiate pyelonephritis from ureteral obstruction.[51-53] A complete abdominal ultrasound examination by a board-certified radiologist interpreted in light of other diagnostic tests is, therefore, required to help differentiate between ureteral obstruction and pyelonephritis. Pyelonephritis, ureteritis, and ureteral obstruction can also coexist, and therefore serial ultrasound assessment may be required to for improvement or worsening of the condition.

POINT-OF-CARE ULTRASOUND EXAMINATION AND LOWER URINARY TRACT DISEASE

Lower urinary tract emergencies include urosepsis, urethral obstruction, and uroabdomen. Scanning the cystocolic view identifies the urinary bladder, its luminal content and any surrounding fluid and this assessment can help distinguish between different causes of lower urinary tract disease (**Table 2**).

Cystoliths appear as dependent, hyperechoic, and variably shaped structures with distal shadowing (**Fig. 8A**).[54] Detection can be enhanced by scanning the cystocolic view while the animal is standing, because the calculi will move to the ventral aspect of the bladder. Urinary bladder neoplasms usually have a broad-based attachment to the bladder wall with variable echogenicity and no acoustic shadowing. Transitional cell carcinomas are the most common urinary bladder neoplasm in older dogs and are usually located in the trigone region (see **Fig. 8C**). Blood clots and urinary sediment are commonly seen in cats with urethral obstruction. Blood clots can be mistaken for cystoliths or neoplasia by the novice ultrasonographer. They are hyperechoic structures that localize to the dependent potion of the bladder, but usually lack distal acoustic shadowing (see **Fig. 8B**).[54] Color Doppler ultrasound examination may also be used to assess for pulsatile flow. In general, no flow supports a thrombus (or artifact), positive flow supports a mass, and a twinkling artifact is sometimes seen distal to a cystolith.[55] Urine sediment, composed of cellular debris and crystalline matrix, also tends to settle in the dependent portion of the bladder, with variable acoustic shadowing depending on the relative mineral content of the sediment, and can be moved with gentle agitation.

Ultrasound findings compatible with cystitis include bladder wall thickening and echogenic urine. However, bladder filling should be considered when assessing wall thickness, and echogenic urine is not a reliable indicator of a urinary tract infection,

Table 2
Ultrasound characteristics of mural and intraluminal bladder changes of common lower urinary tract disorders

	Mural Changes		Intraluminal Changes		
	Cystitis	Neoplasia	Blood Clot	Sediment	Urolith
Location	Cranial Focal or diffuse	Caudodorsal	Gravity dependent	Gravity dependent	Gravity dependent
Echogenicity	Hypoechoic	Variable	Hyperechoic	Variable	Hyperechoic
Acoustic shadowing	No	No unless mineralized	No	Variable	Yes
Mobility	No	No	Variable	Yes	Yes

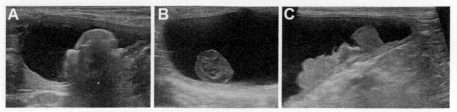

Fig. 8. (*A*) Collection of large calculi in the bladder of a dog, showing a smooth hyperechoic interface and marked distal shadowing (***). (*B*) Rounded amorphous echogenic blood clot within the dependent aspect of the bladder of a cat with cystitis. Note the absence of a distal shadow. (*C*) Sagittal image of the urinary bladder neck of a dog showing an irregular mass in the region of the trigone confirmed as a transitional cell carcinoma on cytology.

also being seen in disease states including dehydration, hemorrhage, and systemic inflammation.[56] Considering the urinary tract is one of the most common septic foci in dogs and cats,[57–59] cystocentesis and urine sediment examination should be performed in animals with signs of sepsis or clinical signs of a urinary tract infection, irrespective of their POCUS findings.

Urethral obstruction in dogs most commonly occurs secondary to uroliths, bladder or urethral masses, or, rarely, blood clots. The animal's signalment, history, diet, and comorbidities can help to differentiate between these causes; for example, an older female neutered dog is more likely to have neoplasia and a young dog with a portosystemic shunt is more likely to have a urolith. Urethral obstruction in cats is most commonly caused by a urethral plug composed of a matrix of organic material, blood cells, and aggregates of crystalline minerals and less commonly by uroliths, strictures, or neoplasia.

Animals with a urethral obstruction usually have a large firm bladder that is difficult to express. However, in some larger overweight animals, abdominal palpation may prove difficult. POCUS findings compatible with urethral obstruction include a large bladder, dilation of the proximal urethra (**Fig. 9**A), bladder wall thickening, echogenic

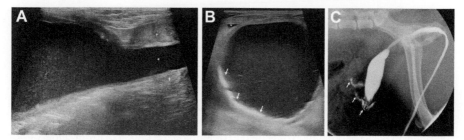

Fig. 9. (*A*) Sagittal image of the bladder neck of a male Bulldog with urethral obstruction by cystine calculi. Note the marked dilation of the proximal urethra (***)that is surrounded by prostatic tissue (†). The urine is mildly echogenic. (*B*) Transverse view of the bladder of a cat with a urethral obstruction by a mucoid plug, showing hyperechoic sediment in the dependent aspect (*arrows*), a small volume of anechoic pericystic fluid (***) adjacent to the body wall, and hyperechoic surrounding peritoneal fat. (*C*) Lateral radiograph of the caudal abdomen of a dog with surgically confirmed bladder rupture following a road traffic accident. A positive contrast retrograde urethrocystogram outlines a normal urethra and a small bladder, with streaks of contrast leaking from the bladder apex into the adjacent peritoneal cavity (*arrows*).

Table 3
Guidelines for diagnosing a uroabdomen, reported as ratios of creatinine and potassium in the fluid relative to blood

	Creatinine Fluid: Blood	Potassium Fluid: Blood
Dog	>2:1	>1.4:1
Cat	>2:1	>1.9:1

material in the bladder, pericystic fluid, hyperechoic pericystic fat, and perinephric fluid (see **Fig. 9**B).[60] A small to medium volume of peritoneal effusion, not biochemically compatible with a uroabdomen (thought to be a sterile inflammatory fluid), has been reported in one-third of cats with urethral obstruction before cystocentesis, with fluid most commonly identified at the cystocolic view and rarely in any other AFAST views.[61] A complete AFAST and abdominal fluid score should be performed before cystocentesis or urethral de-obstruction, with serial monitoring if fluid is identified. Scores should be recorded at each respective view in addition to the total score as locations may be clinically relevant. If the fluid volume or score is increasing or not resolving as expected, the fluid should be aspirated to rule out the presence of a uroabdomen (**Table 3**).

Uroabdomen may occur secondary to urethral obstruction as a result of urinary bladder or urethral injury secondary to increased pressure owing to the urethral obstruction itself or owing to iatrogenic damage caused by decompressive cystocentesis or urinary catheterization. However, blunt trauma is the most common cause of uroabdomen in small animals, most commonly due to bladder rupture.[62,63] The absence of a bladder on abdominal palpation and evidence of perineal or caudoventral abdominal bruising should alert the clinician to the possibility of a bladder rupture and urethral rupture, respectively. In those cases, a positive contrast retrograde urethrocystogram can confirm the diagnosis, revealing leakage of contrast material at the site of the rupture (see **Fig. 9**C).

CLINIC PEARLS

- Owing to the variation in canine and feline kidney size, assessing symmetry of the kidneys alongside their shape and architecture is more useful than assessing size alone.
- Renal asymmetry with pyelectasia (>13 mm) should increase the index of suspicion for a ureteral obstruction.
- Renal ultrasound examination may be normal in animals with AKI and is a poor predictor of function.
- Renal POCUS examination may help to determine the cause of lower urinary tract obstruction including uroliths, neoplasia and blood clots.

SUMMARY

Emergency urinary tract POCUS examination is a useful noninvasive tool for the assessment of unstable animals with azotemia and electrolyte and/or acid–base abnormalities. These initial ultrasound findings may help to guide further investigations, including expediting the diagnosis of specific causes of azotemia, such as urethral obstruction or ureteral obstruction and specific causes of AKI like renal lymphoma.

However, in light of the variability in normal renal size, architecture, and the difficulties of assessing the ureters and interpreting the clinical relevance of bladder and urethral abnormalities, a complete abdominal ultrasound examination may also be beneficial.

DISCLOSURE

The authors have no relevant conflicts of interest.

SUPPLEMENTARY DATA

Supplementary data to this article can be found online at https://doi.org/10.1016/j.cvsm.2021.07.007.

REFERENCES

1. Moore CL, Carpenter CR, Heilbrun ME, et al. Imaging in suspected renal colic: systematic review of the literature and multispecialty consensus. J Am Coll Radiol 2019;16(9 Pt A):1132–43.
2. Ng C, Tsung JW. Avoiding computed tomography scans by using point-of-care ultrasound when evaluating suspected pediatric renal colic. J Emerg Med 2015;49(2):165–71.
3. Alerhand S, Choi A, Ostrovsky I, et al. Integrating basic and clinical sciences using point-of-care renal ultrasound for preclerkship education. MedEdPORTAL 2020;16:11037.
4. Boysen SR, Rozanski EA, Tidwell AS, et al. Evaluation of a focused assessment with sonography for trauma protocol to detect free abdominal fluid in dogs involved in motor vehicle accidents. J Am Vet Med Assoc 2004;225(8):1198–204.
5. Lisciandro GR, Lagutchik MS, Mann KA, et al. Evaluation of an abdominal fluid scoring system determined using abdominal focused assessment with sonography for trauma in 101 dogs with motor vehicle trauma. J Vet Emerg Crit Care (San Antonio) 2009;19(5):426–37.
6. McMurray J, Boysen S, Chalhoub S. Focused assessment with sonography in nontraumatized dogs and cats in the emergency and critical care setting. J Vet Emerg Crit Care (San Antonio) 2016;26(1):64–73.
7. Berent AC. Ureteral obstructions in dogs and cats: a review of traditional and new interventional diagnostic and therapeutic options. J Vet Emerg Crit Care (San Antonio) 2011;21(2):86–103.
8. D'Anjou MA, Bédard A, Dunn ME. Clinical significance of renal pelvic dilatation on ultrasound in dogs and cats. Vet Radiol Ultrasound 2011;52(1):88–94.
9. d'Anjou M. Kidneys and ureters. In: Penninck D, d'Anjou M, editors. Atlas of small animal ultrasonography. 1st edition. Philadelphia: Blackwell Publishing; 2008. p. 339–64.
10. Nyland TG, Widmer WR, Mattoon JS. Urinary tract. In: Nyland TG, Mattoon JS, editors. Veterinary diagnostic ultrasound. 3rd edition. New Jersey: WB Saunders; 2015. p. 557–608.
11. Lamb CR, Dirrig H, Cortellini S. Comparison of ultrasonographic findings in cats with and without azotaemia. J Feline Med Surg 2018;20(10):948–54.
12. Debruyn K, Paepe D, Daminet S, et al. Comparison of renal ultrasonographic measurements between healthy cats of three cat breeds: Ragdoll, British Shorthair and Sphynx. J Feline Med Surg 2013;15(6):478–82.
13. Barella G, Lodi M, Sabbadin LA, et al. A new method for ultrasonographic measurement of kidney size in healthy dogs. J Ultrasound 2012;15(3):186–91.

14. Mareschal A, d'Anjou MA, Moreau M, et al. Ultrasonographic measurement of kidney-to-aorta ratio as a method of estimating renal size in dogs. Vet Radiol Ultrasound 2007;48(5):434–8.

15. Lisciandro S. Focused or COAST3 – urinary bladder. In: Lisciandro GR, editor. Focused ultrasound techniques for the small animal practitioner. 1st edition. New Jersey: Wiley and Sons; 2014. p. 99–109.

16. Finn-Bodner ST. The urinary bladder. In: Cartee RE, Selcer BA, Hudson JA, et al, editors. Practical veterinary ultrasound. 1st edition. Philadelphia: Lea and Febiger; 1995. p. 210–35.

17. Sislak MD, Spaulding KA, Zoran DL, et al. Ultrasonographic characteristics of lipiduria in clinically normal cats. Vet Radiol Ultrasound 2014;55(2):195–201.

18. Cowgill L. Grading of acute kidney injury. International Renal Interest Society website; 2016. Available at: http://www.iris-kidney.com. Accessed February 16, 2021.

19. Sonet J, Barthélemy A, Goy-Thollot I, et al. Prospective evaluation of abdominal ultrasonographic findings in 35 dogs with leptospirosis. Vet Radiol Ultrasound 2018;59(1):98–106.

20. Cole LP, Mantis P, Humm K. Ultrasonographic findings in cats with acute kidney injury: a retrospective study. J Feline Med Surg 2019;21(6):475–80.

21. Forrest LJ, O'Brien RT, Tremelling MS, et al. Sonographic renal findings in 20 dogs with leptospirosis. Vet Radiol Ultrasound 1998;39(4):337–40.

22. Mantis P. Kidneys and ureters. In: Mantis P, editor. Practical small animal ultrasonography. 1st edition. Zaragoza: Servet; 2016. p. 61–76.

23. Holloway A, O'Brien R. Perirenal effusion in dogs and cats with acute renal failure. Vet Radiol Ultrasound 2007;48(6):574–9.

24. Levine S, Saltzman A, Branch C. A model for perinephric fluid accumulation in uremic rats with toxic nephrosis. Toxicol Lett 2003;146(1):9–15.

25. Haddad MC, Medawar WA, Hawary MM, et al. Perirenal fluid in renal parenchymal medical disease ('floating kidney'): clinical significance and sonographic grading. Clin Radiol 2001;56(12):979–83.

26. Adams WH, Toal RL, Breider MA. Ultrasonographic findings in dogs and cats with oxalate nephrosis attributed to ethylene glycol intoxication: 15 cases (1984-1988). J Am Vet Med Assoc 1991;199(4):492–6.

27. Banzato T, Bonsembiante F, Aresu L, et al. Relationship of diagnostic accuracy of renal cortical echogenicity with renal histopathology in dogs and cats, a quantitative study. BMC Vet Res 2017;13(1):24.

28. Mantis P, Lamb CR. Most dogs with medullary rim sign on ultrasonography have no demonstrable renal dysfunction. Vet Radiol Ultrasound 2000;41(2):164–6.

29. Ferreira A, Marwood R, Batchelor D, et al. Prevalence and clinical significance of the medullary rim sign identified on ultrasound of feline kidneys. Vet Rec 2020;186(16):533.

30. Cordella A, Pey P, Dondi F, et al. The ultrasonographic medullary "rim sign" versus medullary "band sign" in cats and their association with renal disease. J Vet Intern Med 2020;34(5):1932–9.

31. McAloney CA, Sharkey LC, Feeney DA, et al. Diagnostic utility of renal fine-needle aspirate cytology and ultrasound in the cat. J Feline Med Surg 2018;20(6):544–53.

32. Taylor A, Finotello R, Vilar-Saavedra P, et al. Clinical characteristics and outcome of dogs with presumed primary renal lymphoma. J Small Anim Pract 2019;60(11):663–70.

33. Taylor AJ, Lara-Garcia A, Benigni L. Ultrasonographic characteristics of canine renal lymphoma. Vet Radiol Ultrasound 2014;55(4):441–6.

34. Valdés-Martínez A, Cianciolo R, Mai W. Association between renal hypoechoic subcapsular thickening and lymphosarcoma in cats. Vet Radiol Ultrasound 2007;48(4):357–60.

35. Parry NMA. Pyelonephritis in small animals. UK Vet 2005;10(6):1–5.

36. Paepe D, Daminet S, Feline CKD. Diagnosis, staging and screening - what is recommended? J Feline Med Surg 2013;15(Suppl 1):15–27.

37. Dunaevich A, Chen H, Musseri D, et al. Acute on chronic kidney disease in dogs: etiology, clinical and clinicopathologic findings, prognostic markers, and survival. J Vet Intern Med 2020;34(6):2507–15.

38. Chen H, Dunaevich A, Apfelbaum N, et al. Acute on chronic kidney disease in cats: etiology, clinical and clinicopathologic findings, prognostic markers, and outcome. J Vet Intern Med 2020;34(4):1496–506.

39. Lisciandro GR, Fosgate GT. Use of urinary bladder measurements from a point-of-care cysto-colic ultrasonographic view to estimate urinary bladder volume in dogs and cats. J Vet Emerg Crit Care (San Antonio) 2017;27(6):713–7.

40. Kendall A, Keenihan E, Kern ZT, et al. Three-dimensional bladder ultrasound for estimation of urine volume in dogs compared with traditional 2-dimensional ultrasound methods. J Vet Intern Med 2020;34(6):2460–7.

41. DiFazio MR, Thomason JD, Cernicchiaro N, et al. Evaluation of a 3-dimensional ultrasound device for noninvasive measurement of urinary bladder volume in dogs. J Vet Intern Med 2020;34(4):1488–95.

42. Berent AC, Weisse CW, Bagley DH, et al. Use of a subcutaneous ureteral bypass device for treatment of benign ureteral obstruction in cats: 174 ureters in 134 cats (2009-2015). J Am Vet Med Assoc 2018;253(10):1309–27.

43. Lamb CR, Cortellini S, Halfacree Z. Ultrasonography in the diagnosis and management of cats with ureteral obstruction. J Feline Med Surg 2018;20(1):15–22.

44. Berent AC, Weisse CW, Todd K, et al. Technical and clinical outcomes of ureteral stenting in cats with benign ureteral obstruction: 69 cases (2006-2010). J Am Vet Med Assoc 2014;244(5):559–76.

45. Lulich JP, Berent AC, Adams LG, et al. ACVIM small animal consensus recommendations on the treatment and prevention of uroliths in dogs and cats. J Vet Intern Med 2016;30(5):1564–74.

46. Niyyar VD, O'Neill WC. Point-of-care ultrasound in the practice of nephrology. Kidney Int 2018;93(5):1052–9.

47. Pathan SA, Mitra B, Mirza S, et al. Emergency physician interpretation of point-of-care ultrasound for identifying and grading of hydronephrosis in renal colic compared with consensus interpretation by emergency radiologists. Acad Emerg Med 2018;25(10):1129–37.

48. Beeston D, Cole L. Evaluation of the utility of point-of-care ultrasound in detecting ureteral obstruction in cats [abstract]. Ultrasound J 2020;45:45.

49. Kyles AE, Hardie EM, Wooden BG, et al. Clinical, clinicopathologic, radiographic, and ultrasonographic abnormalities in cats with ureteral calculi: 163 cases (1984-2002). J Am Vet Med Assoc 2005;226(6):932–6.

50. Wormser C, Reetz JA, Drobatz KJ, et al. Diagnostic utility of ultrasonography for detection of the cause and location of ureteral obstruction in cats: 71 cases (2010-2016). J Am Vet Med Assoc 2019;254(6):710–5.

51. Lemieux C, Vachon C, Beauchamp G, et al. Minimal renal pelvis dilation in cats diagnosed with benign ureteral obstruction by antegrade pyelography: a

retrospective study of 82 cases (2012-2018) [published online ahead of print, 2021 Jan 27]. J Feline Med Surg 2021. https://doi.org/10.1177/1098612X20983980.

52. Fages J, Dunn M, Specchi S, et al. Ultrasound evaluation of the renal pelvis in cats with ureteral obstruction treated with a subcutaneous ureteral bypass: a retrospective study of 27 cases (2010-2015). J Feline Med Surg 2018;20(10): 875–83.

53. Quimby JM, Dowers K, Herndon AK, et al. Renal pelvic and ureteral ultrasonographic characteristics of cats with chronic kidney disease in comparison with normal cats, and cats with pyelonephritis or ureteral obstruction. J Feline Med Surg 2017;19(8):784–90.

54. Léveillé R. Ultrasonography of urinary bladder disorders. Vet Clin North Am Small Anim Pract 1998;28(4):799–821.

55. Louvet A. Twinkling artifact in small animal color-Doppler sonography. Vet Radiol Ultrasound 2006;47(4):384–90.

56. Cheng SN, Phelps A. Correlating the sonographic finding of echogenic debris in the bladder lumen with urinalysis. J Ultrasound Med 2016;35(7):1533–40.

57. de Laforcade AM, Freeman LM, Shaw SP, et al. Hemostatic changes in dogs with naturally occurring sepsis. J Vet Intern Med 2003;17(5):674–9.

58. Summers AM, Vezzi N, Gravelyn T, et al. Clinical features and outcome of septic shock in dogs: 37 Cases (2008-2015) [published online ahead of print, 2020 Dec 31]. J Vet Emerg Crit Care (San Antonio) 2020. https://doi.org/10.1111/vec.13038.

59. Babyak JM, Sharp CR. Epidemiology of systemic inflammatory response syndrome and sepsis in cats hospitalized in a veterinary teaching hospital. J Am Vet Med Assoc 2016;249(1):65–71.

60. Nevins JR, Mai W, Thomas E. Associations between ultrasound and clinical findings in 87 cats with urethral obstruction. Vet Radiol Ultrasound 2015;56(4): 439–47.

61. Gerken KK, Cooper ES, Butler AL, et al. Association of abdominal effusion with a single decompressive cystocentesis prior to catheterization in male cats with urethral obstruction. J Vet Emerg Crit Care (San Antonio) 2020;30(1):11–7.

62. Hornsey SJ, Halfacree Z, Kulendra E, et al. Factors affecting survival to discharge in 53 cats diagnosed with uroabdomen: a single-centre retrospective analysis. J Feline Med Surg 2021;23(2):115–20.

63. Grimes JA, Fletcher JM, Schmiedt CW. Outcomes in dogs with uroabdomen: 43 cases (2006-2015). J Am Vet Med Assoc 2018;252(1):92–7.

Focused Ultrasound of the Fetus, Female and Male Reproductive Tracts, Pregnancy, and Dystocia in Dogs and Cats

Robert M. Fulton, DVM

KEYWORDS

- Reproductive tract • Pregnancy • Dystocia • Fetal • Male • Female
- Point-of-care ultrasound

KEY POINTS

- Reproductive tract point-of-care ultrasound offers a noninvasive diagnostic tool for evaluation normalcy and most disorders and conditions of both male and female reproductive tracts.
- Ultrasound is a valuable tool for assessing fetal viability, growth, and maturation as well as evaluating fetal stress.
- Pregnancy diagnosis using ultrasound represents one of the earliest uses of point-of-care ultrasound studies.

INTRODUCTION

Beginning with pregnancy diagnosis, point-of-care ultrasound (POCUS) of the reproductive system has been utilized for nearly as long as ultrasound has been a clinical tool, and pregnancy remains one of the most common indications for a reproductive POCUS study. Ultrasound is a valuable tool for numerous conditions affecting the fetus and the female and male reproductive systems. It is the most sensitive, least invasive tool for diagnosing pregnancy and for the assessment of infectious, inflammatory, structural, and neoplastic conditions of the male and female reproductive tracts. Furthermore, the use of ultrasound during emergency management of dystocia allows for rapid determination of fetal stress to guide medical or surgical interventions.

Clarividus Veterinary Ultrasound and Education, 2500 East Cary Street, Richmond, VA 23223, USA
E-mail address: rmfultondvm@gmail.com

Vet Clin Small Anim 51 (2021) 1249–1265
https://doi.org/10.1016/j.cvsm.2021.07.008
0195-5616/21/© 2021 Elsevier Inc. All rights reserved.

THE FETUS

Although contained within the uterus, the fetuses represents its own structure, and most are found within the uterine horns. From the uterine body, follow each horn toward the ovary as with any uterine study. Fetal structures are located segmentally along the length of each horn. As pregnancy progresses and the uterus enlarges to keep pace with the developing fetuses, it can be difficult to keep each horn separate. Each fetus should be scanned in sagittal and transverse plane. In the sagittal plane, the fetal spine can be used as guide to orientation along the long axis.

The appearance of the fetus changes dramatically as pregnancy progresses. Fetal organogenesis and growth serve as guides to predict parturition and monitor a pregnancy. Using the preovulatory luteinizing hormone (LH) peak as a starting point, canine fetal maturation can be estimated in days from the LH peak for major parts of organogenesis (**Table 1**).[1,2] The gestational sac may be seen consistently by day 20 and the embryo with cardiac activity between day 23 and day 25. The fetal skeleton begins mineralization between day 33 and day 39, with the stomach and urinary bladder developing their sonographic appearance toward the end of this same time frame. The lungs can be visualized as being hyperechoic to the liver beginning between day 38 and day 42, and the kidneys and eyes develop between day 39 and day 47. Cardiac chambers are evident by day 40.[1,2] Prior to this time, cardiac activity is referred to more properly as flutter, because the true heartbeat is dependent on the presence of anatomic chambers.

The intestines are the final organ to develop their ultrasonographic identity, between day 57 and day 63 from the LH peak, and their appearance typically marks the end of fetal organogenesis (see **Fig. 1**).[1–3] There are 4 distinct sonographic phases of fetal intestinal maturation beginning between approximately day 40 from the LH surge with the final phase of fetal intestinal maturation beginning at approximately day 60 (d 57–62) of gestation. This final phase is characterized by intestinal layering and by consistent and frequent peristalsis. The 3 visible bowel wall layers are the hyperechoic mucosal surface (intestinal lumen), the hypoechoic combined mucosa, submucosa, and muscularis and the hyperechoic serosa. Although intestinal peristalsis begins in phase 3, it is only intermittent. Peristalsis in the fourth phase is constant and may begin

Table 1 Markers of fetal organogenesis	
Day	**Structure**
20	Gestational sac
23–25	Cardiac flutter
33–39	Skeletal mineralization
36–39	Stomach
36–39	Urinary bladder
38–40	Lungs hyperechoic to the liver
39–47	Kidneys
39–47	Eyes
40	Cardiac chambers
57–63	Intestinal layers and peristalsis
57–63	Collapse of renal pelvis

Select structures in canine embryologic and fetal development measured in days from the LH peak when they can be visualized with ultrasound.

as far as 4 days before natural delivery.[1,3] The kidneys offer a more objective assessment, with renal length closely associated with gestational age. Similar to intestinal maturation, 4 phases of renal maturation have been described.[4] The fourth phase of renal maturation, noted by collapse of the renal pelvis (**Fig. 1**), has a similar time frame as the development of peristalsis in the intestinal fourth phase.[3,4] Because both constant intestinal peristalsis and kidney development precede normal parturition by several days, ultrasound should not be the sole determinant for cesarean section timing. If these parameters are present, however, then survivability of the delivered puppies or kittens is questionable.

Ultrasound may be used to age fetuses accurately and there are numerous fetal and extrafetal parameters that can be measured with varying degrees of accuracy.[5] Inner chorionic cavity (ICC) and biparietal diameter (BPD) (**Fig. 2**) in bitches of various breeds and sizes can predict parturition within 2 days, with up to 93% certainty level with ICC being more accurate. Accuracy can drop for multiple reasons, including patient movement (both dam and fetus), quality of ultrasound equipment used, and sonographer experience. Calculations using BPD and ICC have been summarized by Lopate[5,6]:

For small dogs:
> Days before parturition = (BPD in millimeters – 25.11)/0.61 or (ICC in millimeters – 68.88)/1.53

For medium dogs:
> Days before parturition = (BPD in millimeters – 29.18)/0.7 or (ICC in millimeters – 82.13)/1.8
> Gestational age = 21.08 + 14.88 × BPD cm – 0.11 BPD cm^2

The fetal heartbeat is the hallmark characteristic of fetal vitality. The rapid flutter easily is seen in the fetal thorax because the ribs offer minimal acoustic shadowing. The fetal heart can be difficult to image in fetal death because of both lack of heart movement and varying degrees of fetal decomposition. Intrauterine gas, typically

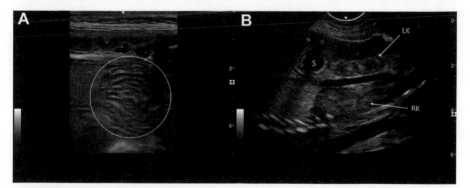

Fig. 1. Fetal markers of organogenesis. These images are of the same fetus and were obtained 3 days prior to parturition. (*A*) The intestines (circled in yellow) are the final organ to develop their sonographic identity with layering evident between day 57 and day 63 from the LH peak. Constant peristalsis marks the final maturation of the intestines. (*B*) The kidney (left kidney [LK] and right kidney [RK]) maturation is similar to intestinal development with closure of the renal pelvis marking final fetal kidney maturation. Also evident is the stomach (S) with fluid in the lumen and thick, hyperechoic wall. (Image used with permission from Robert M. Fulton, DVM.)

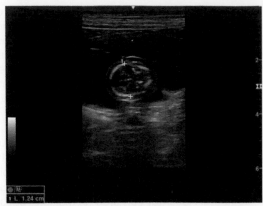

Fig. 2. Fetal BPD. Numerous fetal and extrafetal structures can be measured to estimate gestational age or days before parturition when the LH peak is not known. The BPD (yellow caliper points on either side of the fetal skull) measurement in this fetus. The fetus is estimated to be at just over 39 days (see text for formula), consistent with the known LH peak, and parturition occurred at day 65 post–LH peak. (Image used with permission from Robert M. Fulton, DVM.)

representing fetal death and decomposition, also may be evident during ultrasound by gas shadowing and air reverberation artifacts, which further interfere with fetal cardiac imaging.[1]

DYSTOCIA

The word, dystocia, is from the Greek, *dys*, meaning difficult, and *tokos*, meaning birth—simply put, a difficult birthing.[7] More specifically, dystocia is defined as the inability to expel fetuses through the birth canal during parturition and may result from maternal or fetal factors.[7,8] Two primary pieces of information that ultrasound can help determine during dystocia management are fetal maturation and fetal heart rate. Fetal heart rate is a key indicator of fetal stress: in short, the lower the heart rate, the higher the stress.[7,9]

Fetal Heart Rate

Normal canine or feline fetal heart rates should be greater than 200 beats/min and often are well above 220 beats/min. Normal fetal cat heart rates often are approximately 265 beats/min[7,8] A good rule of thumb has the normal fetal heart rate approximately double the dam's heart rate.[2] Fetal heart rate may be determined by simply counting the beats in real time as they are visualized. This method may be considered an estimate but is easy to perform. More accurately, though technically more challenging, M-mode can be utilized (**Fig. 3**).

Fetal Heart Rates and Fetal Stress

With increasing fetal stress comes decreasing fetal heart rates. From a clinical viewpoint with both dogs and cats, Traas uses the following guidelines[10]:

Fetal heart rates between 150 beats/min and 180 beats/min indicate mild to moderate distress and high risk of fetal death if not delivered within the next 2 hours to 3 hours.

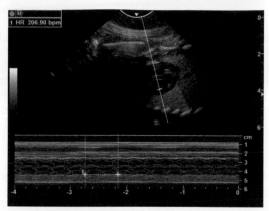

Fig. 3. Fetal M-mode for measuring heart rate. M-mode allows for precise heart rate measurements compared with visually counting heartbeats on the monitor which gives more of an estimate. This machine is set to average 2 beats; the caliper marks are set accordingly. Some machines may measure only 1, and care must be taken not to artifactually over-measure or under-measure heart rates because this can have significant repercussions when assessing fetal health and stress. (Image used with permission from Robert M. Fulton, DVM.)

Fetal heart rates less than 150 beats/min indicate severe distress and that immediate intervention (cesarean section) is required because fetal death is imminent.[7,10]
Zone suggests more conservative values[9]:
Fetal heart rates between 180 beats/min and 220 beats/min indicate mild distress.
Fetal heart rates less than 180 beats/min indicate severe fetal distress.[9]
Variability can exist in litters, where 1 fetus may be severely distressed and another normal. Furthermore, segmental uterine contractions may result in transient reduction of fetal heart rate as they pass over a fetus.[3]
An additional marker of fetal stress is fetal bowel movement. Under severe stress, fetuses exhibit bowel movements,[9] which may be noted as an echogenic character to the amniotic fluid. Similar echogenicity of the amniotic fluid also may be seen with premature placental separation and hemorrhage.[5]

Serial Point-of-Care Ultrasound During Medical Management of Dystocia

The use of ultrasound for monitoring signs of fetal stress during medical management is superior to traditional means. Moreover, its use carries the potential to positively influence the decision-making process regarding medical versus surgical management, thus optimizing the chance for a favorable outcome. During medical management of dystocia, fetal stress can be assessed for by measuring heart rates prior to each oxytocin injection or minimally every 30 minutes.[7]
Clinical intervention, whether surgical or medical, should not be premised solely on ultrasonographic findings, because ultrasound cannot evaluate all forms of dystocia. Abdominal radiography should be used to assess fetal size relative to the mother's pelvic diameter to rule out forms of mechanical dystocia. Bloodwork should be used to rule out metabolic causes of dystocia. History (duration of time between births and duration of hard pushing), physical examination findings, and the owner's observations and expectations all must enter the decision-making process. Fetal POCUS studies to assess fetal development, viability, and stress are a valuable tool to help allow clinicians to make critical choices in the management of dystocia.[7]

FEMALE POINT-OF-CARE ULTRASOUND REPRODUCTIVE SCANS

Imaging both the uterus and ovary may be performed in dorsal recumbency. Dorsal recumbency allows the uterine horns to fall away from each other and allows for a more systematic approach of scanning the entire uterus. Lateral or standing position may be preferred (depending on the sonographer), however, and less stressful for some patients. This is true particularly for the term gravid bitch. A urine-filled bladder provides a convenient acoustic window and can serve as a landmark for caudal abdominal structures.

THE OVARY

The caudal pole of the ipsilateral kidney is the most consistent landmark to find the ovaries.[11] Occasionally, however, they may be located by following the uterine horns cranially from the body. From the caudal pole of the kidney, slide the probe caudally, and then fan toward midline until the aorta is visualized. The aorta serves as the medial landmark and can be used to align the probe along the long axis of the patient. Fan toward the lateral body wall to find the ovary. A linear probe is useful especially because the higher frequency can help differentiate the sometimes subtle difference in echotexture of a quiescent normal ovary from surrounding tissue. During estrus, follicles or cystic changes help with recognition of the ovary. Scan the ovary both in sagittal and transverse planes.

On ultrasonographic appearance, the normal ovary often is difficult to visualize, being nearly isoechoic to hypoechoic to surrounding tissues and often obscured by intestines. A higher-frequency linear probe is useful (**Fig. 4**). Ovarian disease is uncommon in the dog and cat but assessment for changes in size (larger), echogenicity (often hyperechoic), and cysts is possible. Depending on stage of the estrus cycle, follicular cysts normally may be present and typically does not exceed 8 mm.[12]

CONDITIONS OF THE OVARY
Cystic Ovaries

Ovarian cysts account for 80% of ovarian disease, with cysts defined as any fluid-filled structure present outside of physiologic proestrus or estrus.[12] Sonographically, ovarian cysts appear as anechoic, spherical structures. Cysts are prioritized over

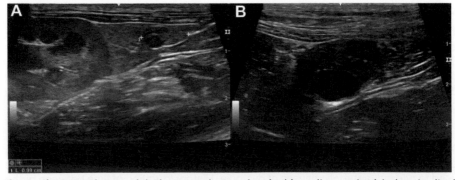

Fig. 4. The normal ovary. (A) The normal ovary (marked by caliper points) in longitudinal plane with a normal follicle. The caudal pole of the ipsilateral kidney, seen in the left portion of the image, serves as the most consistent landmark for locating the ovary. (B) Another normal ovary with an estrus follicle. (Image used with permission from Robert M. Fulton, DVM.)

normal follicles if they exceed 8 mm. There are multiple types of ovarian cysts with the 2 most common primary follicular and luteal cysts. Although follicular cysts typically have thin walls and lutein cysts have thicker walls, tissue sampling is required for definitive diagnosis. Hormone-producing cysts are clinically significant. These patients may present with dermatologic conditions, altered estrus cycles, cystic endometrial hyperplasia (CEH)-pyometra, and bone marrow dyscrasias.[12]

Ovarian Neoplasia

Most primary ovarian neoplasms are epithelial, sex cord–stromal, or germ cell tumors.[12] Like cysts, histopathology is needed for differentiation because the sonographic appearance is not definitive. Most often are mixed echogenic masses of varying sizes. Clinical presentation may vary from signs associated with altered hormone balance (similar to follicular cysts) or abdominal pain if the tumor grows large enough to compress adjacent structures or to pull on associated ligaments.

THE UTERUS

The patient may be scanned in dorsal or lateral recumbency. The urinary bladder trigone and the colon serve as landmarks, with the uterus located between these 2 structures and the cervix near the level of the trigone. When a patient is in dorsal recumbency, the bladder, colon, and uterus often form a triangle, with the uterus located just left of the ventral aspect of the colon. The body for the uterus is scanned in the sagittal and transverse planes. Follow the uterine body cranially to the bifurcation into the uterine horns and caudally to the echogenic cervix. The horns may be easiest followed in transverse orientation; however, they often blend in with surrounding tissues. A linear probe is useful for imaging the uterus, given the improved resolution achievable compared with a curvilinear probe.

On ultrasonographic appearance, the uterine body is of medium, isoechoic homogeneous echogenicity and appears as a tubular structure similar in size or smaller to small intestine. The uterine horns often are difficult to image because they are smaller than the body and blend in with the small intestines and mesentery.[13] The uterine lumen typically is not evident in the anestrous bitch; however, a thin, echogenic stripe within the lumen may be seen during estrus.[11] The cervix is slightly larger than the uterus, with the 2 structures blending into one another (**Fig. 5**). A hyperechoic line

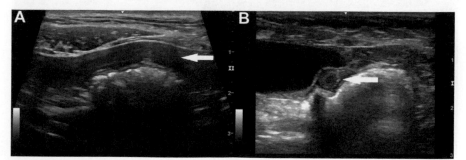

Fig. 5. The normal uterus. (*A*) The uterus in the longitudinal plane. The uterus is the homogeneous isoechoic structure seen draping over the hyperechoic colon (*arrow*). (*B*) The uterus in the transverse plane. The uterine body is the circular structure (*arrow*) located between the urinary bladder (filled with anechoic urine) and the colon (with characteristic hyperechogenicity and gas shadowing). (Image used with permission from Robert M. Fulton, DVM.)

representing the os cervix may be seen at angle within the cervix (**Fig. 6**). The normal, nongravid uterus is distinguished from small bowel by the lack of layering. With the exception of the estrus echogenic stripe, the lumen of the uterus is not appreciated and the walls blend into one structure. Small bowel, on the other hand, is characterized by alternating hypoechoic and hyperechoic layers (lumen, mucosa, submucosa, muscularis, and serosa).

CONDITIONS OF THE UTERUS
Cystic Endometrial Hyperplasia–Pyometra

CEH-pyometra complex is the most frequent and important uterine disorder in bitches, occurring during the luteal phase of diestrus and occasionally during anestrus.[1,12] Ultrasonography has a higher sensitivity for determining the presence of uterine enlargement and fluid accumulation than radiography.[11,14] Careful scanning should be performed along each horn as thoroughly as possible to avoid a false-negative evaluation for pyometra.

Fluid distention of the uterus is the ultrasonographic hallmark of pyometra. The amount and echogenicity of fluid can vary greatly independent of the pyometra being open (cervix open and vaginal discharge) or closed (cervix closed and no vaginal discharge). Echogenicity of intraluminal fluid in pyometra ranges from anechoic (pure black) to viscous and echogenic (**Fig. 7**). In cases of echogenic fluid, fluid movement may be characterized by slow, swirling patterns.[14] Pyometra often is diffuse throughout both uterine horns but may appear compartmentalized as the horns fold on themselves; segmental pyometra to 1 horn, mucometra, and hydrometra also is possible.[15,16]

In pyometra cases, blind cystocentesis carries a high risk of peritonitis.[1] Even with sonographic guidance by an experienced sonographer, it is possible to inadvertently puncture and aspirate the pus-filled uterus during cystocentesis. Thus, free-catch urine sampling with uterine and urine culture occurring at the time of surgical intervention (if elected) may be the safest option. Otherwise, ultrasound always should be used for guided cystocentesis for obtaining urine in suspect pyometra cases while notifying the owner of the potential complication of peritonitis in these patients.

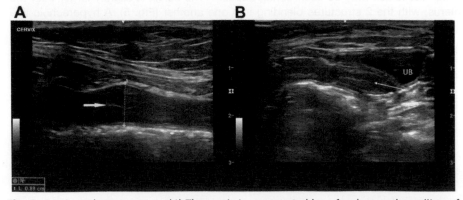

Fig. 6. Cervix and estrus uterus. (*A*) The cervix is represented by a focal, smooth swelling of the uterus without any change in echogenicity. Occasionally, the os cervix is visualized as a central hyperechoic stripe that runs diagonally through the structure (*arrow*). (B) The uterine lumen in normalcy is without fluid in the lumen. During estrus, a thin echogenic stripe may be seen (*arrow*). UB, urinary bladder. (Image used with permission from Robert M. Fulton, DVM.)

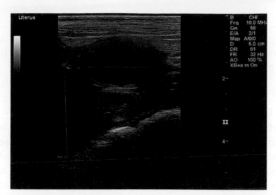

Fig. 7. Pyometra. Pyometra, mucometra, and hydrometra all may have the same sonographic appearance. The hallmark finding is diffuse or segmental fluid distention of the uterine lumen (*yellow dashed lines*). Also evident in this image is hyperechoic luminal debris representing pus. (Image used with permission from Robert M. Fulton, DVM.)

Pseudo-placentational Endometrial Hyperplasia

Appearing like CEH-pyometra, pseudo-placentational endometrial hyperplasia (PEH) occurs during the luteal phase with endometrial remodeling at normal placentation sites.[1,17] Although histologically different, clinical presentation and management of PEH are the same as for CEH-pyometra. PEH is likely to form approximately 2 month post-estrus compared with the typical 2 weeks post-estrus occurrence more common with CEH-pyometra.[1]

Mucometra and Hydrometra

Mucometra and hydrometra appear like pyometra, with varying degrees of fluid distention of the uterine horns and body. These conditions cannot be differentiated from pyometra by the sonographic appearance alone and diagnosis typically is made at the time of surgery.

Uterine Atresia

Atresia, although rare and more common in cats, may involve both or only 1 horn and may be complete or partial.[16]

Stump Pyometra

Typically, stump pyometra may occur following ovariohysterectomy if a portion of the uterine horns or uterine body and ovary are not removed and the animal has increased progesterone concentrations due to the remnant ovarian tissue. Progestins also may come from endogenous sources as sex hormone–secreting adrenal tumors, or exogenous sources, such as progestational compounds used to treat dermatitis or creams used for treatment of menopausal symptoms in women.[1,18]

The female POCUS reproductive scan for stump pyometra is identical as for pyometra; however, the primary area of interest is the caudal abdomen, specifically the region between the trigone of the bladder and colon. Here, search for an area of mixed echogenicity indicative of complex mass effect.[1,19,20] Other local diseases mimicking or causing a stump pyometra include stump granuloma caused by excess residual devitalized uterine body tissue, use of inappropriate suture material, and poor surgical asepsis.

Uterine Torsion

Uterine torsion in the dog and cat is reported uncommonly. The ultrasonographic appearance, however, is similar to that of pyometra. A diagnosis of uterine torsion typically is made at surgery.[1,21,22]

Uterine Neoplasia

Uterine tumors in the dog and cat are rare, accounting for less than 0.5% of all canine tumors.[23] Leiomyomas are the most common, but others include leiomyosarcoma, lipoleiomyoma, polyps, and adenocarcinomas.[13,23] Ultrasound is useful in visualizing uterine tumors but the larger the tumor becomes, the more difficult it becomes to ascertain the tissue of origin.[23] Their sonographic appearance is size, shape, and echogenicity. Tumors may be associated with fluid accumulation within the variable in uterine lumen.[13] There currently are no sonographic markers of identity, and histopathology is required for definitive diagnosis.

Pseudopregnancy

All bitches experience the same progesterone profile whether they become pregnant or not. Because progesterone levels fall at the end of diestrus, some bitches experience overt signs of whelping, including mammary gland development, lactation, nesting behavior, and even abdominal contractions.[1,16] Although rare, the queen also may show signs of pseudopregnancy. Pseudopregnancy easily is differentiated from pregnancy using ultrasound by the absence of fetal structures and uterine distention.

Pregnancy

Pregnancy diagnosis in the dog using ultrasonography first was reported in 1983; and, in that sense, reproductive ultrasound may be considered one of the earliest small animal POCUS studies.[24,25] Pregnancy is characterized sonographically by the gestational sacs appearing as anechoic spherical to ovoid structures with the fetal heartbeat as the hallmark of fetal vitality.[1,26] Fetal vesicles and heartbeats can be seen consistently after day 21 to day 23 post-LH surge.[27] Ultrasound is a relatively inaccurate method for determining litter size but offers an estimate. Litter size determination is best accomplished radiographically 45 days to 50 days post–LH surge.

MALE POINT-OF-CARE ULTRASOUND REPRODUCTIVE SCANS

Most male reproductive ultrasound examinations are performed on dogs, because the tom rarely develops reproductive problems.[28,29] Given breed and size variation across the many breeds, no objective measurements are applicable to the male testes or prostate. Symmetry, rather, is the best rule of thumb. Sonography of the male reproductive tract is indicated in any patient with palpable testicular asymmetry, palpable prostatomegaly, hematuria, abdominal pain or swelling, urinary incontinence, stranguria, dysuria, cryptorchidism, tenesmus, ribbon-like stool, constipation, or prostatic mineralization on survey radiographic evaluation. Symmetry is a key sonographic feature of the male reproductive tract. The testicles and prostate should be smooth in margination and symmetric about their median planes.

THE PROSTATE

The prostate is the dog's only accessory sex gland. It increases in size and weight with age due to glandular hyperplasia in the intact dog and involutes in the castrated dog.[30] The feline prostate is a small structure located along the midurethra to proximal urethra. Due to its small size, intrapelvic location, and rare clinical importance, the feline prostate rarely is imaged.[28,29,31]

The prostate may be imaged with the male dog in dorsal or lateral positions or with the dog standing. The specific position for each patient is determined from individual dynamics (for example, pain, shock, and disposition) and sonographer experience and preference. The urinary bladder serves as initial anatomic landmark. Identify the trigone and follow it into the proximal urethra. The prostate surrounds the proximal urethra and termination of the ductus deferens with most of the gland dorsal and lateral to the urethra. The urethra blends in with the prostatic parenchyma but is evident in cases of distal urethral obstruction. Fan or slide through the prostate both in sagittal and transverse planes.

A healthy prostate is bilobed and symmetric in the sagittal plane. The normal prostate is hyperechoic to the spleen. The parenchyma is homogeneous in appearance, with a finer echotexture than the surrounding tissues.[28] A hyperechoic butterfly pattern, corresponding to ductal tissue, typically is apparent in the transverse view (**Fig. 8**).[5,29] The prostate in the castrated dog after involution appears as a smooth, homogeneous swelling around the proximal urethra, with total width 3-times to 4-times the width of the urethra (**Fig. 9**).[29] The overall echogenicity is like that of the uterine body in the female dog.[29]

CONDITIONS OF THE PROSTATE
Benign Prostatic Hypertrophy

Benign prostatic hypertrophy (BPH) is a common disorder afflicting the prostate in intact male dogs. In patients with BPH, the prostate is sonographically enlarged, uniformly hyperechoic with a smooth margin. The enlargement may be different between dorsal and ventral areas, but the enlargement is symmetric when viewed in the transverse plane (see **Fig. 1**). In time, the expected symmetry and uniform echogenicity of BPH may be lost as the condition progresses into the cystic stage.[28,30]

Prostatitis

The ultrasonographic of prostatitis can vary depending on severity. The shape generally is normal, but the echogenicity may increase or decrease with degree of mottling (mixed echogenicity). A hypoechoic rim may be evident in some dogs. In severe cases, surrounding fat may become hyperechoic.[28–30]

Prostatic Abscesses and Cysts

Abscesses and cysts may be found within or attached to the prostatic parenchyma. Both typically are thin-walled structures, with either anechoic or hypoechoic centers. Septation and echogenic fluid are more suggestive of prostatic abscess.[28,29] Gas may be present with some abscesses and appears as multiple hyperechoic comet tailing foci. This may be confused with parenchymal soft tissue mineralization as may be found with some malignancies. Culture is recommended for suspected bacterial disease.

Paraprostatic Cysts

Paraprostatic cysts, thought be remnants of müllerian ducts, are found adjacent to the gland yet may appear confluent with it. They are thin-walled, typically anechoic structures of varying size, often appearing similar to the urinary bladder. The fluid contained within paraprostatic cysts are of variable echogenicity with or without intraluminal debris.[32–34]

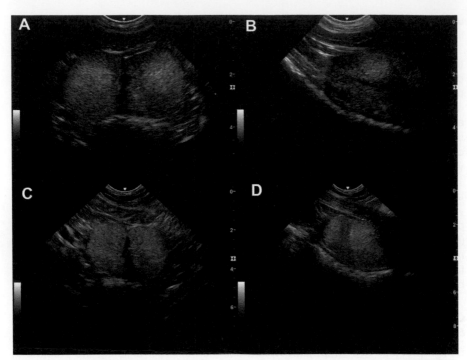

Fig. 8. Normal and BPH prostate. (*A*) The normal prostate in transverse plane. Note the homogenous echogenic parenchymal and centrally hypoechoic pattern resembling butterfly wings. The round central anechoic structure represents the prostatic urethra. (*B*) The normal prostate in longitudinal orientation. The urethra can be seen as the hypoechoic linear structure in the center. (*C*) BPH prostate in the transverse plane. Prostatic lobe symmetry is preserved, but may be lost as the condition advances with development of cysts. (*D*) BPH prostate in longitudinal plane. As the prostate enlarges and becomes heavier, it may be easier to image, because often it is found in the caudal abdomen versus in the pelvic canal. (Image used with permission from Robert M. Fulton, DVM.)

Prostatic Neoplasia

Prostatic neoplasia may show similarities to prostatitis, abscesses, or cysts. Calcification, represented by echogenic foci with acoustic shadowing or comet tailing, severe loss of symmetry or normal architecture, and irregular margination, is suggestive of malignancy (see **Fig. 9**).[28,29] The neutered male dog is more prone to prostatic adenocarcinoma than the intact male dog, and this is a primary differential for any castrated dog with an enlarged prostate.[29,35] Fine-needle aspiration or biopsy easily is performed, typically with no complication, and can diagnose prostatic carcinoma in approximately 50% to 90% of cases, respectively.[30]

THE SCROTUM AND TESTICLES

Given its external location, the scrotum easily is accessible with a patient in dorsal, lateral, or standing position. The testicles are imaged side by side to evaluate symmetry between each. Given the superficial location, a standoff pad may be used; however, it is simpler to use 1 testicle as a standoff pad for the opposite testicle. The testicles are imaged both in sagittal and transverse orientations. The epididymis serves as an

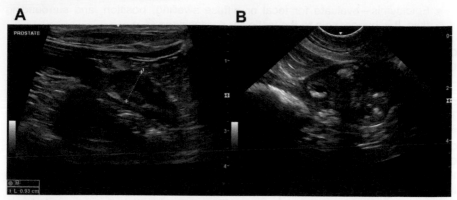

Fig. 9. Common prostatic conditions. (*A*) This is the prostate from a neutered dog. The prostate involutes with the lack of circulating testosterone. (*B*) Prostatic adenocarcinoma. Note how the parenchyma is of a mixed echogenic character with echogenic mineralization (hyperechoic foci, some with acoustic shadowing) and cystic areas. (Image used with permission from Robert M. Fulton, DVM.)

anatomic marker of position, with the head beginning caudally, with the body and tail extending dorsally toward the cranial aspect of the testicle (**Fig. 10**). The scrotum should be imaged systematically for the 3 main areas:

- Scrotal space—evaluate for fluid, intestines (inguinal hernia), or other extratesticular structures.[29]
- Testicle—evaluate for symmetry in size and shape, tumors, overall echogenicity. Position may be assessed based on the epididymis (head caudal, body dorsal, and tail dorsocranial). The testicular parenchyma is hyperechoic and homogeneous like the spleen.[32] The linear mediastinum testis easily is identified in the center of the organ as a bright echodense line, whereas the fibrous hyperechoic tunica albuginea surrounds the testicle.[29,30] Transverse imaging of both testicles side by side allows for assessing differences between the testicles.[29,32]

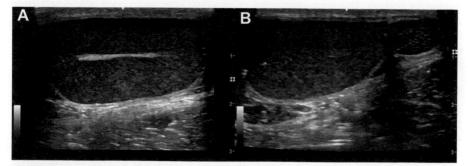

Fig. 10. The normal testicle. (*A*) The normal testicle in the longitudinal plane. Note the homogeneous parenchyma with the mediastinum testes represented by the hyperechoic linear structure in the center. (B) The normal testicle in longitudinal orientation with the normal epididymis in the right near-field region of the image. The head of the epididymis is located at the caudal aspect of the testicle and serves as a reference landmark for position of the testicle. (Image used with permission from Robert M. Fulton, DVM.)

- Epididymis—evaluate for focal or diffuse swelling, position, and surrounding fluid. It is hypoechoic to the testicular parenchyma.[29]

CONDITIONS OF THE SCROTUM AND TESTICLES
Cryptorchidism

Descent of testicles normally occurs by 10 days after birth; however, in the young puppy and kitten, the testicles can move between the scrotum and inguinal canal.[29,36] The inguinal canal closes at approximately 6 months of age, precluding any additional movement. Cryptorchidism is a heritable, developmental defect in which descent of 1 or both testes does not occur by the time of inguinal canal closure.[37] Unilateral cryptorchidism is more common than bilateral. Retained testes are smaller than scrotal testes, with size directly correlated with the degree of retention (abdominal vs inguinal).[29,37] The cryptorchid testes typically retains its normal anatomic appearance but may be smaller than a scrotal testicle. The retained testicle may be located anywhere from the inguinal canal to the ipsilateral kidney, with the inguinal location more common.[29,32,37]

The scan is performed in lateral recumbency with the contralateral side down and the ipsilateral leg raised to allow access to the inguinal region. A systematic scan, in both longitudinal and transverse orientation is advanced from the inguinal canal to the caudal pole of the ipsilateral kidney. The lateral positioning allows for gravity to pull viscera away from the inguinal and retroperitoneal areas.

Orchitis and Epididymitis

Orchitis and epididymitis may occur singly or in combination and typically are painful conditions. Acute orchitis usually is characterized by enlargement of the testicle with the parenchyma taking on a patchy, hypoechoic texture. Epididymitis is associated with testicular enlargement and focal parenchymal changes. Fluid may be present with either condition.[11,29,32] Zoonotic diseases, including brucellosis, should be considered in all sexually active male dogs.[29,38]

Torsion

Dogs with testicular torsion, more appropriately termed torsion of the spermatic cord, typically present with signs of an acute abdomen, including abdominal pain, vomiting, dysuria, hematuria, pyrexia, anorexia, lethargy, and stiff gait.[37] Neoplasia is a common reason for torsion. The intra-abdominal cryptorchid spermatic cord is affected more often in torsions than the scrotal cord.[29,37] The testicle of the affected cord typically is enlarged with diffuse hypoechogenicity. Absence of blood flow using color flow or power doppler imaging is highly suggestive and definitive diagnosis is made at the time of surgery, the treatment of choice.[29,37]

Tumors

Testicular neoplasms are the most common tumors in male dogs, second only to skin tumors. Tumors may be unilateral or bilateral and different tumor types may be present within the same testicle. The 3 most common types of tumor are Sertoli cell, seminoma, and interstitial (Leydig) cell tumors.[37,39] Nearly all interstitial cell tumors are benign, as are most seminomas; however, approximately 5% to 10% of seminomas may metastasize to regional lymph nodes, liver, spleen, kidneys, lungs, and skin.[40] Sertoli cell tumors cause most of their morbidity associated with hormonal production and may metastasize in up to 15% of cases.[41] Although dogs with testicular neoplasia commonly present with testicular enlargement as the only sign, Sertoli cell tumors may present with bone marrow toxicity (anemia), symmetric truncal alopecia, and gynecomastia.[29,39] Testicular tumors may be focal masses with variable echogenicity. Fine-needle aspirate or biopsy is required for a definitive diagnosis but can predispose to infertility, infection, or spermatic granuloma formation.[11,29,32] An enlarged testicle in the older dog without testicular pain prioritizes neoplasia over orchitis.[29,39]

Miscellaneous Scrotal Swellings

Herniation of small bowel into the scrotum may be detected by finding the normal bowel layers adjacent to the teste. Intestinal peristalsis may be present.[29,42] Hematomas, abscesses, and spermatic granulomas all may appear sonographically similar with poorly demarcated margins with variable echogenicity and texture.[29,43] Scrotal fluid may occur in cases of ascites, coagulopathy, and traumatic hemoabdomen.[43]

SUMMARY

Beginning with pregnancy diagnosis as one of the earliest POCUS studies, ultrasound of the reproductive organs has proved an invaluable tool for investigating both normal and abnormal conditions in both male and female dogs. Use of ultrasound in the pregnant animal furthermore allows for monitoring fetal development and prediction of parturition. Reproductive POCUS allows quick image acquisition, and this aspect comes into significant play in the emergent management of the dystocia patient. Using organ development as an indicator of fetal maturation and heart rate as an indicator of fetal stress, critical decisions regarding medical versus surgical management of the dystocia patent may be made more specifically.

DISCLOSURE

The author has no financial relationships or conflicts of interest.

REFERENCES

1. Fulton RM. POCUS: Reproductive – Female. In: Lisciandro GR, editor. Point of care ultrasound Techniques for the small animal Practitioner. 2nd edition. John Wiley & Sons; 2021. p. 255–64.

2. Mattoon JS, Nyland TG. Ovaries and Uterus. In: Nyland TG, Mattoon JS, editors. Small animal diagnostic ultrasound. 3rd edition. St Louis (MO): Elsevier Saunders; 2015. p. 634–54.

3. Gil E, Garcia D, Froes T. In utero development of the fetal intestine: sonographic evaluation and correlation with gestational age and fetal maturity in dogs. Theriogenology 2015;84:681–6.

4. Gil E, Garcia D, Giannico A, et al. Early results on canine fetal kidney development: Ultrasonographic evaluation and value in prediction of delivery time. Theriogenology 2018;107:180–7.

5. Lopate C. Estimation of gestational age and assessment of canine fetal maturation using radiology and ultrasonography: a review. Theriogenology 2008;70: 397–402.

6. Lopate C. Gestational Aging and Determination of Parturition Date in the Bitch and Queen Using Ultrasonography and Radiography. Vet Clin Small Anim 2018;48:617–38.

7. Fulton RM. POCUS: Dystocia. In: Lisciandro GR, editor. Point of care ultrasound Techniques for the small animal Practitioner. 2nd edition. John Wiley & Sons; 2021. p. 265–70.

8. Jutkowitz L. Reproductive emergencies. Vet Clin North Am Small Anim Pract 2005;35:397–420.
9. Zone MA, Wanke M. Diagnosis of canine fetal health by ultrasonography. J Reprod Fertil 2001;57(suppl):215–9.
10. Traas AM. Surgical management of canine and feline dystocia. Theriogenology 2008;40:337–42.
11. Feeney D, Johnston G. The uterus, ovaries, and testes. In: Thrall DE, editor. Textbook of Veterinary diagnostic Radiology. 5th edition. St Louis (MO): Saunders/Elsevier; 2007. p. 735–49.
12. Arlt S, Haimerl P. Cystic ovaries and ovarian neoplasia in the female dog – a systematic review. Reprod Domest Anim 2016;51(Suppl 1):3–11.
13. Pollard R. Ultrasound of the reproductive system: female dog. Clin Theriogenology 2015;7(3):199–202.
14. Bigliardi E, Parmigiani E, Cavirani S, et al. Ultrasonography and cystic hyperplasia-pyometra complex in the bitch. Reprod Domest Anim 2004;39:136–40.
15. Verstegen J, Dhaliwal G, Verstegen-Onclin K. Mucometra, cystic endometrial hyperplasia, and pyometra in the bitch: advances in treatment and assessment of future reproductive success. Theriogenology 2008;70:364–74.
16. Johnston S, Root-Kustriz M, Olson P. Disorders of the feline uterus and uterine tubes (oviducts). In: Johnston S, Root-Kustriz M, Olson P, editors. Canine and feline Theriogenology. Philadelphia: WB Saunders; 2001. p. 463–71.
17. Schlafer DH, Gifford AT. Cystic endometrial hyperplasia, pseudo-placentational endometrial hyperplasia, and other cystic conditions of the canine and feline uterus. Theriogenology 2008;70:349–58.
18. Howe L. Surgical methods of contraception and sterilization. Theriogenology 2006;66:500–9.
19. Davidson A, Baker T. Reproductive ultrasound in the bitch and queen. Top Compan Anim Med 2009;24(2):55–63.
20. England G, Yeager A, Concannon P. Ultrasound imaging of the reproductive tract of the bitch. In: Concannon PW, England G, Verstegen J, et al, editors. Recent advances in small animal reproduction. New York: International Veterinary Information Service; 2003. Available at: https://www.ivis.org/library/recent-advances-small-animal-reproduction/ultrasound-imaging-of-reproductive-tract-of-bitch. Accessed February 27, 2021.
21. Misumi K, Fujiki M, Miura N, et al. Uterine horn torsion in two non-gravid bitches. J Small Anim Pract 2000;41(8):465–71.
22. Chambers B, Laksito M, Long F, et al. Unilateral uterine torsion secondary to an inflammatory endometrial polyp in the bitch. Aust Vet J 2011;59(8):350–4.
23. Percival A, Singh A, Alex Zur Linden R, et al. Massive uterine lipoleiomyoma and leiomyoma in a miniature poodle bitch. Can Vet J 2018;59:845–50.
24. Taverne M, Okkens A, van Oord R. Pregnancy diagnosis in the dog: A comparison between abdominal palpation and linear-array real-time echography. Vet Q 1985;7(4):249–55.
25. Bondestam S, Alitalo I, Karkkainen M. Real-time pregnancy diagnosis in the bitch. J Small Anim Pract 1983;24:145–51.
26. Khatti A, Jena D, Singh S, et al. Application of Ultrasonography in Canine Pregnancy- An Overview. Int J Livestock Res 2017;7(2):20–7.
27. Concannon P. Canine Pregnancy: Predicting Parturition and Timing Events of Gestation. In: Concannon PW, England G, Verstegen J, et al, editors. Recent advances in small animal reproduction. New York: International Veterinary Information Service; 2003. Available at: https://www.ivis.org/library/recent-advances-

small-animal-reproduction/canine-pregnancy-predicting-parturition-and.   Accessed February 27, 2021.

28. Lattimer J, Essman S. The prostate gland. In: Thrall DE, editor. Textbook of Veterinary diagnostic Radiology. 5th edition. St Louis (MO): Saunders/Elsevier; 2007. p. 729–37.

29. Fulton RM. POCUS: Reproductive - Male. In: Lisciandro GR, editor. Point of care ultrasound Techniques for the small animal Practitioner. 2nd edition. John Wiley & Sons; 2021. p. 247–54.

30. Johnston S, Root-Kustriz M, Olson P. Disorders of the canine prostate. In: Johnston S, Root-Kustriz M, Olson P, editors. Canine and feline Theriogenology. Philadelphia: WB Saunders; 2001. p. 337–55.

31. Dimitrov R, Toneva Y. Computed tomographic features of the feline prostate. Acta Morphol Anthropol 2007;12:186–92.

32. Davidson A, Baker T. Reproductive ultrasound of the dog and tom. Top Compan Anim Med 2009;24(2):64–70.

33. Smith J. Canine prostatic disease: a review of anatomy, pathology, diagnosis, and treatment. Theriogenology 2008;70:375–83.

34. Lisciandro GR. What is your diagnosis? Large, round mass with intramural mineralization in the mid-to-caudal portion of the abdominal cavity – prostatomegaly. J Am Vet Med Assoc 1995;206(2):171–2.

35. Root-Kustriz M. Pathogenesis of prostatic neoplasia in castrated dogs: why the increased risk? Clin Theriogenol 2010;2(3):152–4.

36. Hoskins JD, Taboada J. Congenital defects of the dog. Comp Contin Educ Pract Vet 1992;14:873–97.

37. Johnston S, Root-Kustriz M, Olson P. Disorders of the canine testes and epididymes. In: Johnston S, Root-Kustriz M, Olson P, editors. Canine and feline Theriogenology. Philadelphia: WB Saunders; 2001. p. 312–32.

38. Hollett B. Update on canine brucellosis. Clin Theriogenol 2010;1(2):257–95.

39. Root-Kustriz M. Neoplasia of the Reproductive Tract of the Male Dog. Clincal Theriogenology 2009;1(1):93–103.

40. Ontiveros M, Hanlon D, Anderson A, et al. Seminomas and an interstitial cell tumor in an 8 year old male Husky. Clin Theriogenology 2018;10(2):97–106.

41. Withers S, Lawson C, Burton A, et al. Management of an invasive and metastatic Sertoli cell tumor with associated myelotoxicosis in a dog. Can Vet J 2016;57: 299–304.

42. Mattoon J, Nyland T. Prostate and Testes. In: Nyland TG, Mattoon JS, editors. Small animal diagnostic ultrasound. 2nd edition. Philadelphia: WB Saunders; 2002. p. 231–49.

43. Foster R. Pathology of male reproductive organs. Clin Theriogenol 2010;2(4): 531–44.

Section IV: Focused Ultrasound of Vascular Disease

Focused Ultrasound of Vascular System in Dogs and Cats—Thromboembolic Disease

Erin Mays, DVM, DACVECC[a], Kathryn Phillips, DVM, DACVR, DACVR-EDI[b,*]

KEYWORDS

- Thrombosis • Thromboembolism • Clot • Point-of-care ultrasound

KEY POINTS

- Point-of-care ultrasound can be used by nonradiologists to support a diagnosis of thromboembolism in small animals.
- Interrogation of large vessels is easy to accomplish and usually well-tolerated.
- In many cases, vascular ultrasound should be combined with other imaging techniques to optimize diagnostic power.

INTRODUCTION

Thrombosis refers to the formation of an occlusive or partially occlusive clot within a blood vessel that reduces blood flow to downstream tissue and organs. Large occlusive clots (thrombi) can break off and embolize to form secondary thrombi in downstream locations. The process of thrombosis followed by embolism is collectively termed thromboembolism and can culminate in a variety of acute or chronic disorders. Thromboembolic disease frequently affects small animals in critical or chronic disease states and is associated with significant morbidity and mortality.[1–7] Various anatomic sites can be affected in both the arterial and venous circulation including the right atrium/auricular appendage, distal aorta and femoral arteries, cerebrovascular arteries, pulmonary arteries, cranial and caudal vena cava, and splanchnic vessels (eg, portal, splenic, mesenteric).

Several disease conditions in small animals have been linked to a tendency to form clots and many of these risk factors have been identified through retrospective studies.[1–7] At-risk populations of dogs and cats have recently been defined by the CURATIVE guidelines.[8] These include animals with the following prothrombotic conditions: immune-mediated hemolytic anemia (IMHA), protein-losing nephropathy (PLN), pancreatitis, hyperadrenocorticism (as well as those receiving exogenous glucocorticoids), neoplasia,

[a] Veterinary Specialty Services, 1021 Howard George Drive, Manchester, MO 63021, USA; [b] UC Davis, 1275 Med Science Drive, Davis, CA 95616, USA
* Corresponding author.
E-mail address: klphilli@ucdavis.edu

Vet Clin Small Anim 51 (2021) 1267–1282
https://doi.org/10.1016/j.cvsm.2021.07.013

sepsis, and cerebrovascular and cardiac diseases. Dogs with IMHA or PLN, cats with cardiomyopathy, and dogs or cats with *greater than one* of the aforementioned prothrombotic conditions are considered high risk. With the exception of IMHA, PLN, or cats with cardiomyopathy, the presence of a single prothrombotic condition confers a low or moderate risk of thrombosis. Although the mechanisms driving thrombosis vary depending on the specific condition as well as host factors, a combination of hypercoagulability, endothelial disturbance, and blood stasis (Virchow's Triad) remain fundamental to the pathologic formation of blood clots.[9]

Types of Blood Clots

Venous and arterial blood clots differ in their constitution and, to some degree, in the factors that favor formation.[10] In people, the primary trigger for arterial thrombosis is the rupture of an atherosclerotic plaque in the artery wall. Arterial thrombi are rich in platelets and, owing to high-flow dynamics of the arterial circulation, occur under high shear stress. Much of the pathophysiology of arterial clot formation is mediated by platelet activation and aggregation. Thrombi that form in veins develop in the low shear, low-flow venous circulation. These clots are rich in fibrin and trapped red blood cells and are often referred to as "red clots." Fibrin generation plays a key role in the formation of venous clots. The primary therapeutic strategies can differ depending upon clot type and location. Similarly, clinical signs differ based on clot type. For example, femoral artery thrombosis tends to result in a cold, pulseless, and sometimes necrotic limb, whereas venous limb thrombosis often tends to lead to swelling, erythema, and heat. Clinical signs may also vary based on temporal factors. Clinical signs associated with chronic thrombosis may be insidious, whereas acute thrombosis (particularly when associated with embolism) often results in sudden and severe clinical signs.

Although some thromboembolic events are catastrophic, those that are survivable are more likely to result in favorable outcomes if met with prompt diagnosis followed by appropriate pharmacologic intervention. Therefore, examination of the arteries and veins via point-of-care ultrasound offers an early opportunity to support the clinical index of suspicion of thrombosis for the nonradiologist sonographer.

Point-of-Care Ultrasound as a Diagnostic Tool

Ultrasound is an excellent tool for targeted vascular evaluation. Small animal veterinary patients are particularly amenable to the use of ultrasound, given their size and the ease with which one can trace abdominal, cervical, and larger vessels of the limbs. Ultrasound investigation of some anatomy is limited by overlying bone and gas, which obscures direct investigation of much of the intrathoracic vasculature as well as the vessels of the skull. Other factors that limit the utility of ultrasound for vascular interrogation include the small size and sheer number of blood vessels throughout the body. As the vessels taper to smaller diameters the ability to trace these vessels becomes lost. Given the vast number of blood vessels and the amount of time it would take to perform a comprehensive examination, a targeted approach to vascular ultrasound is best. Contrast-enhanced CT is a much better imaging modality for broad screening of thrombosis as it allows large areas including small vessel diameters to be imaged in a short time and it inherently overcomes problems with superimposed structures including gas and bone. However, ultrasound is more readily available and minimally invasive, making it a valuable tool when evaluating specific vessels for thrombosis. Furthermore, ultrasound can discern different causes of occlusion including compression by adjacent masses, tumor thrombosis where the tumor extends into the vascular lumen, in situ or embolized thrombi, phlebitis, and other intraluminal objects such as worms or catheters.[11] (**Fig. 1**)

Appearance of Thrombi Over Time

The ultrasonographic appearance of a thrombus changes over time. Acute thrombi tend to be hypoechoic to anechoic and can be easily missed on B-mode imaging. Color flow Doppler is useful to identify filling defects created by the otherwise hard to identify thrombus. Duplex imaging is convenient for this purpose, wherein B-mode imaging and color flow Doppler are integrated to investigate a vascular structure (**Fig. 2**). Compression techniques are also useful in identifying these hypoechoic, easily missed thrombi. Compression techniques take advantage of the fact that normal veins are easily compressed compared to their paired artery. The sonographer increases and decreases the amount of pressure applied to the structure with the ultrasound probe while imaging and failure to compress normally suggests that thrombosis might be present.. Thrombi increase in echogenicity rapidly with noticeable changes within 6 hours after the induction of experimentally induced thrombi, correlating with increases in fibrin content.[12] Over time, recanalization occurs with small tracks of blood flow re-establishing passage through or around the thrombus as the thrombus contracts or is lysed by fibrinolytic enzymes (**Fig. 3**).

Aortic Thrombosis and Thromboembolism

Feline aortic thromboembolism (ATE) is a life-threatening complication of cardiac disease in cats that carries a poor prognosis. Many cats are euthanized on presentation and those that are treated experience less than 50% survival.[3,13,14] The risk for development of ATE in cats with preclinical cardiomyopathy was recently assessed at 11.3% in the 10 years after diagnosis.[15] It is theorized that blood stasis, endocardial injury, and a hypercoagulable state may all contribute to the formation of the thrombus within the left atrium and its appendage.[16,17] The clot will sometimes embolize and "lodge" at the aortic trifurcation, but it can also terminate in an artery supplying a

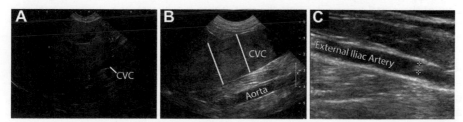

Fig. 1. (*A*) Porta hepatis of a 7-year-old MC Australian Shepherd images of the right cranial abdomen obtained with small 4.2 to 10.2 MHz probe, longitudinal view via right intercostal window with a large liver mass marked with blue calipers, compressing the CVC and (*B*) A 10-year-old MC Pug imaged using a 4.2 to 10.2 MHz curvilinear probe with an adrenal mass extending into the caudal vena. The portion of the tumor thrombosis imaged is distending and occluding the caudal vena cava. (*C*) A 4-year-old FS cat presented for clinical signs of a thromboembolism with right pelvic limb including monoparesis, pain, and no right femoral pulse. Ultrasound of the right external iliac artery using an 18 MHz linear transducer revealed a luminal structure with parallel walls compatible with an aberrant heartworm. Ultrasound was used to guide surgical cutdown and remove the worm. This case was published in JVIM. From Oldach MS, Gunther-Harrington CT, Balsa IM, et al. Aberrant migration and surgical removal of a heartworm (dirofilaria immitis) from the femoral artery of a cat. *Journal of veterinary internal medicine.* 2018;32(2):792-796.

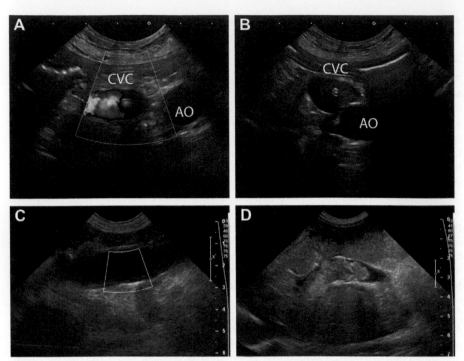

Fig. 2. A 9-year-old Bloodhound with oligoanuric acute renal failure, imaged with a 4.2 to 10.2 MHz curvilinear probe. (*A*) At presentation, a catheter extending into the caudal vena cava with an extrinsic thrombus creating a partial filling defect on color Doppler interrogation. (*B*) 4 days later, the thrombus persists and is more echoic allowing identification of all margins. (*C*) An 11-year-old Shar Pei with multifocal thromboembolic disease and protein-losing enteropathy. Ultrasound image of an acute portal vein thrombus. The prehepatic portal vein is distended with a hypoechoic occlusive thrombus and no evident flow on color flow Doppler interrogation. (*D*) A 4-year-old FS French Bulldog. An intercostal longitudinal view of the portal vein as it enters the liver. There is a hyperechoic chronic portal vein thrombus with rounded undulating margins. Images were acquired for both patients using a 5 to 8 MHz curvilinear probe.

forelimb or other major organ systems (eg, kidney, brain, splanchnic). Following embolization, the blood clot and associated vasoactive response frequently causes complete limb ischemia resulting in paresis/paralysis and severe pain, and occasionally limb necrosis. In a minority of cases, ATE can be associated with noncardiac disease, most commonly pulmonary neoplasia.[18,19] In the minority of cats that do survive ATE, prompt diagnosis and treatment are important. Fortunately, this clinical presentation is seldom ambiguous. Cats often present acute onset of hindlimb paresis/paralysis, pain and vocalization, pale or cold limb(s), and in many cases, signs of congestive heart failure.

Thrombosis of the aorta can also occur in dogs. However, in dogs, the aorta is more commonly obstructed by a clot that has formed in situ rather than an embolized clot.[20–26] Unlike feline ATE, cardiac disease is not often associated with aortic thrombosis in the dog. Instead, comorbidities such as protein-losing nephropathy, neoplasia, steroid administration, endocrinopathy, and inflammatory/infectious disease are thought to contribute to aortic thrombosis in up to 77% of affected dogs.[27] Acute clinical signs such as pain, neurologic deficits, and nonambulatory status are

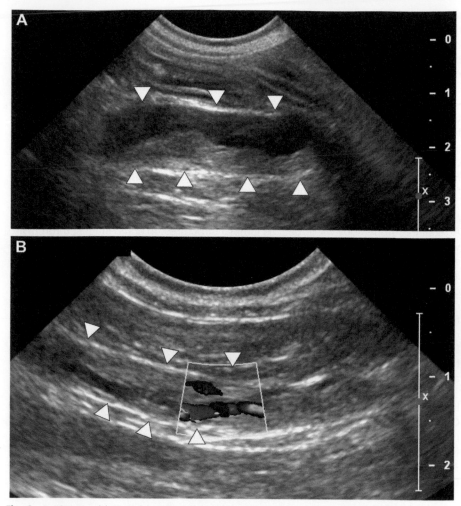

Fig. 3. A 10-year-old FS Golden-Doodle. Ultrasound images using a 5 to 8 MHz curvilinear probe, 12 months after initial diagnosis of an aortic thrombus. (*A*) Within the distal intraabdominal aorta, a broad-based undulant in margination nonocclusive thrombus is seen along the dorsal endothelium. (*B*) Is the left external iliac artery, (*arrowheads*) with a path of recanalized flow identified using color Doppler through the middle of the chronic thrombus.

less common than more gradual or chronic clinical signs such as progressive lameness or weakness.[21,26,27]

In both canine and feline aortic thrombosis, prompt identification and treatment are important to prevent clot extension. Point-of care ultrasound has the potential to further support this differential in suspected cases.

Imaging Technique

The distal aorta and aortic trifurcation is a common site of aortic thrombosis/thromboembolism. Ultrasound evaluation of this region requires identification of the caudal abdominal aorta and tracing of the large branches extending toward the limbs. This is easily done from the ventral inguinal region or lateral abdomen placing the probe just ventral to the transverse processes in the paralumbar fossa. A mid-range curvi-linear abdominal probe (~5–12 MHz) will suffice for cats and dogs. The examination begins with identification of the aorta and lumbar vertebra at the level of the urinary bladder. The caudal vena cava will be flaccid and easily compressible, so you may not identify it right away because of this compression. The major branches of the caudal aorta are the right and left external iliac arteries, which extend at approximately 45-degree angles from the distal aorta. These can be traced down the pelvic limb to the femoral arteries. The next set of branches are the much smaller internal iliac ar-teries. The sacral artery extends caudally from the aorta just ventral to the sacrum and is often not seen on examination due to small size. Because the most common cause of ATE in cats is thrombosis within the left atrium and auricular appendage, focused cardiac ultrasound (FCU) with special attention to the left atrium is of value for supporting the diagnosis of ATE in cats (**Fig. 4**).

Findings
Arterial thromboemboli will appear as luminal structures. In acute stages, thrombi are very hypoechoic to anechoic and easily missed. Thus, the use of color Doppler can be extremely helpful to identify occult thrombi, particularly when luminal obstruction is incomplete. As thrombi age, they become more hyperechoic and firm and are more conspicuous on B-mode imaging. Depending on the extent of the thrombus and oc-clusion, you may recognize that the paired venous structures are under distended from decreased blood flow. With late stage, or mature thrombi, you can start to recog-nize recanalization with small tracts of blood flow through the thrombus. Using B-mode imaging, recanalization will appear as small, hypoechoic striations within the thrombus but these small pathways of flow are best observed using color flow and power Doppler.

In cats only, FCU can be used to support the diagnosis of an arterial thromboembo-lism due to association of cardiac disease with this phenomenon (see Chapter FCU Cats). Paired with clinical signs of ATE, the presence of a thrombus and/or sponta-neous echoes within a dilated left atrium or its appendage support the diagnosis. More advanced techniques can be used to assess contraction of the auricle as well as auricular flow velocity whereby decreased contractions and slow flow can increase the probability of the presence of feline ATE.

Portal and Splenic Vein Thrombosis
Portal and splenic vein thrombosis (PVT, SVT) can arise in hypercoagulable states. Conditions that have been associated with portal and splenic vein thrombi in dogs include neoplasia and inflammatory disease (eg, pancreatitis, sepsis).[4] When splenic vein thrombi are identified in isolation, it should raise clinical suspicion of thrombo-philia, but clinical signs seldom arise. However, in rare cases, acute clinical signs have been attributed to SVT.[28,29] In contrast, portal vein thrombosis, particularly acute PVT, frequently causes clinical signs associated with portal hypertension and conse-quences can be severe. Sudden onset of abdominal pain and shock, peritoneal fluid, vomiting, and/or diarrhea are clinical signs associated with acute PVT. Peritoneal fluid can resolve to some degree with the development of acquired shunting vessels. Although any prothrombotic condition can contribute to PVT or SVT formation, local disease appears to be particularly important.[4,6,30]

Imaging technique
Ultrasound evaluation of the portal system is an advanced technique as it requires identification and tracing of the vessels throughout the abdomen. To do this

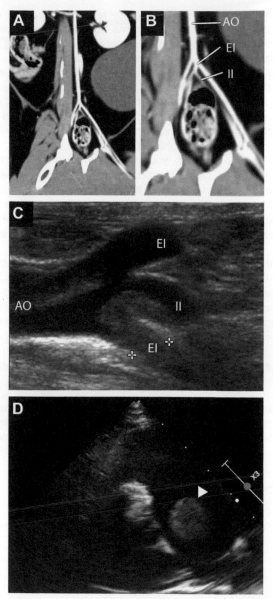

Fig. 4. (A) Dorsal CT image demonstrating normal anatomy of the aorta at the level of the external iliac arteries in a feline patient. AO, aorta; EI, external iliac artery; II, internal iliac arteries. (B) Longitudinal ultrasound image of the caudal aorta in a dog with a partial thrombus of the caudal aorta, internal iliac artery, and occlusive thrombus in the left external iliac artery. (C) An echocardiographic image of feline patient with a large, round left atrial thrombus and left atriomegaly.

thoroughly, this examination takes time, skill, and an ideal environment for the sonographer. Evaluation of the entire portal system is not typically a POCUS examination; even if the sonographer is concentrating on this anatomic system, it covers a large anatomic region and is a time and skill-intensive examination. During this examination, the patient must be able to lie in dorsal or lateral recumbency for an extended period and must tolerate pressure applied to the cranial abdomen. No matter the skill level of the sonographer, tracing vessels requires concentration. Optimizing the environment to have as few distractions as possible is recommended.

To evaluate the portovascular system, prep the entire ventral abdomen as you would for a complete abdominal examination including shaving, cleaning of the skin, and applying coupling gel. When evaluating the portal vein as it enters and branches in the liver, it helps to shave and prep further cranially on the right side of the patient, up over the caudal ribs and dorsal to match the abdominal shaved region. Extend dorsally to the level of the right kidney.

For the majority of dogs and cats, you will use a mid-range MHz curvilinear probe (~5–12 MHz). For very large, deep-chested dogs or dogs in which the abdomen is distended with peritoneal effusion, a lower frequency large curvilinear probe may be beneficial (~1–6 MHz). When evaluating for subtle findings such as luminal thrombi, it is important to remember that if a lower frequency is required to penetrate and visualize deeper structures, this benefit comes at the expense of a loss of spatial resolution.

The major branching tributaries to the portal vein include the cranial and caudal mesenteric veins, the splenic vein, and the gastroduodenal vein (**Fig. 5**). Tracing these vessels will require moving over the entire abdomen. The porta hepatis is the point of convergence of the major hepatic vessels and bile duct at the margin of the liver. This region can be seen from a ventral approach but investigation can be obscured by gas in the transverse colon, duodenum, or a distended stomach. The porta hepatis can also be identified from a right lateral intercostal approach[31] (**Fig. 6**). From this intercostal window, the portal vein can be seen in both transverse and longitudinal planes.

Findings

Imaging findings that should prompt evaluation for a portal vein thrombus include peritoneal effusion, acquired shunting vessels, and edema of multiple organs such as the gastrointestinal wall and pancreas.[6] When there are numerous acquired

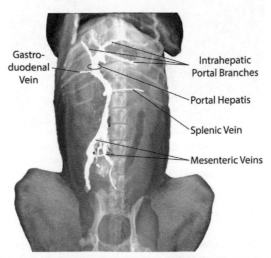

Fig. 5. Maximum intensity projection dorsal reformatted vascular image of a CT angiogram of the portal vein overlying a canine abdominal radiograph demonstrating the anatomy of the portal tributaries to be evaluated when examining the portal vein.

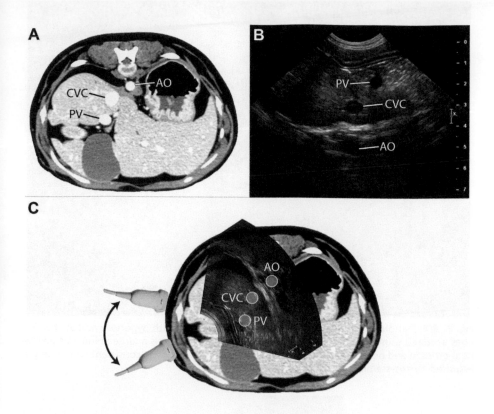

Fig. 6. (*A*) Transverse postcontrast CT image, (*B*) ultrasound, and (*C*) composite images demonstrating the anatomy of the porta hepatis using a right intercostal window. The 2 probes show the region to examine to find the porta hepatis.

portosystemic shunting vessels, they can appear as nests of tortuous vessels, typically in the region of the mesenteric root or caudal to the left kidney (**Fig. 7**).

Evaluation of the portal vein for a thrombus is the same as in other vessels; one should attempt to identify a luminal structure or filling defects (**Fig. 8**). Color flow Doppler interrogation of the portal vein is valuable because it provides information on the direction of flow. Portal vein flow reverses when there is an upstream occlusion and subsequent opening of remnant alternative blood flow pathways via acquired shunts. Portal blood flow is normally toward the liver, or hepatopedal flow. When abnormal, reversed, and moving away from the liver, it is called hepatofugal flow.

Portal vein velocities can be used to evaluate for portal hypertension which could occur with complete or partially occlusive thrombi. In cases of portal hypertension, the velocity of flow in the portal vein slows. Obtaining portal vein velocities requires an ultrasound machine capable of pulse wave Doppler. There are inherent obstacles to obtaining accurate measurements (such as angle to laminar flow and motion from breathing). To obtain the most accurate measurement of velocity, the Doppler angle, the angle of the ultrasound waves relative to the blood flow should be between 30° and 60°. For each degree that the probe is angled away from the direction of flow (closer to 90°), the measured velocity will be falsely decreased. To get the appropriate angle of the ultrasound beam to the portal vein, the sonographer must angle the probe and apply a moderate amount of pressure to the abdominal wall, as the portal vein courses

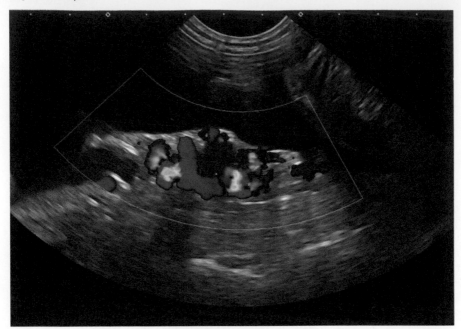

Fig. 7. A 4-year-old Black Russian Terrier that was presented with hyporexia and ascites, images acquired using a 4.2 to 10.2 MHz curvilinear probe. There is a large volume of peritoneal effusion and nests of tortuous vessels caudal to the left kidney consistent with multiple acquired portosystemic shunts.

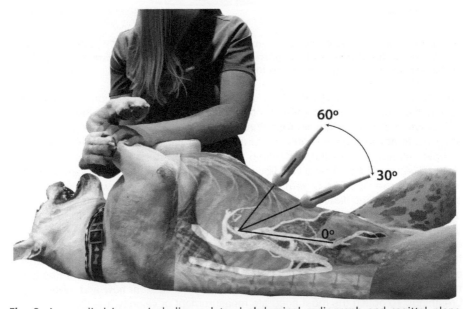

Fig. 8. A complied image including a lateral abdominal radiograph and sagittal plane maximum intensity projection of a CT angiogram of the great vessels to demonstrate anatomy of the portal vein. To accurately measure portal vein velocities, the ultrasound probe needs to be between 30° and 60° from the portal vein. Obtaining the appropriate angle of insonation can be a limiting factor if the abdomen is distended with ascites, the patient has a deep-chested confirmation or a painful abdomen.

under the ribcage. Patient resistance, abdominal pain, or a turgid abdomen from peritoneal effusion can greatly limit the sonographer's ability to perform this examination (**Fig. 9**).

Up to 55% of canine patients with pancreatitis also had portal vein thrombi identified with contrast-enhanced CT. All of those patients had ultrasound examinations performed by senior radiology residents or a boarded radiologist. Contrast-enhanced CT was significantly better at diagnosing concomitant portal vein thrombi ($P = .003$) when compared with ultrasound examinations.[32,33] This demonstrates how regional pancreatic inflammation and abdominal pain can create technical challenges that limit sonographic assessment and sensitivity for identifying PVT in patients with this proinflammatory, prothrombotic condition.

Imaging technique (splenic vein)
The splenic vein is a tributary to the portal vein. Multiple small splenic veins emerge at the splenic hilus and converge to form the splenic vein, which also receives branches from the left gastric and left gastroepiploic veins. The splenic veins at the hilus are readily visualized in the left cranial abdomen. The primary ultrasound probe for imaging the splenic vein is a mid-range MHz small curvilinear probe (~5–12 MHZ). Because the spleen is a superficial organ, this probe will be sufficient for even large dogs.

Findings
It is common to see spontaneous echoes (smoke) in the splenic veins near the splenic hilus, attributable to slow flow in this region. The identification of splenic thrombi at the splenic hilus is not uncommon and can be seen in patients with no attributable clinical signs (**Fig. 10**). However, if a splenic thrombus is identified, underlying risk factors for hypercoagulability should be considered. If a splenic thrombus is identified, the splenic vein should be traced along its length to the portal vein to evaluate the extent of the thrombus and for concurrent portal vein thrombosis.

Regions of acute infarction may also be detected within the splenic parenchyma. In these cases, there is usually a sharp, often linear demarcation within the splenic parenchyma between normal spleen and a more hypoechoic region. This is usually at the peripheral margin of the spleen. In addition to being hypoechoic, this area of the spleen may bulge and appear thicker. The infarcted region will have less blood flow compared to the remainder of the splenic parenchyma. In these cases, the thrombus itself is not usually identified.

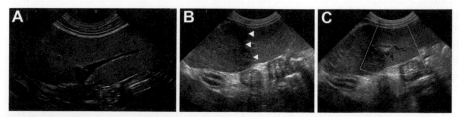

Fig. 9. (*A*) A 9-year-old FS German shepherd dog being staged for mammary carcinoma. View of the splenic hilus using a 4.2 to 10.2 MHZ curvilinear transducer. There is a rounded, hyperechoic thrombus in one of the splenic veins. (*B & C*) An 11-year-old MI Scottish Terrier. There is a well-demarcated hypoechoic region in the tail of the spleen (*arrowheads*), without blood flow identified using color flow Doppler representing a splenic infarct. Images were acquired with a 5 to 8 MHz curvilinear probe.

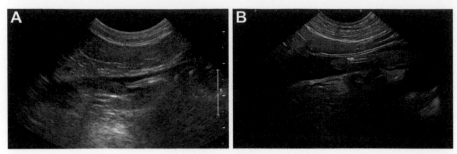

Fig. 10. (*A*) A 7-year-old male castrated Border Collie with immune-mediated hemolytic ane-mia. A sessile-shaped mural thrombus is along the endothelial surface of the caudal vena cava at the end of the catheter. The image was acquired using a 5 to 8 MHz curvilinear probe. (*B*) A 9-year-old female spayed Bloodhound with oligoanuric renal failure and a thrombus surrounding the catheter within the caudal vena cava. The image was acquired using a 4.2 to 10.2 MHz curvilinear probe.

Pulmonary Thromboembolism

Pulmonary thromboembolism (PTE) is a term that represents the presence of a thrombus formed in a pulmonary arterial vessel (pulmonary thrombosis) or the mobi-lization of a thrombus or clot fragment from a distant site to the pulmonary vasculature (pulmonary embolism, or PE). The two can be difficult to differentiate. The true prev-alence of this condition is unknown but is suggested to be near 1% for dogs (over a 10-year period) and 0.06% in cats (over a 24-year period).[2,7] This is almost certainly an underestimate because the diagnosis is infrequently considered and can be diffi-cult to confirm. The severity of pulmonary and cardiac compromise that results from PTE can vary dramatically. Massive PTE (defined as PTE causing hypotension and shock) is a life-threatening emergency and these dogs and cats are hemodynamically very unstable. Any patient with undifferentiated shock should be promptly evaluated for acute PTE using FCU and an integrative approach such as Global FAST, which in-cludes Vet BLUE lung ultrasound.

Imaging

The best imaging modality to evaluate for PTE is computed tomography pulmonary angiography (CTA) wherein an iodinated contrast agent is administered intravenously and tomographic slices through the thorax are acquired in a pulmonary, arterial, venous, and delayed phases to evaluate the enhancement of the pulmonary vascular system. Although this technique is best performed under general anesthesia to limit breathing motion artifact, CTA has been described in critically ill canine patients hav-ing a clinical suspicion for PTE using only light sedation.[34] Regardless, this modality is not always available or feasible because of equipment limitations, costs, or patient stability factors. Thus, FCU, TFAST, and Vet Blue lung ultrasound can be used as screening tests for PTE. Using FCU, dilation of the right ventricle, interventricular septal flattening, right atriomegaly, and elevated velocity of tricuspid regurgitant jets can indicate an acute change in pulmonary arterial pressure, consistent with (although not specific for) massive PTE. In some cases, a visible thrombus is observed in the main pulmonary artery or a principal division, confirming diagnosis. Using Vet Blue lung ultrasound, the finding of a pulmonary "wedge sign" in non–gravity-dependent caudodorsal region supports a diagnosis of PTE (see Chapter 2 Lung Ultrasound). It is important to realize when performing this examination that a lack of findings on FCU does not exclude the possibility of PTE.[34]

Caval and Device-Associated Thrombosis and Phlebitis

Cranial caval thrombosis is almost always device-associated and has been described in 8 dogs following pacemaker implantation and in 17 dogs with risk factors for thrombosis combined with history of central venous catheter placement.[5,35–38] Mediastinal lymphoma has been documented as the cause of cranial caval thrombosis in one cat.[39] Clinical signs associated with cranial caval thrombosis include chylous or non-chylous pleural effusion, facial or forelimb edema, and jugular venous distension.[33,34] The caudal vena cava can also be affected by device-associated thrombosis via placement of peripherally inserted central catheters (commonly referred to as PICC lines). However, caudal caval thrombosis is more commonly reported in association with adrenal neoplasia.[40,41]

Imaging technique

Probe placement and technique will depend on the target vessel. For the most superficial structures, the highest frequency probe should be used (linear probes will have the highest frequencies). For very superficial vessels, a linear probe and stand-off pad can be used to move the structure of interest into the optimized region for improved lateral resolution and to overcome near field artifact. Superficial veins are very compressible making them challenging to image.

Interrogation of pelvic limb PICC lines requires imaging of the caudal vena cava within the abdomen, ideally using a mid-range curvilinear probe ($\sim$5–12 MHz). Evaluation should include tracing the caudal vena cava through the liver, from the porta hepatis to the aortic trifurcation. If tracing the entire length of the vessel is not possible, investigation of vessel segments at the level of the liver, renal veins, and aortic trifurcation should be attempted. To view the caudal vena cava at the level of the liver, the sonographer could use a right intercostal window by identifying the right kidney and then moving cranially over the ribs.

The external jugular vein can be traced from the neck to the thoracic inlet. One then encounters a segment of the cranial vena cava that is obscured by overlying gas in the lungs and cannot be traced until the level of the heart where one can evaluate for thrombi extending from the cranial vena cava into the right atrium. For evaluation of the jugular vein, use either a linear or small curvilinear probe. The jugular vein lies just under the skin and when normal, is very compressible. This examination often begins by finding the carotid artery and then lightning probe pressure and (if needed) moving slightly lateral to find the jugular veins. The cranial portion of the cranial mediastinum can be evaluated from the neck by angling the probe caudally into the thoracic inlet. The cranial mediastinum can also be evaluated from the ventrolateral thorax via an intercostal window.

Findings

In the limbs, the vessels tend to travel in vascular bundles with the artery and associated vein. Normal veins should be easily compressible, to the point where a sonographer might only identify the artery initially, after which intentional lightning of pressure will allow filling and identification of the vein. This compressibility characteristic can be exploited to better recognize early, hypoechoic, or anechoic venous thrombi when vessels do not compress as one would expect.

Catheter-related thromboses can be intraluminal or extraluminal.[42,43] Intraluminal thrombi form within the catheter lumen and cannot be detected using ultrasound. Extraluminal thrombi are also undetectable via ultrasound if they exist as a thin fibrin sheath covering the external surface of the catheter. However, more conspicuous forms of echogenic extraluminal thrombi are easily detected using ultrasound. These include complete or partial venous thrombosis encircling the catheter or mural thrombosis, which occurs on only one side of the catheter where it interacts with a vessel wall. Occasionally, a fibrin "flap" will form at the tip of the catheter, which blocks aspiration but still allows infusion. This type of clot may be observed using ultrasound, particularly if the dynamics of the clot are challenged by infusion and aspiration during imaging.

SUMMARY

Point-of-care ultrasound is a useful tool to further investigate clinical suspicion of thrombotic disease in small animals. Using the techniques described, clinicians have the potential to identify clinically relevant thrombosis but should acknowledge that the sensitivity of this tool for detection of thrombosis has not been described described, particularly in nonradiologist sonographers. The ultrasonographic appearance of thrombi can change over time, potentially impacting detection in early stages. However, given the increasing availability of point-of-care ultrasound in small animal practice and the ease-of-use for this modality, clinicians should consider familiarizing themselves with these techniques to interrogate small animal patients with risk factors or clinical signs consistent with thrombosis.

DISCLOSURE STATEMENT

The authors have nothing to disclose.

REFERENCES

1. Carr AP, Panciera DL, Kidd L. Prognostic factors for mortality and thromboembolism in canine immune-mediated hemolytic anemia: A retrospective study of 72 dogs. J Vet Intern Med 2002;16(5):504–9.
2. Johnson LR, Lappin MR, Baker DC. Pulmonary thromboembolism in 29 dogs: 1985–1995. J Vet Intern Med 1999;13(4):338–45.
3. Laste NJ, Harpster NK. A retrospective study of 100 cases of feline distal aortic thromboembolism: 1977-1993. J Am Anim Hosp Assoc 1995;31(6):492–500.
4. Laurenson MP, Hopper K, Herrera MA, et al. Concurrent diseases and conditions in dogs with splenic vein thrombosis. J Vet Intern Med 2010;24(6):1298–304.
5. Palmer KG, King LG, Van Winkle TJ. Clinical manifestations and associated disease syndromes in dogs with cranial vena cava thrombosis: 17 cases (1989-1996). J Am Vet Med Assoc 1998;213(2):220–4.
6. Respess M, O'Toole TE, Taeymans O, et al. Portal vein thrombosis in 33 dogs: 1998-2011. J Vet Intern Med 2012;26(2):230–7.
7. Schermerhorn T, Pembleton-Corbett JR, Kornreich B. Pulmonary thromboembolism in cats. J Vet Intern Med 2004;18(4):533–5.
8. deLaforcade A, Bacek L, Blais M, et al. Consensus on the rational use of antithrombotics in veterinary critical care (CURATIVE): Domain 1—defining populations at risk. J Vet Emerg Crit Care 2019;29(1):37–48.
9. Furie B, Furie BC. Mechanisms of thrombus formation. N Engl J Med 2008;359(9):938–49.
10. Previtali E, Bucciarelli P, Passamonti SM, et al. Risk factors for venous and arterial thrombosis. Blood Transfus 2011;9(2):120.
11. Oldach MS, Gunther-Harrington CT, Balsa IM, et al. Aberrant migration and surgical removal of a heartworm (dirofilaria immitis) from the femoral artery of a cat. J Vet Intern Med 2018;32(2):792–6.

12. Fowlkes JB, Strieter RM, Downing LJ, et al. Ultrasound echogenicity in experimental venous thrombosis. Ultrasound Med Biol 1998;24(8):1175–82.

13. Borgeat K, Wright J, Garrod O, et al. Arterial thromboembolism in 250 cats in general practice: 2004–2012. J Vet Intern Med 2014;28(1):102–8.

14. Guillaumin J, Gibson RM, Goy-Thollot I, et al. Thrombolysis with tissue plasminogen activator (TPA) in feline acute aortic thromboembolism: A retrospective study of 16 cases. J Feline Med Surg 2019;21(4):340–6.

15. Fox PR, Keene BW, Lamb K, et al. International collaborative study to assess cardiovascular risk and evaluate long-term health in cats with preclinical hypertrophic cardiomyopathy and apparently healthy cats: The REVEAL study. J Vet Intern Med 2018;32(3):930–43.

16. Stokol T, Brooks M, Rush JE, et al. Hypercoagulability in cats with cardiomyopathy. J Vet Intern Med 2008;22(3):546–52.

17. Payne JR, Borgeat K, Connolly DJ, et al. Prognostic indicators in cats with hypertrophic cardiomyopathy. J Vet Intern Med 2013;27(6):1427–36.

18. Guarino AL, Jeon AB, Abbott JR, et al. Pulmonary sarcomatoid carcinoma associated with arterial thromboembolism in a cat. Case Rep Vet Med 2021.

19. da Cruz Schaefer G, Veronezi TM, da Luz CG, et al. Arterial thromboembolism of non-cardiogenic origin in a domestic feline with ischemia and reperfusion syndrome–a case report. Semina Ciências Agrárias 2020;41(2):717–24.

20. Williams TP, Shaw S, Porter A, et al. Aortic thrombosis in dogs. J Vet Emerg Crit Care 2017;27(1):9–22.

21. Lake-Bakaar GA, Johnson EG, Griffiths LG. Aortic thrombosis in dogs: 31 cases (2000–2010). J Am Vet Med Assoc 2012;241(7):910–5.

22. Winter RL, Budke CM. Multicenter evaluation of signalment and comorbid conditions associated with aortic thrombotic disease in dogs. J Am Vet Med Assoc 2017;251(4):438–42.

23. Winter RL, Sedacca CD, Adams A, et al. Aortic thrombosis in dogs: Presentation, therapy, and outcome in 26 cases. J Vet Cardiol 2012;14(2):333–42.

24. Santamarina G, Vila M, Lopez M, et al. Aortic thromboembolism and retroperitoneal hemorrhage associated with a pheochromocytoma in a dog. J Vet Intern Med 2003;17(6):917–22.

25. Kirberger RM, Zambelli A. Imaging diagnosis–aortic thromboembolism associated with spirocercosis in a dog. Vet Radiol Ultrasound 2007;48(5):418–20.

26. Van Winkle TJ, Bruce E. Thrombosis of the portal vein in eleven dogs. Vet Pathol 1993;30(1):28–35.

27. Ruehl M, Lynch AM, O'Toole TE, et al. Outcome and treatments of dogs with aortic thrombosis: 100 cases (1997-2014). J Vet Intern Med 2020;34(5):1759–67.

28. Kim J. A case of acute splenic vein thrombosis in a dog. J Vet Med Sci 2019; 81(10):1492–5.

29. Clements CA, Rogers KS, Green RA, et al. Splenic vein thrombosis resulting in acute anemia: An unusual manifestation of nephrotic syndrome in a chinese shar pei with reactive amyloidosis. J Am Anim Hosp Assoc 1995;31(5):411–5.

30. Rogers CL, O'Toole TE, Keating JH, et al. Portal vein thrombosis in cats: 6 cases (2001-2006). J Vet Intern Med 2008;22(2):282–7.

31. D'Anjou M, Penninck D, Cornejo L, et al. Ultrasonographic diagnosis of portosystemic shunting in dogs and cats. Vet Radiol Ultrasound 2004;45(5):424–37.

32. French JM, Twedt DC, Rao S, et al. Computed tomographic angiography and ultrasonography in the diagnosis and evaluation of acute pancreatitis in dogs. J Vet Intern Med 2019;33(1):79–88.

33. French JM, Twedt DC, Rao S, et al. CT angiographic changes in dogs with acute pancreatitis: A prospective longitudinal study. Vet Radiol Ultrasound 2020; 61(1):33–9.
34. Goggs R, Chan DL, Benigni L, et al. Comparison of computed tomography pulmonary angiography and point-of-care tests for pulmonary thromboembolism diagnosis in dogs. J Small Anim Pract 2014;55(4):190–7.
35. Van De Wiele, Carrie M, Hogan DF, et al. Cranial vena caval syndrome secondary to transvenous pacemaker implantation in two dogs. J Vet Cardiol 2008;10(2): 155–61.
36. Murray JD, O'Sullivan ML, Hawkes KC. Cranial vena caval thrombosis associated with endocardial pacing leads in three dogs. J Am Anim Hosp Assoc 2010;46(3): 186–92.
37. Mulz JM, Kraus MS, Thompson M, et al. Cranial vena caval syndrome secondary to central venous obstruction associated with a pacemaker lead in a dog. J Vet Cardiol 2010;12(3):217–23.
38. Cunningham SM, Ames MK, Rush JE, et al. Successful treatment of pacemaker-induced stricture and thrombosis of the cranial vena cava in two dogs by use of anticoagulants and balloon venoplasty. J Am Vet Med Assoc 2009;235(12): 1467–73.
39. Sottiaux J, Franck M. Cranial vena caval thrombosis secondary to invasive mediastinal lymphosarcoma in a cat. J Small Anim Pract 1998;39(7):352–5.
40. Jaffe MH, Grooters AM, Partington BP, et al. Extensive venous thrombosis and hind-limb edema associated with adrenocortical carcinoma in a dog. J Am Anim Hosp Assoc 1999;35(4):306–10.
41. Scavelli TD, Peterson ME, Matthiesen DT. Results of surgical treatment for hyper-adrenocorticism caused by adrenocortical neoplasia in the dog: 25 cases. J Am Vet Med Assoc 1986;189:1360–4.
42. Wall C, Moore J, Thachil J. Catheter-related thrombosis: A practical approach. J Intensive Care Soc 2016;17(2):160–7.
43. Beathard GA. The use and complications of catheters for hemodialysis vascular access: Introduction 2001;14(6):410.

Focused Ultrasound of Superficial–Soft Tissue Swellings, Masses, and Fluid Collections in Dogs and Cats

Susanne Stieger-Vanegas, Dr med vet, PhD

KEYWORDS

- Imaging • Superficial • Cellulitis • Abscess • Foreign body • Hernia • Neoplasia
- Point-of-care ultrasound

KEY POINTS

- Ultrasound allows further characterization of superficial soft tissue masses and identification of internal fluid collections.
- Several benign and malignant superficial soft tissue masses can have a similar sonographic appearance, and early differentiation is critical for treatment planning and prognosis.
- Ultrasound-guided fine needle aspirates or biopsies can assist in differentiating various masses, for example, hematoma versus soft tissue sarcoma or superficial hemangiosarcoma.
- Ultrasound of superficial masses can be helpful to identify and localize foreign bodies. Furthermore, it can be a helpful localizing tool to assist during surgical removal of the foreign body.
- Real-time ultrasound with application of external transducer pressure and subsequent release of pressure during the examination can help to detect and localize abscesses or while changing the position of the patient can assist in identification of displaced abdominal organs.

INTRODUCTION

Superficial subcutaneous palpable masses occur commonly in small animal patients and are a common reason small animals are seen by veterinarians. Likely many of these masses are ultimately benign in nature and may represent lipomas, fluid collections, cysts, or foreign bodies; however, some of these masses will be malignant tumors and may represent life-altering or threatening lesions. It is therefore often

Department of Clinical Sciences, Carlson College of Veterinary Medicine, Oregon State University, Magruder Hall, 700 Southwest 30th Street, Corvallis, OR 97331, USA
E-mail address: Susanne.stieger@oregonstate.edu

Vet Clin Small Anim 51 (2021) 1283–1293
https://doi.org/10.1016/j.cvsm.2021.07.009
0195-5616/21/© 2021 Elsevier Inc. All rights reserved.

critical to know what these masses are to optimize treatment planning. Especially in malignant lesions, early diagnosis and treatment planning are critical. Although some of these superficial palpable masses are easily diagnosed and managed based on history and clinical examination, frequently additional imaging is required, as these masses are nonspecific on presentation.

Ultrasound is an attractive modality for evaluating soft tissue masses because of its low cost, lack of ionizing radiation, and high spatial resolution, while providing real-time point-of-care information. In addition, ultrasound offers the ability to assess blood flow without contrast agent administration. Furthermore, when soft tissue masses are large or deep within the muscles and fascia, ultrasound can be an effective initial technique to assist obtaining tissue samples by way of fine needle aspiration or biopsy. However, cross-sectional imaging techniques, such as contrast-enhanced computed tomography or MRI, typically offered in combination with sonographic interventions (eg, fine needle aspiration or biopsy), are better suited to evaluate the extent of the mass, mass margination, and involvement of adjacent anatomic structures.

ULTRASOUND TECHNIQUE AND CLINICAL HISTORY

Ultrasound of a superficial soft tissue mass is usually targeted and focused on the area of the palpable mass or symptoms. A complete history is often critical to assess the mass sonographically and should include information about when the mass was first observed, any change of size of the mass, pain at the site, drainage from the site, skin lesion and a history of trauma, travel, or any other malignancy being present. In addition, the history should include prior treatments and if (and when) aspirates or biopsies have been previously performed.

Ultrasound of superficial masses requires usually minimal preparation and should be performed with a high-frequency transducer. Dependent on location, a linear transducer with a small contact surface is preferred. It is important to use the highest frequency possible, which still provides adequate depth. In thicker body areas and when soft tissue masses are located deeper within superficial tissues, a lower-frequency transducer is needed to assess the full extent of the lesion.

The major soft tissue structures observed using ultrasound to assess masses usually include the dermis, subcutaneous tissue, fascial layers, muscle, vascular structures, and adjacent osseous surfaces.

Doppler ultrasound of the soft tissues can be used to assess blood flow; however, as masses are often hypovascular or when only low vascular flow is present, careful adjustment of the color and power Doppler settings is necessary to obtain high-quality images and maximize detection of slow moving or minimal blood flow:

- Use the highest frequency transducer that provides adequate visualization and depth.
- Minimize the size of the Doppler color box to maximize frame rate.
- Minimize applying pressure on the mass during the ultrasound examination. Increasing the pressure with the transducer or the hand can result in an increased pressure within the mass, which can reduce or eliminate seeing blood flow within a superficial mass.[1]
- Decrease the color Doppler scale (pulse repetition frequency).
- Increase the color Doppler gain until you see flash artifacts and then slowly decrease it.
- If color Doppler signal is noted within a mass, use spectral Doppler to assess if the signal represents venous versus arterial flow.[1]

SOFT TISSUE SWELLINGS
Edema and Cellulitis

Edema and cellulitis are common pathologic conditions of the skin and superficial fascia, which are usually diagnosed and differentiated clinically. In skin and soft tissue infections, including cellulitis, an abscess may be present (**Fig. 1**), and the physical examination alone may not be sufficient to rule out an abscess. In these cases, ultrasound can be an excellent option to evaluate the superficial soft tissues. Edema (**Fig. 2**) and cellulitis have a similar sonographic appearance, including the following:

- Thickening of the skin and adjacent fat
- Heterogeneity of the skin and fat owing to mixed echogenicity tissue consisting of hypoechoic to anechoic areas with hyperechoic striations
- Nonlocular perifascial fluid
- Hypervascularity

FLUID COLLECTIONS
Seroma

A seroma is a local fluid accumulation that can occur secondary to trauma or after a surgical procedure (**Fig. 3**). To differentiate between sterile and infected seroma, aseptical ultrasound-guided fluid aspiration may be necessary. Sonographic features of seroma include the following:

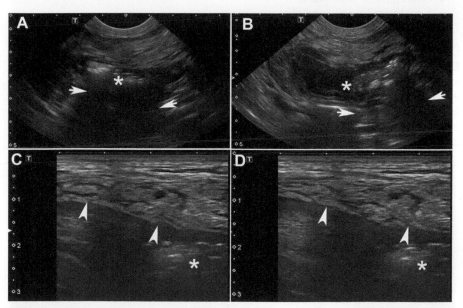

Fig. 1. Cellulitis with abscess. Longitudinal (A) and transverse (B) ultrasound images of the neck of a 5-year-old golden retriever with swelling and a right forelimb lameness revealed a cavitary mass (*asterisk*) with fluid and gas as noted by the hyperechoic material with associated reverberation artifacts (*arrows*) and lack of Doppler signal. The adjacent soft tissues, best seen on higher-frequency ultrasound images (C, D), demonstrate thickened, lobular, and hyperechoic soft tissue (*arrowheads*), which is septated by thin hypoechoic to anechoic strands of tissue. Sonographically, an abscess with regional cellulitis was suspected and confirmed at surgery. No foreign body was identified with ultrasound or at the time of surgery.

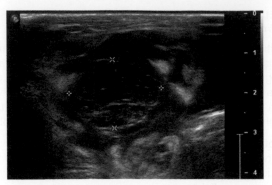

Fig. 2. Lymphoma and edema. Longitudinal ultrasound image of a neck swelling in a 12-year-old Lhasa apso with known T-cell rich B-cell lymphoma. A large mass with a central ovoid hypoechoic area (*outlined by calipers*) and surrounding mixed echogenic tissues with bands of anechogenicity is noted. Ultrasound-guided fine needle aspirates of the central aspect of the mass revealed lymphoma cells surrounded by edema. No signs of infection were documented.

- Thin-walled cavitary structure with internal anechoic fluid and deep acoustic enhancement
- Small internal septations
- No internal Doppler signal

Hematoma

Superficial and intramuscular hematoma can occur because of a wide range of causes, including trauma, surgical interventions, and coagulopathies. The sonographic appearance of hematomas can vary over time. In addition, there is an overlap of sonographic features that can be seen with sarcoma (eg, hemangiosarcoma or histiocytic sarcoma), which can have intralesional bleeding and fluid-filled cavities similar to what is seen in a

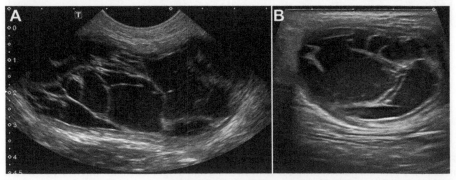

Fig. 3. Abdominal wall seroma. Longitudinal (*A*) and transverse (*B*) ultrasound images of the left inguinal subcutaneous region of an 11-year-old spayed female cat with a history of a firm palpable, partially encapsulated mass at the site of surgical resection of inguinal lymph nodes 1 month prior. A well-defined, thin-walled mass having internal anechoic fluid, multiple echogenic septations, and mobile echogenic particles is present in the postoperative left inguinal space. Sonographically, a seroma was suspect and confirmed with fluid analysis and negative culture.

hematoma. It is crucial to assess the history of the patient to make sure there is a potential cause for hematoma to not incorrectly misdiagnose a sarcoma for a hematoma.

Sonographic features of acute hematoma can include the following:

- Hyperechoic with variable linear hyperechogenicities or anechoic similar to seroma
- May have Doppler signal and sonographically change size when active bleeding is present

Sonographic features of chronic hematoma can include the following:

- Hypoechoic with variable degree of linear hyperechogenicities
- No Doppler signal

Abscess

Soft tissue infections are a common reason animals are seen by a veterinarian. Abscesses can be well defined (**Fig. 4**) or ill-defined from the surrounding tissue and have anechoic to hyperechoic content (**Fig. 5**). When an abscess is superficial, gentle compression of the soft tissue while real-time ultrasound scanning can allow assessing for mobile fluid within the mass; this can help to differentiate an abscess from a soft tissue mass.

Common sonographic features of an abscess include the following:

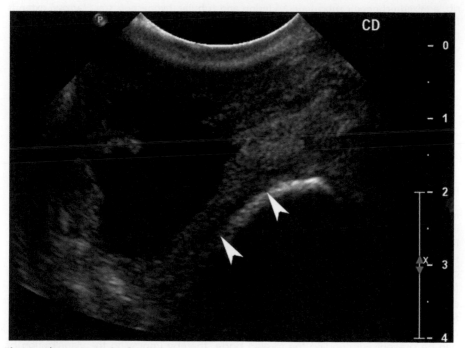

Fig. 4. Abscess. Longitudinal ultrasound image of a 12-year-old spayed female Labrador retriever with a history of a recurrent swelling on the dorsal aspect of the head. A well-defined, irregularly marginated, encapsulated mass with a thick wall and central fluid-attenuating area is noted. The adjacent bone (*arrowheads*) is well defined, smooth, and normal. An abscess was sonographically suspected and confirmed with fine needle aspiration.

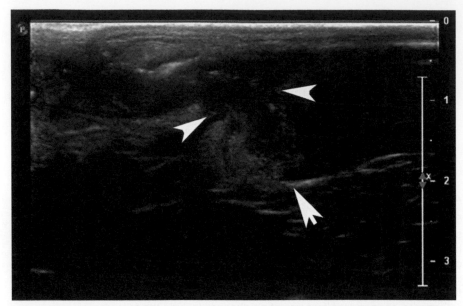

Fig. 5. Abdominal wall abscess with sinus tract. Longitudinal image of the left dorsolateral abdominal wall. In the lateral abdominal subcutaneous soft tissues caudal to the thirteenth rib, a mixed echogenic subcutaneous lesion and tubular, hypoechoic tract (*arrow*) extends from the subcutaneous tissue to the craniolateral abdominal body wall, displacing the peritoneum (*arrowheads*) medially. No perforation into the peritoneal cavity was identified, which was significant to the surgical planning for this patient.

- Well- or ill-defined from surrounding soft tissue
- A peripheral hyperechoic capsule may be seen
- Variable shape
- Anechoic to hypoechoic mobile content
- No internal vascular flow
- Peripheral hypervascularity

FOREIGN BODY

Foreign bodies in superficial structures occur commonly and are often not identified on initial clinical examination. Ultrasound is an excellent imaging technique to identify these foreign bodies. In addition, ultrasound can be used to assist in surgical retrieval of these foreign bodies.[2,3] Foreign bodies are typically echogenic without or with acoustic shadowing. The echogenicity and pattern of the foreign body are very dependent on the foreign body type. Glass and metal foreign bodies are usually echogenic, may produce a comet-tail artifact (**Fig. 6**), and can cause acoustic shadowing. Plant (**Fig. 7**) and wood foreign bodies may have a characteristic shape, are echogenic, and may have partial or complete acoustic shadowing.[4,5] Fluid or a small hypoechoic rim of granulation tissue can be present surrounding the foreign body, thereby improving the visualization of the foreign body. In addition, the adjacent soft tissue is often heterogenous in echogenicity because of foreign body reaction or migration.[6] When extensive cellulitis is present, identification of a foreign body can be challenging and hindered by the hyperechoic strands of tissue commonly present with cellulitis or subcutaneous emphysema (because of penetrating wound or gas-producing bacteria).

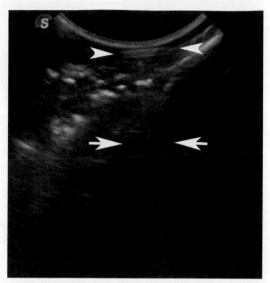

Fig. 6. Metal foreign body. Longitudinal ultrasound image of the soft palate after previous surgical procedure to localize a fragmented small metallic medical device. In the thickened soft palate, a linear hyperechoic foreign body (*arrowheads*) causing a comet-tail artifact (*arrows*) is noted in the near field. Cranial to this linear foreign body, the soft tissues contain multiple small hyperechoic focal areas with small reverberation artifacts consistent with gas likely owing to the recent surgical intervention. Ultrasound was used to guide successful surgical removal of the metallic foreign body.

NEOPLASMS

Superficial subcutaneous tumors occur commonly in dogs and cats, and differentiating the type and extent of the tumor is crucial in treatment planning and prognosis. Superficial tumors can easily be imaged using ultrasound.

Lipoma

Lipomas are one of the most common benign soft tissue tumors. They are frequently located in the skin or muscles, and less commonly within the thorax or abdomen. On palpation, lipomas tend to be soft to rubbery, mobile, and not painful. Common sonographic features of lipomas include the following:

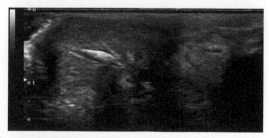

Fig. 7. Grass awn foreign body. Longitudinal image of the soft tissues on the palmar aspect of the metacarpus of a 5-year-old dog. A spindle-shaped, hyperechoic structure with thin linear hyperechoic strands is noted in the soft tissues palmar to the metacarpal bones. This is classic for a grass floret with awns foreign body. The foreign body was surgically removed using ultrasound guidance.

- Smooth margination, frequently oval to lobulated in shape and well-defined form surrounding soft tissue (**Fig. 8**)
- Often longer than wide
- Frequently hypoechoic to isoechoic[7] to adjacent normal subcutaneous fat and contain wavy hyperechoic striations
- Homogenous echotexture with wavy to linear internal striations and otherwise uniform internal echogenicity[7]
- No acoustic shadowing is present
- Minimal or no deep enhancement
- Usually no or very minimal Doppler signal

Malignant Neoplasms

A wide range of superficial malignancies are reported with sarcomas, and mast cell tumors are more commonly reported in some canine breeds; fibrosarcoma, squamous cell carcinoma, mast cell tumors, and basal cell tumors are more commonly reported in cats.[8] Malignant neoplasms, including sarcomas, are often sonographically a mixed group of mass lesions with variable echogenicity, shape, and vascularity (**Fig. 9**); additionally, they can be solid or can have internal fluid-filled areas. The following sonographic features should raise concern that the mass is malignant and should prompt further investigation:

- Larger size
- Deep or intramuscular location
- Extending across tissue planes
- Rapid growth
- Heterogenous echogenicity[9]
- Pain
- Fluid collections without history of trauma or other good clinical cause

Abdominal Wall Injury or Hernia

The diagnosis of abdominal wall injuries and hernias is not always straightforward, especially when patients are obese, and various imaging modalities can be used to

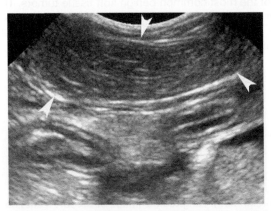

Fig. 8. Subcutaneous lipoma. In the subcutaneous tissue of the caudal abdominal wall, a well-defined, heterogeneous, hypoechoic, small mass with fine linear hyperechoic striations consistent with lipoma is noted (*arrowheads*). Fine needle aspiration supported the index of suspicion for lipoma.

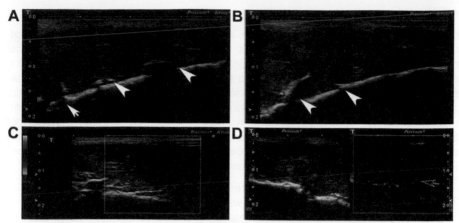

Fig. 9. Hemangiosarcoma. Longitudinal B-mode (*A, B*) images of the medial aspect of the left tibia illustrating a heterogeneous, indistinctly defined soft tissue mass with adjacent periosteal remodeling (*arrowheads*) and permeative cortical lysis (*arrow*) of the tibia. Using color Doppler ultrasound (*C*), no vascular flow, and with microvascular imaging, a highly sensitive new Doppler imaging technique (*D*) minimal vascular flow (*dotted arrow*) is noted. Ultrasound-guided fine needle aspirates revealed a sarcoma. Full-thickness biopsies confirmed hemangiosarcoma.

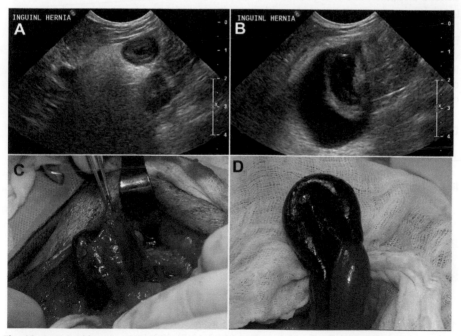

Fig. 10. Inguinal hernia with displacement and wall necrosis of a segment of jejunum. Transverse ultrasound image (*A*) reveals that the inguinal canal is increased in width, and a loop of jejunum and mesenteric fat is extending through the inguinal canal into the peri-inguinal subcutaneous tissue. (*B*) The segment of jejunum after passing through the inguinal canal has a moderately reduced wall layer definition, is increased in width, amotile, and surrounded cranially by anechoic fluid. (*C*) In surgery, a widened inguinal canal with fat and jejunum passing through the canal and into the subcutaneous tissue is noted. (*D*) The segment of jejunum in the subcutaneous tissue is severely hyperemic and was resected.

gain additional information. Ultrasound is a great real-time technique to further evaluate hernias. Displacement of abdominal organs into these abdominal wall defects may only be seen when the abdominal pressure is increased, for example, during coughing or with manual pressure applied externally to the afflicted body cavity. While performing the examination, gentle abdominal compression, or changing the patient's position during the ultrasound examination can cause dynamic displacement of herniating abdominal structures, which may then be observed and can allow further assessment of the abdominal wall defect. Using ultrasound, the layers of muscles and fascia of the abdominal wall can be delineated[9] and allow for visualization of defects (**Fig. 10**). Ultrasound criteria for a hernia include the following:

- Widening of the inguinal canal or presence of an abdominal wall defect
- Abnormal separation of abdominal wall layers
- Displacement of omentum, peritoneal fat, or intestines into the hernia

SUMMARY

Ultrasound is an effective initial imaging technique to evaluate superficial soft tissue swellings and masses. Ultrasound offers several unique advantages compared with other imaging techniques, including real-time dynamic imaging during compression to assess for the presence of an abscess or alternating the position of the animal to assess displacement of organs in a hernia as well as the use of ultrasound during surgical foreign body removal. In addition, ultrasound provides a minimally invasive means of obtaining image-guided fine needle or biopsy samples. Furthermore, Doppler ultrasound imaging can assist in the noninvasive assessment of blood flow, which can aid in delineating cysts, lipomas, and abscesses from neoplasms given differences in blood flow pattern. Ultrasound is an excellent modality to identify fluid accumulations, but the diagnosis of hematoma should be made with caution to not delay diagnosis of a malignant neoplasia, such as a sarcoma.

DISCLOSURE

The author has nothing to disclose.

REFERENCES

1. Wagner JM, Lamprich BK. Ultrasonography of lumps and bumps. Ultrasound Clin 2014;9(3):373–90.

2. Della Santa D, Rossi F, Carlucci F, et al. Ultrasound-guided retrieval of plant awns. Vet Radiol Ultrasound 2008;49(5):484–6.

3. Stades FC, Djajadiningrat-Laanen SC, Boroffka SA, et al. Suprascleral removal of a foreign body from the retrobulbar muscle cone in two dogs. J Small Anim Pract 2003;44(1):17–20.

4. Gnudi G, Volta A, Bonazzi M, et al. Ultrasonographic features of grass awn migration in the dog. Vet Radiol Ultrasound 2005;46(5):423–6.

5. Armbrust LJ, Biller DS, Radlinsky MG, et al. Ultrasonographic diagnosis of foreign bodies associated with chronic draining tracts and abscesses in dogs. Vet Radiol Ultrasound 2003;44(1):66–70.

6. Frendin J, Funkquist B, Hansson K, et al. Diagnostic imaging of foreign body reactions in dogs with diffuse back pain. J Small Anim Pract 1999;40(6): 278–85.

7. Nyman HT, Kristensen AT, Lee MH, et al. Characterization of canine superficial tumors using gray-scale B mode, color flow mapping, and spectral Doppler ultrasonography–a multivariate study. Vet Radiol Ultrasound 2006;47(2):192–8.
8. Ho NT, Smith KC, Dobromylskyj MJ. Retrospective study of more than 9000 feline cutaneous tumours in the UK: 2006–2013. J Feline Med Surg 2018;20(2):128–34.
9. Stieger-Vanegas SM. POCUS: Musculoskeletal – soft tissue. Point-of-care ultrasound techniques for the small animal practitioner 2021:647-661.

Section V: Focused Ultrasound of the Eye

Ocular Ultrasound Abnormalities and Optic Nerve Sheath Diameter in Dogs and Cats

Jane Cho, DVM, DACVO

KEYWORDS

- Point-of-care • Ocular ultrasound • Hyphema • Retinal detachments
- Exophthalmos • Secondary glaucoma • Ocular tumors

KEY POINTS

- Ocular ultrasonography can be a helpful and sometimes essential adjunct to eye examination when the globe itself is opaque or not directly visible. A good ophthalmic examination is needed to correlate all findings.
- Ocular ultrasonography is relatively easy and generally can be done awake under topical anesthesia only.
- Results of ocular ultrasonography can help determine whether a case ultimately is medical or surgical, the prognosis for the eye and life, and whether and when specialty referral is needed.
- Comparison to the fellow or normal eye can be helpful in understanding ultrasound findings.
- Orbital disease can be defined better and, in some cases diagnosed, utilizing ocular ultrasound with or without additional testing (eg, fine needle aspiration).

INTRODUCTION

All veterinary ocular complaints necessitate a good ocular examination,[1] but a diagnosis cannot always be reached with clinical examination alone. If an eye is opaque or is not visible or there is suspicion of orbital disease or trauma, ocular ultrasound can be helpful in narrowing a differential list and arriving at a more accurate diagnostic and treatment plan. In many cases, a diagnostic ocular ultrasound can provide enough information to avoid more costly imaging methods, help provide an initial prognosis for vison and the globe, and decide if a surgical or medical plan is most appropriate.[2] Ocular ultrasound cannot substitute for a full ocular examination[1] and a basic

Veterinary Eye Specialists PLLC, 620 Commerce Street, Thornwood, NY 10594, USA
E-mail address: jcdacvo@gmail.com
Website: https://www.vesny.com

Vet Clin Small Anim 51 (2021) 1295–1314
https://doi.org/10.1016/j.cvsm.2021.07.010
0195-5616/21/© 2021 Elsevier Inc. All rights reserved.

vetsmall.theclinics.com

understanding of ophthalmic anatomy and disease still always is required to utilize imaging information correctly.

Discussion of treatment of ocular pathology is beyond the scope of this article. Readers are referred to clinical ophthalmology texts for further diagnostic and therapeutic steps.[3]

INDICATIONS FOR OCULAR ULTRASOUND

- Opaque or cloudy eye: cannot visualize through the ocular media (**Fig. 1**A-1F)
- Ocular or orbital trauma: to evaluate (cautiously) for globe integrity in cases of severe trauma (**Fig. 1**G)
- Bulging eye: to differentiate exophthalmos (the protruding normal-sized globe) from buphthalmos (the enlarged globe) and to sonographically define a suspected space-occupying orbital lesion (**Fig. 1**H, 1I)
- Swollen periocular tissues: lids and/or conjunctival swelling prevents viewing the globe directly
- To evaluate other orbital conditions: in cases of the globe itself not visible (apparent microphthalmos, anophthalmos,[4] and phthisis), to evaluate for other orbital disease (cellulitis, foreign bodies,[5] and so forth) (**Fig. 1**J-1L)

OBJECTIVES OF OCULAR ULTRASOUND

To identify the location, size, and shape of normal and abnormal ocular and periocular structures and to better identify the existence of pathology warranting specific treatment, thus optimizing preservation of vision and the globe.

ULTRASOUND SETTINGS

For imaging the globe, the ultrasound probe with the highest frequency available should be used.

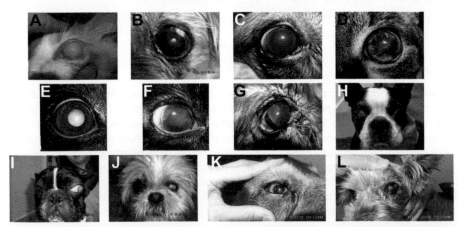

Fig. 1. Indications for ultrasound. Opacity in the visual axis can prevent directly viewing the intraocular structures, including (*A*) corneal edema, (*B*) corneal pigmentation and scarring, (*C*) hyphema, (*D*) synechia, (*E*) cataract, (*F*) other structures in the anterior chamber, and (*G*) severe trauma. Ultrasound also can help distinguish between (*G*) exophthalmos and (*I*) buphthalmos and help better define (*J*) a small eye, (*K*) orbital cellulitis, or (*L*) suspected orbital foreign body. (Courtesy of Dr Jane Cho, Veterinary Eye Specialists, PLLC, Thornwood, New York, and Point-of-care Ultrasound Techniques, Wiley-Blackwell ©2021)

- A 7.5-MHz probe is adequate for imaging deeper structures (orbit). A 5-MHz probe may be acceptable for detecting deeper large lesions at the expense of losing detail. A probe 7.5-MHz or higher provides better detail in the nearer fields.
- A probe with a small scan head diameter (linear or sector) is preferred.
- A "small parts" or "eye" setting or other adjustments in the settings of the machine should be made to optimize focus in the near field (1–5 cm).
- A foot pedal, if available, is helpful for hands-free freezing of images.
- Gain can be adjusted during the examination to highlight certain structures.

PATIENT EYE PREPARATION

1. Topical anesthesia is required for placement of the probe on the ocular surface. Several drops of ophthalmic proparacaine, tetracaine, or another appropriate topical ophthalmic anesthetic over 1 minute to 2 minutes (may be in the refrigerator) are usually adequate.
2. If adequate topical anesthetic effect is not achieved with 5 drops to 6 drops over 2 minutes, chemical restraint may be needed (or use of the retrobulbar view might be considered). If sedation is used, this should be adjusted to the lightest anesthetic plane needed. Resulting changes in globe position may make scanning more difficult.
3. A sterile, viscous, aqueous-based ultrasound gel without alcohol that is nontoxic to the eye and ocular surfaces should be used. The author routinely uses Aquasonic 100 (Parker Laboratories, Fairfield, New Jersey) brand ultrasound gel, a commonly used and readily available ultrasound gel, on the intact ocular surface, with no ill effects.[5] Aquasonic also is available in sterile form. Gels, such as K-Y (Reckitt Benckiser, Slough, Berkshire, England), ophthalmic 2.5% methylcellulose gel, and other forms of over-the-counter gel-type artificial tears (not ointment) can be used; however, these are much less viscous and may be more difficult to use. In cases of possible globe rupture, a sterile gel should be used; or, use a transpalpebral or retrobulbar view.
4. The probe should be cleaned well and dried according to manufacturer's instructions before placement on the eye.
5. If a standoff is needed for imaging the anterior, most superficial parts of the eye, either a thicker layer of gel or a water-filled glove may be used, although the latter can be unwieldy.
6. All gel should be flushed gently and completely off the ocular surfaces with sterile saline eyewash immediately after the examination. Fluorescein staining of the cornea after the examination is recommended.

PERFORMING OCULAR ULTRASOUND

The animal should be able to sit, lie sternal, or stand normally in a comfortable position (**Fig. 2**). If sitting or standing, make sure the animal is not allowed to scoot or slide backwards (see **Fig. 2**A). At least 1 assistant is needed to hold the animal's head still. Additional assistance holding the eyelids open and working the freeze button may be needed.

Ascertain the probe orientation to obtain the view desired (discussed later). If using a vertical view, align the top of the probe dorsally. Place a dollop of ultrasound gel on the probe and (for direct globe imaging) and place the dollop directly on the cornea (see **Fig. 2**B), taking care to maintain a layer of gel 3-mm to 10-mm thick between the probe and the cornea. Avoid pressing the probe into the eye.

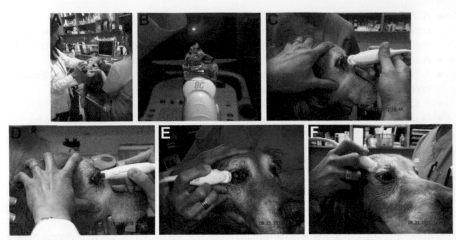

Fig. 2. Ultrasound procedure. (*A*) Ocular ultrasound setup. The patient and screen should face the same direction. Be ready to freeze images using a freeze pedal or assistant. (*B*) Apply a large amount of eye-safe gel to the probe first, and maintain a 3-mm to 10-mm standoff layer of gel. (*C*) The vertical probe position divides the globe into lateral and medial parts. (*D*) The horizontal probe position divides the globe into upper and lower sections. (*E*) The equatorial/lateral probe position divides the globe into anterior and posterior sections. (*F*) The retrobulbar probe position directs the probe from back to front. Images obtained using this view will not be of as good quality as those obtained with corneal contact. The room lights may be dimmed according to sonographer preference. (Courtesy of Dr Jane Cho, Veterinary Eye Specialists, PLLC, Thornwood, New York, and Point-of-care Ultrasound Techniques, Wiley-Blackwell ©2021)

Be mindful of the direction of the patient's gaze. Look at the position of the other eye and the facial muscles for help in orienting the images of the eye being evaluated.

Performing the scan first at higher gain, then at lower gain, allows for differentiation of smaller, more subtle, and lower-intensity lesions.[2]

If images are saved, make sure to correctly label which eye was imaged and for orientation.

VIEW OPTIONS

Vertical (bisecting the globe into medial and lateral halves): place the probe on the central cornea such that the top of the screen shows the dorsal aspect of the globe (see **Fig. 2**C) to image the globe from the anterior to the posterior pole. Sweep the probe, moving the point of contact from one side of the cornea to the other, imaging the entire globe. Alternately, pivot the angle of the probe while keeping the probe contact point stationary.

Horizontal (bisecting the globe into top and bottom halves): place the probe on the central cornea with the "top" of the probe either medial or lateral. The probe then is swept/angled from top to bottom (see **Fig. 2**D).

Equatorial/lateral (bisecting the globe into anterior and posterior halves) (see **Fig. 2**E): place the probe parallel to the iris from the lateral aspect of the globe, sweeping/angling the probe from front to back. This may not be possible to do in eyes that are deep-set, and ability to use this may depend on the angle of gaze; this view is not as commonly used as the Vertical or Horizontal views.

Transpalpebral: any of these views may be performed with the probe on the closed eyelids rather than directly on the cornea. Topical anesthesia is less necessary with any view where the probe is placed on the skin than with any view where the probe is placed directly on the globe due to the lack of eyeball contact, and injury to the cornea less likely, but image quality likely is reduced, and direct visualization of globe position is not possible, making orientation of images less certain. The closed lid may serve as a standoff, which may be helpful in some instances.

Retrobulbar (from behind the orbital ligament, directed from the back to the front of the eye) (see **Fig. 2**F): palpate the orbital ligament and feel for the slight depression behind it. Palpating the other side to locate the ligament may be needed, because orbital injury often is what necessitates this view. Thoroughly wet down or clip the haired skin behind the orbital ligament and place the probe there pointing toward the front of the eye. A thick layer of gel is not needed. Although this view produces an inferior quality image, it may be safer than directly imaging on the globe if the cornea or globe might be ruptured.

In cases of suspected globe rupture (gross hyphema, hypotony [low intraocular pressure (IOP)], or visible globe deformation/deflation), if imaging is required, a transpalpebral or retrobulbar view is preferred, to prevent contamination of the intraocular space. Do not press on the globe or lids, to prevent further damage.

ULTRASONOGRAPHIC FINDINGS IN A NORMAL EYE

When imaging using the vertical or horizontal view, under the layer of gel, the most superficial structure seen is the cornea, represented by 2 very thin bright parallel curved lines (the anterior and posterior corneal surfaces) about 1 mm apart (**Fig. 3**B)[6] or a single bright 1-mm thick curved line. If there is not enough standoff space, it may not be visible at all (**Table 1**).[2,7–10]

Just posterior to this is the anterior chamber. This always should be anechoic because it is filled with the aqueous humor, an acellular solution, and normally is approximately 3-mm to 5-mm deep in the central axis.[8] It is bordered posteriorly by the iris and axial anterior lens capsule and peripherally by the iridocorneal angle (which typically is not seen in any detail).

The iris might be visible as an area of increased echogenicity at the peripheral anterior aspect of the lens but often is not distinguishable. It should be thin with an approximately flat anterior surface. Pupil size may affect how easily it can be imaged.

The lens is directly behind the iris, and the anterior lens capsule may not be distinguishable from the iris where they are in contact. The lens capsule is a thin bright line surrounding the lens in an oval shape. It should be smooth and curvilinear and appears brightest along the central axis of the eye (axially) and image due to specular reflection and often disappears toward the periphery. The ability to see even a part of the lens capsule with its characteristic appearance allows the lens to be reliably located, especially when the lens is not in a normal position. The lens material inside the capsule generally is fairly anechoic, but it often is more hyperechoic than the aqueous humor in front of it and the vitreous body behind it and may not be uniform. Nuclear sclerosis and cataracts are variably echogenic structures within the normally hypoechoic lens. The lens normally always should be centered in the visual axis.

The lens zonules generally are not visible on standard ultrasound (this would require ultrahigh frequency). The ciliary body may be seen as a small mound of echogenic tissue behind the iris and peripheral to the lens equator but is also often not distinguishable.

Posterior to the lens is the vitreous body, composed mainly of water and collagen fibers. The vitreous normally is uniformly anechoic. Various vitreal abnormalities

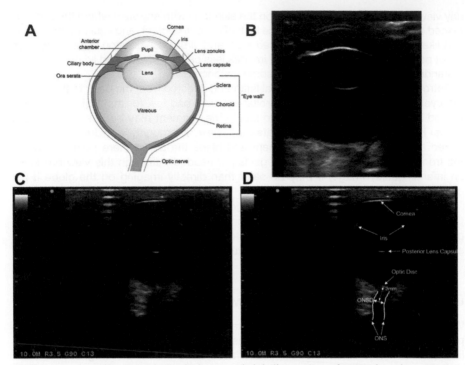

Fig. 3. Normal ocular anatomy and ultrasound. (*A*) Illustration of normal ocular anatomy. (*B*) Ultrasound image of a normal eye. Note the bright concave cornea anteriorly (*top*), the anechoic anterior chamber, the bright iris (*left*), the bright thin curved anterior and posterior lens capsules (axially), the anechoic vitreous, the convex posterior eye wall, and cone-shaped retrobulbar tissues. (*C, D*) The optic nerve. Just ventral to the posterior pole of the globe is the uniformly hypoechoic or anechoic, straight to slightly curved optic nerve, with hyperechoic parallel sides (*arrowheads* [*D*]) comprised by the thin optic nerve sheath and fat. The ONSD is measured as the distance between these two parallel sides at 3 mm posterior to the optic disc, as shown. This view was obtained with a standardized temporal transpalpebral view. (Courtesy of Dr Jane Cho, Veterinary Eye Specialists, PLLC, Thornwood, New York, and Point-of-care Ultrasound Techniques, Wiley-Blackwell ©2021. C) and D) From Smith et al. Transpalpebral ultrasonographic measurement of the optic nerve sheath diameter in healthy dogs. *J Vet Emerg Crit Care* 2018; 28(1): 31-38; with permission)

(asteroid hyalosis [**Fig. 4**D] and vitreal strands), however, may be present without being a clinically significant cause for disease.

Posterior to the vitreous is the posterior eye wall, a smooth and echogenic curved line representing the back of the globe. The posterior eye wall is made up of 3 thin layers (the retina, choroid, and sclera) that normally are so closely opposed to each other as not to be distinguishable from each other. In the vertical and horizontal views, all intraocular structures should be symmetric within the globe; asymmetry within the globe is abnormal.

Behind the globe, it may be possible to identify the hypoechoic optic nerve, originating just ventral to the back of the globe with a hyperechoic border made up of the optic nerve sheath and surrounding fat. This is surrounded by the broader hypoechoic extraocular muscle bellies oriented as a cone pointing toward the posterior orbit. Machine settings should be adjusted to image this deeper area, and no standoff is required. The optic nerve sheath diameter (OSND) is discussed further later.

Table 1
Normal findings

	Structure	Echo Appearance
Should always see	Anterior chamber	Should be anechoic
	Aanterior and posterior lens capsule	Thin bright line(s) of specular reflection curving backwards and forwards most visible along the central axis of the image (although where they meet peripherally often cannot be seen)
	Vitreous	Should be anechoic
	Posterior eye wall	Smooth curved bright white line with no hyperechoic adjoining structures most visible along the central axis of the image
Will often see	Cornea	Linear, uniform, moderately echogenic structure forming anterior eye wall—usually not visible without a thick layer of gel or a standoff
	Retrobulbar extraocular muscle cone	Hypoechoic muscle bellies originating around the optic nerve and converging at the back of the orbit, forming a cone
	Frontal bone	A bright hyperechoic angled line behind and ventromedial to globe
Might see	Iris	A very thin hyperechoic linear structure peripheral and anterior to, but not often distinguishable from, the anterior lens surface
	Optic nerve	A straight or curved hypoechoic linear structure from just below the globe's posterior pole with parallel linear borders, surrounded by the hyperechoic optic nerve sheath, fat, and the retrobulbar extraocular muscle cone
Should not see		Any hyperechoic structures in the anterior chamber or vitreous
		Any anechoic structures in the orbit (behind the globe)

Finally, a bright line representing the ventromedial bony wall of the orbit may be seen behind these retrobulbar soft tissue structures. This is a smooth and bright line that curves away from the globe ventrally.

Imaging the other eye for comparison often is helpful for distinguishing lesions and better identifying what is normal for that animal.[8,11]

INDICATIONS FOR OCULAR ULTRASOUND AND ABNORMAL FINDINGS
Anterior Lens Luxation

Clinical findings

- History: acute change in the eye (trauma not required); variable (**Table 2**)
- Signalment: terrier breeds but can occur in any dog or cat
- Eye examination: corneal edema—(usually central cornea); mydriasis; poor pupillary light response (PLR); may be unable to visualize intraocular structures; and high IOP, often over 30–40 mm Hg). Directing focal light from the side and across the anterior chamber may highlight a brightly reflective rim of the luxated lens in the peripheral anterior chamber. Signs of glaucoma may be present (scleral injection, negative menace and/or dazzle, diffuse corneal edema, blepharospasm, pain, and so forth).
- IOP elevation may be absent in some chronic cases

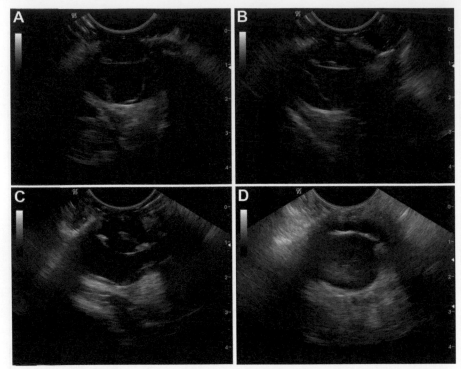

Fig. 4. Posterior segment: retinal detachments and asteroid hyalosis. (*A*) The hyperechoic detached retina is still attached at the optic nerve and has a gull wing shape, in this case with an anechoic subretinal space. (*B*) A different view of this same eye shows the detached retina extending toward the ora serrata, the other natural anatomic attachment point. (*C*) The detached retina may be close and/or parallel to the posterior eye wall, a so-called flat detachment. (*D*) Asteroid hyalosis typically appears as an amorphous, fairly uniform, semi-mobile echogenic material anywhere in the normally anechoic vitreous, often in the central vitreous. (Courtesy of Dr Jane Cho, Veterinary Eye Specialists, PLLC, Thornwood, New Yor,k and Point-of-care Ultrasound Techniques, Wiley-Blackwell ©2021)

Ultrasonographic findings

- No lens in normal location
- Lens in anterior chamber: sometimes can see an anechoic lens-shaped structure with its thin bright capsule in the anterior chamber; anterior chamber may be abnormally deep (see **Figs. 5**C and **7**B).
- Mobile, thin, amorphous strands in vitreous might be present.
- Possible retinal detachment

Because acute anterior lens luxation causing acute glaucoma may be treatable with a chance to save vision, this can be an emergent situation requiring immediate referral for possible surgery. Do not give mydriatics (tropicamide, atropine) or miotics (latanoprost, pilocarpine) because these may exacerbate glaucoma; refer to clinical texts for further information. Note that if the globe already is buphthalmic and blind; the glaucoma has been chronic and is not an emergency.

Hyphema

Clinical findings

- History: red color noted; vision loss; trauma not required

Table 2
Types of abnormal ultrasonographic findings and possible causes[2]

Deep Anterior chamber	• Buphthalmos • Posterior lens (sub)luxation (**Fig. 5D**) • Prior lens removal surgery (aphakia)
Shallow anterior chamber	• Mass in anterior chamber (**Fig. 6A–C**) • Anterior synechiae • Intumescent cataract (see **Fig. 5A**) • Iatrogenic (compressing cornea with probe) • Ruptured cornea with loss of aqueous humor • Aqueous misdirection syndrome (rare and only in cats)
Echogenic material in anterior chamber	• Anterior lens luxation (see **Figs. 5C; Fig. 7C**) • Blood, fibrin, and/or cells in anterior chamber • Cyst(s) in anterior chamber[12] • Anterior synechiae • Iris (or other) mass (see **Fig. 6A–C**) • Foreign body (rare)
Echogenic lens material within lens capsule	• Cataract (varying degrees and distribution of echogenicity possible)[2] • Nuclear sclerosis • Gain turned too high • Artificial intraocular lens implant due to prior cataract surgery (lens implant would be thinner than a normal lens, and hyperechoic)
Abnormal lens shape or size	• Hypermature cataract (lens smaller than normal) • Intumescent cataract (lens larger than normal) (see **Fig. 5A**) • Cells or other material adherent to lens surface (eg, as occurs with lens capsule rupture or persistent hyaloid remnant) • Lenticonus (rare)
Abnormal lens location	• Lens subluxation or luxation (see **Fig. 5D** and **7B**)
Echogenic structure(s) in posterior segment	• Vitreal degeneration • Asteroid hyalosis (see **Fig. 4D**) • Vitreal hemorrhage and fibrin • Posterior lens luxation (see **Fig. 5D**) • Retinal detachment (see **Fig. 4A–C**) • Retinal hemorrhage • Mass or other abnormal accumulation of cells in posterior segment • Foreign body[5] • Hyaloid vessel remnant • Marked optic nerve head swelling
Abnormal globe shape	• Scleral or corneal rupture (see **Fig. 1G; Fig. 8**) • Phthisis bulbi (see **Fig. 1J**)

(continued on next page)

Table 2 (*continued*)	
	• Large intraocular or scleral mass deforming globe • Retrobulbar mass (indenting posterior globe) (**Fig. 9**) • Staphyloma or coloboma • Scleral thickening
Abnormal globe size	• Buphthalmos due to chronic glaucoma (see **Figs. 1I and 7**) • Phthisis bulbi or microphthalmos (see **Fig. 1J**)
Masslike structure in or around eye	• Neoplasia (see **Fig. 6**) • Inflammation/granuloma • Blood clots and hemorrhage (**Fig. 8**) • Foreign body (rare)[5] • Displaced, enlarged, or swollen normal tissue • Cystic structure
Poor image quality	• Air under lids or in gel • Eye or patient motion • Inadequate amount of gel • Settings on machine (gain, probe type, zoom, etc.) require adjustment • Technical probe or machine issues

- Signalment: variable
- Eye examination: reduced or absent PLR, menace, and dazzle; blood in anterior chamber obscuring iris; variable mydriasis; anisocoria; conjunctival hyperemia; possible retinal hemorrhages, generalized red color from behind pupil, or retinal detachment; signs of trauma; IOP elevation

Ultrasonographic findings

- Diffuse echogenic material in the anterior chamber, obscuring the iris and/or lens
- Possible iris or ciliary body mass possibly displacing the lens (see **Fig. 6**)
- Echogenic areas in the vitreous, which could be vitreal hemorrhage, vitreal degeneration, retinal detachment, mass, foreign body, posteriorly luxated lens, or other structures.[5,13,14]
- If gross trauma is present, carefully evaluate the integrity of the eye wall[15] (discussed later).
- In the absence of trauma, 2 of the most common causes for spontaneous unilateral hyphema in older dogs are retinal detachment and intraocular neoplasia.

Retinal Detachment

Clinical findings

- History: possible acute or subacute vision loss; anisocoria; trauma not required
- Signalment: variable.
- Eye examination: unilateral or bilateral reduced or absent PLR, menace and dazzle; hyphema; mydriasis; possible retinal hemorrhages or generalized red color from behind pupil; visible retinal detachment on fundic examination; anterior uveitis.

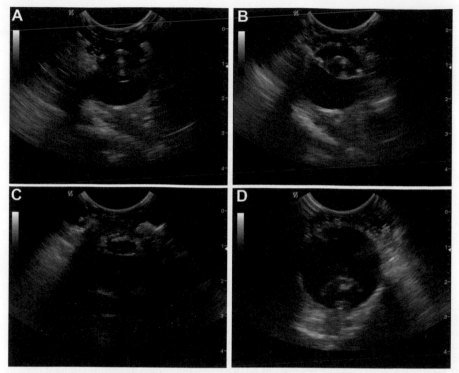

Fig. 5. Lens abnormalities. Shallow anterior chamber. (*A*) A swollen lens due to an intumescent cataract can cause the anterior chamber to look shallow, compared with (*B*), the fellow eye of the same dog with a normal sized cataractous lens. (*C*) Anterior lens luxation. The hyperechoic lens capsule is absent from its normal location, and is right behind the cornea. (*D*) Posterior lens luxation. The hyperechoic lens capsule is absent from its normal location and is clearly visible along the posterior eye wall. The globe also is buphthalmic.

Ultrasonographic findings

- Retinal/vitreal hemorrhages appear as indistinct echogenic areas of variable size and location anywhere within the normally anechoic vitreous.
- The retinal detachment itself appears as a thin bright continuous curvilinear structure in the posterior segment that can be followed back to the optic nerve head—often making a V-shape or Y-shape (a "gull wing" appearance) (see **Fig. 4**A). The shape is variable, because detachments may be partial, or more separated from the eye wall in some places than others, making a variably wavy line. In the author's experience, it always is attached at the optic nerve head.
- The retina often remains attached at the ora serrata (junction between retina and ciliary body) (see **Fig. 4**B).
- Retinal detachments may be bullous (retina widely separated from the posterior eye wall) or flat (retina close to and parallel to the posterior eye wall) (see **Fig.** 4C).
- Uncommonly, there may be discontinuities (tears or holes) in the detached retina.
- Often accompanied by other echogenic structures (vitreal strands, hemorrhage, and asteroid hyalosis) (see **Fig. 4**B) in the posterior segment.
- The subretinal space is more often hypoechoic (serous retinal detachment) than echogenic (indicating subretinal blood, cells or a mass) and usually is more hypoechoic than either the retina or the posterior eye wall.

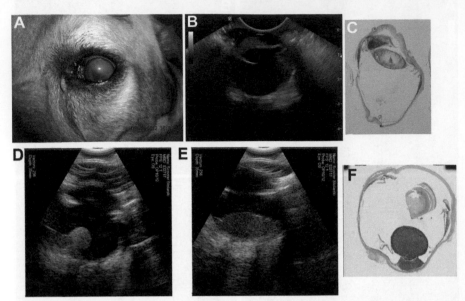

Fig. 6. Anterior chamber mass in a dog. (*A*) Focal corneal edema obscures the intraocular contents of the left eye of this 9-year-old dog, which is blind and glaucomatous. (*B*) A large, uniformly echogenic mass is in the anterior chamber, originating from the iris and slightly displacing the lens. The mass has rounded, distinct borders but the rest of the eye is normal. (*C*) Histopathology revealed the mass to be uveal melanocytoma. Posterior segment mass in a dog. (*D, E*) A large, uniformly echogenic, lobulated, broad-based structure is seen along the posterior eye wall in the eye of this 7-year-old dog. Different probe angles used in (*D*) and (*E*) reveal different aspects of its shape. (*F*) Histopathology revealed the mass to be a lobulated choroidal melanocytoma. The complete lens is not present due to processing artifact. (Courtesy of Dr Jane Cho, Veterinary Eye Specialists, PLLC, Thornwood, New York, and Point-of-care Ultrasound Techniques, Wiley-Blackwell ©2021)

Intraocular Masses

Clinical findings

- History: variable; may be incidental finding unless glaucoma or hyphema present
- Signalment: variable but generally middle-aged to older animals
- Eye examination: findings can include outward focal bulging of eye wall; intraocular hemorrhage; dyscoria, iris discoloration and/or thickening; visible mass; lens subluxation; retinal detachment; secondary glaucoma.

Ultrasonographic findings can include

- An outward bulge in the normally spherical eye wall with a solid hyperechoic mass just underneath
- Vitreal hemorrhage, vitreal strands, retinal detachment, and/or rarely a foreign body[5]
- Iris thickening if the mass is primary iridal neoplasia
- Masses often are broad-based (typically originating on or near the eye wall), sessile, uniformly echogenic, rounded with a distinct border, and often not pedunculated, although depending on the mass shape, may appear pedunculated at a particular viewing angle (**Fig. 6**D, 6E).[16]

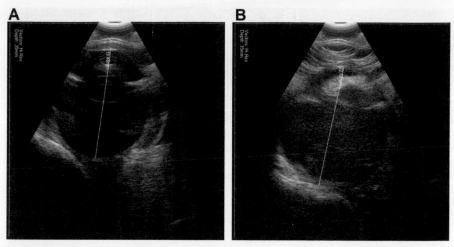

Fig. 7. Measuring globe size. Measure the globe at the widest front-to-back diameter and comparing to the normal/fellow eye. (*A*) The normal eye, this anteroposterior diameter is 19.48 mm. (*B*) The larger fellow eye (which has an anterior lens luxation) is 22.02 mm. Note that the posterior lens capsule is visible in the normal position in (*A*) but not in (*B*).

- The most common type in dogs (uveal melanoma) originates at the iris or ciliary body, possibly causing lens subluxation (see **Fig. 6**B).
- The most common type in cats (diffuse iris melanoma) may be seen as generalized or multifocal iris thickening and less like a focal mass.
- Differentiate masses from uveal cysts, which are thin-walled, anechoic within the cyst, possibly multiple, free-floating in the anterior chamber or vitreous, or attached to the posterior iris, pupil margin or peripheral retina.[12]
- Color flow or power Doppler might show blood flow within a mass.

Vitreal Hemorrhage

Clinical findings

- History: variable (trauma not necessary).
- Signalment: variable.
- Eye examination: hyphema, red or red-black haze from posterior segment; fundus not visible; variable pupil size and PLR. Variable clinical signs depending on cause

Ultrasonographic findings

- Variably sized and variably shaped structure(s) within the vitreous with poorly defined borders that quiver with eye motion but not necessarily gravity-dependent; may be densely and uniformly hyperechoic or heterogenous; may be near eye wall (where the original bleeding occurred)
- Often associated with thin, indistinct vitreal strands
- Differentiate from asteroid hyalosis (see **Fig. 4**D) and a solid intraocular mass (see **Fig. 6**).
- May be associated with retinal detachment, intraocular masses and/or scleral rupture (see **Figs. 6 and 8**)

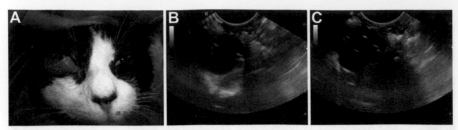

Fig. 8. Retrobulbar mass/exophthalmos. (*A*) This 10-year-old cat has had progressive exophthalmos for 3 weeks to 4 weeks. Note the exophthalmos, elevated nictitans, chemosis, and globe deviation dorsally. (*B*) A distinct rounded echogenic mass is behind and indenting the globe. (*C*) At another angle, a larger more hypoechoic area extends from the mass, causing further distortion to the normal globe contour. (Courtesy of Dr Jane Cho, Veterinary Eye Specialists, PLLC, Thornwood, New York, and Point-of-care Ultrasound Techniques, Wiley-Blackwell ©2021)

Asteroid Hyalosis

Clinical findings

- History: usually no problems noted by owner
- Signalment: often 10+ years.
- Eye examination: multiple (dozens to hundreds) of tiny white dots suspended in the vitreous; ay be regional in the eye and unilateral or bilateral

Ultrasonographic findings

- Indistinct, uniform, mildly echogenic structure(s) usually in the central vitreous, usually with an anechoic peripheral vitreal border (see **Fig. 4**D). Higher gain may reveal multiple tiny hyperechoic dots within the larger less echoic mass of asteroid. Often quivers when the eye moves; also may be seen with vitreal strands.
- Must be differentiated from other, more pathologic causes of hyperechoic structures in the vitreous

THE BULGING EYE: EXOPHTHALMOS VERSUS BUPHTHALMOS

Distinguishing between exophthalmos (globe being pushed out of orbit) and buphthalmos (globe enlargement), which clinically can look similar, is key to choosing the right treatment plan when the eye is bulging (see **Fig. 1**H, I).

Exophthalmos

Clinical findings

- History: variable, may be acute or gradual onset
- Signalment: variable
- Eye examination findings include globe protrusion, reduced globe retropulsion compared to normal side; globe same size as other eye; globe deviation, often without strabismus; reduced ocular motility; elevated nictitans; secondary lagophthalmos and central corneal exposure; focal fundic indentation; variable changes in vision and IOP (often normal); intact menace, PLR, and vision.
- Physical examination abnormalities can include facial asymmetry, palpable abnormalities of the orbital rim and bridge of the nose; ipsilateral dental or nasal

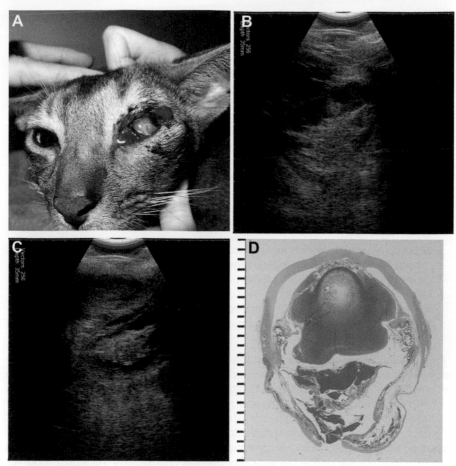

Fig. 9. Globe trauma. (*A*) This 3-year-old male Abyssinian sustained unknown trauma out-doors, causing a central corneal rupture and hyphema. (*B, C*) Extensive disorganized echogenic material mixed with smaller anechoic areas fill the globe, and neither the lens nor posterior eye wall is distinguishable. These two images were scans taken of the eye in (*A*) and (*D*) with the probe held at different angles. (*D*) Histopathology confirms retinal detachment, expulsive vitreal and subretinal hemorrhage, posterior scleral rupture, cataract, and lens capsule rupture. A ballistic foreign body was suspected. (Courtesy of Dr Jane Cho, Veterinary Eye Specialists, PLLC, Thornwood, New York, and Point-of-care Ultrasound Techniques, Wiley-Blackwell ©2021)

disease, distortion or inflammation in caudal soft palate; pain on opening mouth; local lymphadenopathy.

Ultrasonographic findings

- Affected globe is normal size (discussed later). Compare with the other eye.
- Possible globe indentation posteriorly (see **Fig. 9**) (more consistent with a mass or cyst than cellulitis)
- Mass effect of variable echotexture with variably discrete borders behind the globe.[17] Hyperechogenicity versus hypoechogenicity is not necessarily predictive of the etiology of a retrobulbar mass.[18]

- o Cellulitis/abscesses usually have indistinct borders and variable echogenicity and echotexture and obliterate/obscure normal structures.
- o Cystic structures typically are marginated more sharply with anechoic interior
- o Neoplastic masses tend to be more discrete (than cellulitis/abscess) and more uniform but may have cavitation, indistinct borders, and variable echogenicity and even be occult via ultrasonography.[18]
- Masses often are medial, ventral, and dorsomedial to the globe; they are less commonly lateral or anteroventral to the globe. A lateral orbital location may be more suggestive of abscess than neoplasm.
- Orbital masses may or may not be attached to the globe and this may be visible ultrasonographically or on fundic examination. If nonadherent to the globe, neoplasia or cyst is more likely than an inflammatory mass.
- Doppler may be able to identify blood flow within a neoplastic mass or a vascular anomaly.
- Bony destruction is more indicative of neoplasia (better detected using other imaging modalities).
- Most common differentials include abscesses (generally acute onset and painful on opening mouth) and neoplasia (generally gradual onset and of varying degrees of pain). Most primary orbital/periorbital neoplasia is malignant.[17,19]
- Other differentials include cysts (including sialoceles), foreign bodies, cellulitis or inflammation of retrobulbar tissues (sialoadenitis and extraocular muscle myositis), bony orbital masses, hamartomas, vascular anomalies, and parasitic disease.

Fine-needle aspiration of suspected retrobulbar masses carries the risk of hemorrhage, iatrogenic globe puncture, or nerve damage but can be diagnostic for neoplasia and infection,[20] and risk is reduced with ultrasound guidance.[21] Aspiration not always is possible, depending on location, and may require general anesthesia. Vascular anomalies, although extremely rare, may develop significant bleeding when aspirated or biopsied and may not be amenable to typical hemorrhage control maneuvers. Advanced imaging (computed tomography or magnetic resonance imaging) may be needed to both better define the extent of disease and identify the safest route for sample acquisition.

Buphthalmos

Clinical findings

- History: gradual onset
- Signalment: for dogs, a breed predisposed to primary glaucoma but variable for secondary glaucoma
- Eye examination: enlarged globe; signs of chronic glaucoma, including blindness, episcleral injection, diffuse corneal edema, corneal striae, negative menace and PLR, mydriasis, lens subluxation, high IOP, hyperreflective tapetum, and dark optic nerve head; secondary lagophthalmos; intact ocular motility

Ultrasonographic findings

- Measure the globe at the widest front-to-back diameter (freeze image) and compare with the normal/fellow eye (see **Fig. 7**). A thick layer of standoff gel is required to clearly image the anterior cornea.
- Normal intraocular structures other than possible lens subluxation
- Normal orbital structures

Buphthalmos is caused only by glaucoma and thus is distinctly different in pathology and prognosis from exophthalmos. Ultimately, buphthalmos is nonemergent and requires treatment of chronic glaucoma.

Suspected Globe Rupture

Clinical findings

- History: suspected or known trauma
- Signalment: variable
- Eye examination: acute ocular pain; globe deformation (a smaller globe), gross hypotony (a deflated look to the globe) if fairly acute; chemosis, subconjunctival hemorrhage; other periocular injuries, lid swelling, and bruising; hyphema and/or anterior uveitis (see **Figs. 1G and 8**); blood, fibrin (gray, clear, or tan), and uveal tissue (dark brown or black) may be mounded externally at site of rupture (may not be visible from front); orbital or skull fractures

Ultrasonographic findings

Extreme care should be used in utilizing ocular ultrasonography in these cases. Novice sonographers likely should consider referral. The patient should be evaluated for other significant trauma and systemically stabilized if needed before addressing an ocular injury. Avoid any direct contact with the suspected ruptured area; use sterile gel and adequate topical and anesthesia and/or utilize the retrobulbar view; avoid any pressure to the globe and avoid excessive restraint. In some cases, ultrasound cannot be done safely without general anesthesia.

Ultrasound findings may include

- Globe not spherical or smaller than the other eye
- Eye wall may not clearly visible in all views—intraocular structures may seem to blend in with adjacent extraocular structures consistently in 1 location.
- Often accompanied by sonographic evidence of retinal detachment, vitreal hemorrhage, and/or lens luxation or loss.[15]
- The interior of the whole globe may appear heterogeneously echogenic (due to the presence of blood and fibrin) except for the lens, which remains hypoechoic (or hyperechoic if cataractous) and identifiable. The absence of vitreal hemorrhage (ie, a normal, uniformly anechoic vitreous) is unlikely with a ruptured globe.

If a fixed mass of mucus-like material, fibrin, blood, and/or brown uveal-type tissue is on the ocular surface, do not aggressively try to remove this because it may be sealing a defect in the eye wall. Many cases of suspected globe rupture ultimately require enucleation, but timely referral to an ophthalmologist may best identify all options.

OPTIC NERVE SHEATH DIAMETER

Increased OSND may support the suspicion of increased intracranial pressure (ICP) in animals (without ocular disease).[22–27] A standardized transpalpebral approach has been used and a reference range developed for ultrasound-measured ONSD in dogs.[27] Placing the probe on the closed eyelids slightly temporally to the globe on a transverse plane with the probe indicator medial, the probe then is fanned up and down until the hypoechoic to anechoic optic nerve emanating from the optic disc at the posterior eye wall is seen. The ONSD, representing the optic nerve and CSF within the hyperechoic borders (sheath and fat), is measured transversely at its maximal width at a point 3-mm posterior to the optic disc (see **Fig. 3D**). ONSD values increase with body weight and decrease with age and body condition in dogs and a formula for prediction intervals has been determined utilizing these variables in normal dogs.[27] The ratio of ONSD to the transverse globe diameter may be fairly consistent across varying body weight, head size, body condition score, and other variables.[28]

The ability to image and reliably measure the optic nerve sheath may require practice and a fair amount of patient cooperation. Theoretically, the OSND should be increased bilaterally in cases of increased ICP, whereas unilaterally increased ONSD may be more indicative of optic nerve disease.[29] Serial ONSD measurement has been used to monitor changes in presumptive ICP in humans.[30,31]

SUMMARY

Ocular ultrasound can aid greatly in diagnosis of ocular disease when the tissues in question cannot be visualized, providing information not always obtainable with ophthalmic examination alone. It is critical to correlate ultrasound findings with clinical ophthalmic signs. If disease is not limited to the eye, consider surveying other areas using an integrative point-of-care ultrasound approach, such as Global FAST. If the correct diagnosis and plan still are not clear, referral to an ophthalmologist always should be considered.

CLINICS CARE POINTS

- If an eye is opaque for any reason, and especially if there is glaucoma, an ocular ultrasound can be very helpful to more precisely diagnose the nature of the pathology.
- Correlating the ophthalmic exam findings and history to ocular ultrasound results is critical to arriving at the most correct diagnosis. Always do a full ophthalmic exam on both eyes when presented with an ophthalmic complaint.
- Maintaining a thick layer of standoff gel is important to discerning structures in the anterior globe.
- Intraocular structures should be symmetrical within the globe.
- Remember to adjust both magnification and gain to try to discern ultrasonographic lesions.
- Unless you are very comfortable with your diagnosis and treatment plan, if should be noted that if an eye is diseased enough to warrant ultrasound, it most likely should be referred to an ophthalmologist.

DISCLOSURE

None.

REFERENCES

1. Cho J. Ophthalmic examination. In: Cote E, editor. Veterinary clinical advisor. 3rd edition. St. Louis: Elsevier Mosby; 2015. p. 1202–4.
2. Dietrich UM. Ophthalmic examination and diagnostics part 3: diagnostic ultrasonography. In: Gelatt KN, editor. Veterinary ophthalmology. 5th edition. Ames: Blackwell Publishing; 2013. p. 669–83.
3. Slatter's Fundamentals of Veterinary Ophthalmology. 5th edition. St. Louis: Elsevier Saunders; 2013.
4. Saraiva I, Delgado E. Congenital ocular malformations in dogs and cats: 123 cases. Vet Ophthalmol 2020;20:064 78.

5. Shank A, Texiera L, Dubielzig R. Ocular porcupine quilling in dogs: Gross, clinical and histopathologic findings in 17 cases (1986-2018). Vet Ophthalmol 2021;24: 114–24.

6. Dziezyc J, Hager DA. Ocular ultrasonography in veterinary medicine. Semin Vet Med Surg (Small Animal) 1988;3(1):1–9.

7. Spaulding K. Eye and orbit. In: Penninck D, D'anjou MA, editors. Atlas of small animal ultrasonography. Iowa: Blackwell Publishing; 2008. p. 49–90.

8. Cottrill NB, Banks WJ, Pechman RD. Ultrasonographic and biometric evaluation of the eye and orbit of dogs. Am J Vet Res 1989;50(6):898–903.

9. Gonzalez EM, Rodriguez A, Garcia I. Review of ocular ultrasonography. Vet Radiol Ultrasound 2001;42(6):485–95.

10. Williams J, Wilkie DA. Ultrasonography of the eye. Comp Cont Educ Pract Vet 1996;18:667–78.

11. Chiwitt CLH, Baines SJ, Mahoney P, et al. Ocular biometry by computed tomography in different dog breeds. Vet Ophthalmol 2017;20(5):411–9.

12. Delgado E, Pissarra H, Sales-Luís J, et al. CASE REPORT: Amelanotic uveal cyst in a Yorkshire terrier dog. Vet Ophthalmol 2010;13(5):3430347.

13. Bayón A, Tovar MC, Fernández del Palacio MJ, et al. Ocular complications of persistent hyperplastic primary vitreous in three dogs. Vet Ophthalmol 2001; 4(1):35–40.

14. Book BP, van der Woerdt A, Wilkie DA. Ultrasonographic abnormalities in eyes with traumatic hyphema obscuring intraocular structures: 33 cases (1991-2002). J Vet Emerg Crit Care 2008;18(4):383–7.

15. Rampazzo A, Eule C, Speier S, et al. Scleral rupture in dogs, cats and horses. Vet Ophthalmol 2006;9(3):149–55.

16. Badanes Z, Espineihra Gomes F, Ledbetter E. Choroidal melanocytic tumors in dogs: a retrospective study. Vet Ophthalmol 2020;23:987–93.

17. Attali-Soussay K, Jegou J, Clerc B. Retrobulbar tumors in dogs and cats: 25 cases. Vet Ophthalmol 2001;4(1):19–27.

18. Mason DR, Lamb CR, McLellan GJ. Ultrasonographic findings in 50 dogs with retrobulbar disease. J Am Anim Hosp Assoc 2001;37:757–62.

19. Kern TJ. Orbital neoplasia in 23 dogs. J Am Vet Med Assoc 1985;186:489–91.

20. Isaza D, Robinson N, Pizzirani S, et al. Evaluation of cytology and histopathology for the diagnosis of feline orbital neoplasia: 81 cases (2004-2019) and review of the literature. Vet Ophthalmol 2020;23:682–9.

21. Flaherty E, Robinson N, Pizzirani S. Evaluation of cytology and histopathology for the diagnosis of canine orbital neoplasia: 112 cases (2004-2019) and review of the literature. Vet Ophthalmol 2020;23:259–68.

22. Evangelisti MA, Carta G, Burrai GP, et al. Repeatability of ultrasound examination of the optic nerve sheath diameter in the adult cat: comparison between healthy cats and cats suffering from presumed intracranial hypertension. J Feline Med Surg 2020;22(10):959–65.

23. Giannasi S, Kani Y, Hsu F-C, et al. Comparison of direct measurement of intracranial pressures and presumptive clinical and magnetic resonance imaging indicators of intracranial hypertension in dogs with brain tumors. J Vet Intern Med 2020; 34(4):1514–23.

24. Ilie LA, Thomovsky EJ, Johnson PA, et al. Relationship between intracranial pressure as measured by an epidural intracranial pressure monitoring system and optic nerve sheath diameter in healthy dogs. Am J Vet Res 2015;76(8):724–31.

25. Lodzinska J, Munro E, Shaw DJ, et al. MRI of the optic nerve sheath and globe in cats with and without presumed intracranial hypertension. J Feline Med Surg 2020. https://doi.org/10.1177/1098612X20976106.

26. Scrivani PV, Fletcher DJ, Cooley SD, et al. T2-weighted magnetic resonance imaging measurements of optic nerve sheath diameter in dogs with and without presumed intracranial hypertension. Vet Radiol Ultrasound 2013;54:263–70.

27. Smith JJ, Fletcher DJ, Cooley SD, et al. Transpalpebral ultrasonographic measurement of the optic nerve sheath diameter in healthy dogs. J Vet Emerg Crit Care 2018;28(1):31–8.

28. Dupanloup A, Osinchuk S. Relationship between the ratio of optic nerve sheath diameter to eyeball transverse diamteter and morphological characteristics of dogs. Am J Vet Res 2021;82:667–75.

29. Lochner P, Leone MA, Fassbender K. Transorbital sonography and visual outcome for the diagnosis and monitoring of optic neuritis. J Neuroimaging 2017;27(1):92–6.

30. Ertl M, Aigner R, Krost M, et al. Measuring changes in the optic nerve sheath diameter in patients with idiopathic normal-pressure hydrocephalus: a useful diagnostic supplement to spinal tap tests. Eur J Neurol 2017;24(3):461–7.

31. Sik N, Erbas IM, Demir K, et al. Bedside sonographic measurements of optic nerve sheath diameter in children with diabetic ketoacidosis. Ped Diabetes 2021. https://doi.org/10.1111/pedi.13188.

Section VI: Integrating POCUS Information

Global FAST for Patient Monitoring and Staging in Dogs and Cats

Gregory R. Lisciandro, DVM, DABVP, DACVECC[a],
Stephanie C. Lisciandro, DVM, DACVIM (SAIM)[a,b],*

KEYWORDS

- Global FAST • POCUS • Monitoring • Staging Disease • CPR • Shock

KEY POINTS

- Global FAST is a standardized integrative approach as a FAST ultrasound examination of the abdomen (AFAST) and thorax (TFAST), including heart and lung (Vet BLUE), with exact clarity to its 15 views that prevents imaging interpretation errors, such as satisfaction of search error and confirmation bias error, through selective imaging.

- Global FAST may be used for patient monitoring, incorporating AFAST for soft issue abnormalities of its target organs, detection of ascites and semi-quantitating volume through the abdominal fluid scoring system and its small-volume versus large-volume principle, volume assessment through characterization of the caudal vena cava and hepatic veins, urinary bladder volume estimation formula, pneumoperitoneum, and gastrointestinal motility.

- Global FAST may be used for patient monitoring, incorporating TFAST for soft issue abnormalities of the heart and thorax, detection of pleural and pericardial effusion, detection and semi-quantification of pneumothorax through the TFAST thirds rule, cardiac assessment by its fundamental echocardiography views, and volume assessment through characterization of the caudal vena cava and hepatic veins.

- Global FAST may be used for patient monitoring, incorporating Vet BLUE and its regional, pattern-based approach, wet lung versus dry lung assessment, B-line scoring system, and visual lung language with lung ultrasound signs of consolidation, and the echelon of its lung language signs may be used for tracking respiratory disease.

- Global FAST is used in combination with physical examination and laboratory findings for rapidly detecting treatable forms of by and evaluating the Hs and Ts of cardiopulmonary resuscitation.

- Global FAST may be used for differentiating localized versus disseminated disease and locating potential sampling sites for a cytologic and histopathologic diagnosis.

---

[a] Hill Country Veterinary Specialists and FASTVet.com, Spicewood, TX, USA; [b] Oncura Partners, Fort Worth, TX, USA
* Corresponding author.
E-mail address: FastSavesLives@gmail.com

Vet Clin Small Anim 51 (2021) 1315–1333
https://doi.org/10.1016/j.cvsm.2021.07.011
0195-5616/21/© 2021 Elsevier Inc. All rights reserved.

INTRODUCTION

Veterinary point-of-care ultrasound (POCUS), which includes FAST examinations, has been defined as a goal-directed ultrasound examination(s) performed by a health care provider to answer a specific diagnostic question(s) or guide performance of an invasive procedure(s) cageside (**Fig. 1**).[1] An unbiased set of data imaging points, however, is important to prevent imaging interpretation errors, such as satisfaction of search error, by stopping imaging at the first major abnormality, and confirmation bias error, through selective POCUS imaging.[2] The use of Global FAST should be considered an extension of the physical examination, because it rapidly rules in and rules out important obvious abnormalities, including effusions and soft tissue abnormalities in both cavities.[3] By seeing the problem list, diagnostics are streamlined, and treatment is directed with more evidence-based information over traditional work-ups of physical examination, laboratory testing, and plain radiography. Global FAST can answer many clinical questions without any additional views and search for treatable forms of shock, the Hs and Ts of cardiopulmonary resuscitation (CPR), when minutes count, similar to approaches in human medicine.[4–6] The Global FAST fallback views gain cardiac information without TFAST echocardiography views, especially when they are unavailable due to limited acoustic windows (respiratory distress/lung interference) and patient risk (time and restraint).[7,8]

Global FAST should be considered an "ultrasound physical examination" because it provides an unbiased set of data through its 15 defined views of the abdomen and thorax.[4,8] After Global FAST, then clinicians can perform focused or targeted POCUS on additional systems of interest. Examples of the shortcomings of traditional work-ups

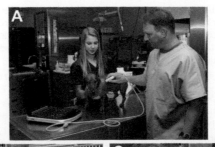

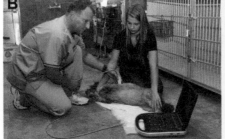
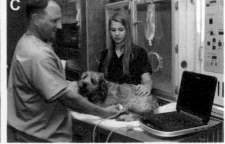

Fig. 1. POCUS techniques premise themselves on bringing the ultrasound to the patient and making imaging evaluation low impact, especially for critically ill patients. Examples are shown in being cageside in (*A*) standing, (*B*) right laeral recumbency, and (*C*) modified lateral recumbency. Note that when possible, the patient, assistant, and sonographer should be looking at the screen, as in (*A*), for patient and personal safety. (© 2021 Gregory R. Lisciandro.)

without ultrasound and the limitations of plain radiography are endless. Examples that help illustrate the importance of the integrative Global FAST approach are herein described.

GLOBAL FAST PERFORMED IN LATERAL RECUMBENCY AND STANDING, THE BLEND

Global FAST may be performed within minutes and efficiently using a blended methodology of AFAST, TFAST, and Vet BLUE (Video 1).[4,8–10] In patients presenting in right lateral recumbency (and it can be figured analogously if in left lateral recumbency), start with the TFAST-AFAST diaphragmatico-hepatic (DH) view and then rapidly do the AFAST splenorenal (SR), cystocolic (CC), and spleno-intestino umbilical (SIU) views and then the focused spleen before moving to the Vet BLUE of the left thorax, the TFAST left pericardial site view to the right TFAST right pericardial site view, and then moving the patient to access the right Vet BLUE and hepatorenal fifth bonus view (**Fig. 2**). The advantages for right lateral include TFAST echocardiography, because the heart falls against the thoracic wall at the cardiac notch, electrocardiography, and the spleen lies left of midline.[4,8–10] Thus, for the focused spleen, the probe does not have to be positioned under the patient, which is not only difficult for probe manipulation because of the weight of the patient but also causes patient discomfort of probe pressure.

In patients that are standing (or sternal), the sonographer stands on the patient's left side and perform the left Vet BLUE, followed by the TFAST left pericardial site view, followed by AFAST and the focused spleen, and then, physically move to the other side of the patient and perform right TFAST pericardial site views, and then complete the study with the hepatorenal fifth bonus view (see **Fig. 2**). The advantage is that from the left side the sonographer is "looking" at the spleen because it courses from approximately midline to the left kidney. Thus if the sonographer does not locate the spleen at the umbilical view, they should sweep dorsally and slide the probe cranially and caudally repeating this until the find the spleen along the left body wall. Also, this order allows getting all the easy Global FAST information before TFAST echocardiography, the most time-consuming views for most. With this order, however, the sonographer already knows if there is lung pathology, pleural effusion (PE), pericardial effusion (PCE), ascites, and volume status and can assess patient stability and their ability to tolerate different forms of restraint, if needed.

Additional videos on how to perform Global FAST efficiently are available at FASTVet.com under the Free Resources category. In summary, perfecting Global FAST image acquisition requires standardized repetition.

GLOBAL FAST AND INTEGRATING INFORMATION

Global FAST consists of 15 views that provide an unbiased data imaging points and thus prevent common imaging interpretation errors (eg, satisfaction of search and confirmation bias errors).[2,4–6] For example, during a focused cardiac ultrasound, the patient is determined to be hypovolemic and administered a crystalloid challenge; however, the cause is marked intra-abdominal hemorrhage. It has to be wondered when would the attending clinician figure out that the hypovolemia was due to intra-abdominal hemorrhage and be treated more accurately? Will the clinician figure out this cause before the patient decompensates or dies? Through Global FAST, the clinician automatically searches for other rule-outs similar to imaging strategies, such as extended FAST (EFAST) and the rapid ultrasound for shock and hypotension examination (RUSH).[4–6,8,11]

As another example, a clinician incorrectly concludes that the collapsed canine with gallbladder wall edema has anaphylaxis, referred to as an anaphylactic gallbladder, when in fact the patient has PCE or dilated cardiomyopathy (DCM), referred to as a

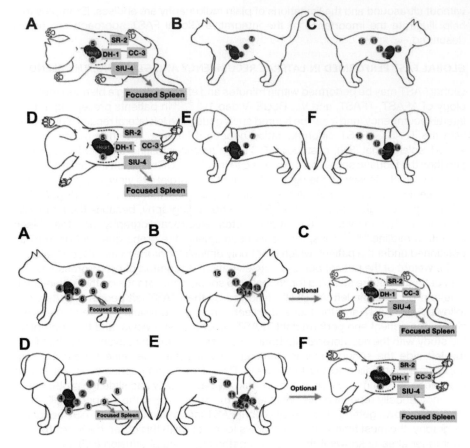

Fig. 2. The most efficient ways the authors have found to perform Global FAST are blending the AFAST, TFAST, and Vet BLUE, dependent on patient positioning. Most often, patients either are standing or in right lateral recumbency, so examples are shown for each. In the top boxed area, the Global FAST blend is shown in cats (*A-C*) and dogs (*D-F*) and numbered in their order of performance (1-15). The first view is the DH view because it gives immediate information regarding both the abdomen and thorax that also includes characterization of the CVC and hepatic veins. The focused spleen is performed after the SIU view. The TFAST left and right pericardial site views are performed next then the left Vet BLUE and moving the patient to sternal or standing the right Vet BLUE followed by the hepatorenal fifth bonus view. In the bottom boxed area, the Global FAST blend is shown in both dogs and cats and begins with the left Vet BLUE followed by the left TFAST pericardial site view, AFAST, and the focused spleen. Then moving to the right side of the patient, right Vet BLUE followed by the TFAST right pericardial site views, including their echocardiography and ending at the hepatorenal fifth bonus view. For experienced Global FAST sonographers, the blending of views takes 5-7 minutes. The goal-directed templates should follow these orders as well. These may be acquired at FASTVet.com in it Free Resources category (https://fastvet.com/most-updated-global-fast-goal-directed-templates/). (© 2021 Gregory R. Lisciandro.)

cardiac gallbladder.[2,12] The Global FAST approach prevents this error by mandating TFAST and directs more appropriate and often lifesaving therapy.

A final example is considered. A cat has a flash or POCUS thorax and is found to have PE; however, by recognizing there is concurrent PCE, congestive heart failure, a treatable disease, moves to the top of the differential diagnosis list.[13,14] The clinician, however, failed to look beyond the first major POCUS abnormality. The authors do not recommend risking patient death assessing TFAST echocardiography in real time; however, by saving cine clips during the standardized TFAST views, the captured images may be evaluated more closely after the feline patient has been placed in oxygen post–initial treatment. In this case, the finding of PCE pushes a treatable disease to the top of the differential and neoplasia further down. Thus, the presentation to the client may be more optimistic prognostically and for continued work-up. Furthermore, treatment may be performed more accurately based on evidence-based information, giving the patient a better chance at survival. As a final point, Global FAST always should be repeated because status changes and serial examination give the clinician the opportunity to reassess.[15–17] Often, after the initial POCUS examination, the clinician delays further evaluation by scheduling more advanced imaging that may be delayed until the following day(s).

Performing for Global FAST makes it likely to miss important clinical information, as summarized in **Fig. 3**.

GLOBAL FAST FOR VOLUME STATUS AND LEFT-SIDED AND RIGHT-SIDED CARDIAC PROBLEMS

Global FAST integrates TFAST echocardiography views and its fallback views for left-sided and right-sided congestive failure by incorporating lung (Vet BLUE) and

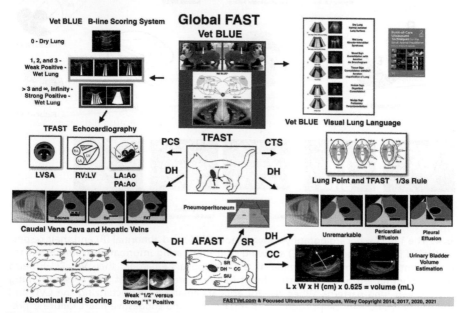

Fig. 3. The graphic shows, although not comprehensively, examples of how much clinical information may be gained through the standardized 15 views of Global FAST that include AFAST, TFAST, and Vet BLUE. CTS, chest tube site; H, height; L, length; LVSA, LV short axis; PA, pulmonary artery; W, width. (© 2021 Gregory R. Lisciandro.)

characterization of the caudal vena cava (CVC) and hepatic venous distension (AFAST-TFAST DH view) **(Fig. 4)**.[8–11,18–27] When TFAST echocardiography views are obtained, the fallback views provide additional evidence for left-sided (wet lung vs dry lung on Vet BLUE) and right-sided (FAT-distended CVC with hepatic venous distension [tree trunk sign] vs a bounce or flat CVC) congestive heart failure (see **Fig. 4**). Conversely, if TFAST echocardiography views cannot be obtained because they are too risky because of restraint or the patient is too critical, fallback views help rule in and rule out left-sided and right-sided congestive heart failure without echocardiography.[8–11,18–27] For example, dry lung all views on Vet BLUE rules out any clinically relevant left-sided congestive heart failure and TFAST echocardiography, or more complete echocardiography can wait until the patient is more stable.[20–24] Moreover, loop diuretics generally are not indicated when there is no evidence-based information for any form of pulmonary edema (no B-lines).[20–24,28] As for right-sided congestive heart failure, a bounce of flat CVC rules out any clinically relevant right-sided congestive heart failure and, again, TFAST echocardiography or more complete echocardiography often can wait until the patient is more stable.[12,27,29–31]

These Global FAST fallback views also provide additional information regarding the interpretation of TFAST echocardiography findings. For example, if the left atrium (LA) appears enlarged, Vet BLUE helps screen for left-sided congestive heart failure versus

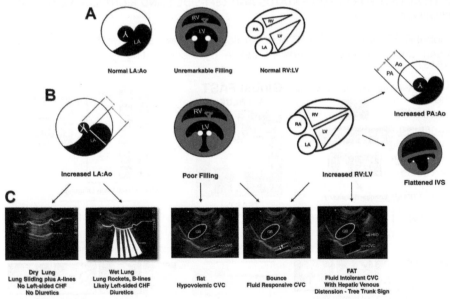

Fig. 4. The TFAST echocardiography views as normal (A) and abnormal (B) and their respective Global FAST fallback views (C) showing that integrating information is important for best patient assessment. For example, if the LA appears enlarged, then Vet BLUE helps sort out whether left-sided congestive heart failure is present by wet lung versus dry lung (and the wet lung pattern). When the RV appears enlarged, characterizing the CVC and associated hepatic veins helps support whether right-sided congestive heart failure is present by a FAT CVC with distended hepatic veins (tree trunk sign). Volume and contractility can be assessed further by both Vet BLUE and CVC characterization. Lastly, when the RV is enlarged, the pulmonary artery and interventricular septum can help screen for pulmonary hypertension. (© 2021 Gregory R. Lisciandro.)

other wet lung conditions by using its regional, pattern-based approach. If Vet BLUE in combination with TFAST echocardiography supports left-sided congestive heart failure (and not pneumonia), then the client is better advised for a timelier work-up and treatment plan, including complete echocardiography, versus the finding of a suspect enlarged LA with dry lung. Regarding the right heart, the same Global FAST fallback view strategy is helpful. For example, if the right ventricle (RV) appears enlarged, the characterization of the CVC and hepatic veins at the AFAST-TFAST DH view is used for assessing the presence of right-sided congestive heart failure. A FAT (distended) CVC along with hepatic venous distension (tree trunk sign) pushes the client recommendation for a timelier work-up and treatment plan, including complete echocardiography, versus an enlarged RV with an unremarkable CVC and no hepatic venous distension. Through this approach, cardiac disease can be better characterized and assessed, lowering the probability of inadvertently sending a patient home risking a cardiac crisis.

GLOBAL FAST FOR MONITORING

The combined use of its 3 components provides a tremendous amount of information, with AFAST and its target organ approach, fluid scoring system, urinary bladder volume estimation formula, pneumoperitoneum, gastrointestinal motility, gallbladder wall edema, and examination of the retroperitoneal space; TFAST for PE, PCE, pneumothorax (PTX), and its PTX thirds rule and its echocardiography views for chamber and soft tissue abnormalities; and Vet BLUE and its regional, pattern-based approach, B-line scoring system, and visual lung language for a working diagnosis and monitoring tool (see **Fig. 2**).[12,15,22,28,31–40]

AFAST and Abdominal Fluid Scoring

The small-volume versus large-volume concept is impactful for patient care for both the bleeding and nonbleeding patient (see AFAST videos).[11,15,19] The system (1) helps categorize small-volume versus large-volume bleeder/effusion to anticipate both transfusion need (hemoglobin support) and volume replacement, (2) may help with the location of the origin of the problem in lower scoring patients, (3) provides an opportunity to sample free fluid when scores increase dependent on skill level, and (4) serves as a tracking tool for static, worsening, and resolving cases (see **Fig. 5**).

AFAST Cystocolic View and Estimating Urinary Bladder Volume and Urine Output

There have been several approaches to estimating urinary bladder volume but only one that evaluated both dogs and cats that is also easy to remember. The formula is length × height measured in the longitudinal plane and the width measured in the transverse plane without extending into the trigone at the CC view multiplied by 0.625 (**Figs. 5 and 6**).[33] When measurements are made in centimeters, the volume is in milliliters and over time urine output may be estimated noninvasively.

AFAST for Free Air

The use of ultrasound is extremely sensitive for detecting small amounts of free intraabdominal air. The principle is that air rises and fluid falls into gravity-dependent regions. Thus, the SR view is the optimal view in a patient in right lateral recumbency. The enhanced peritoneal stripe sign identifies free air, pneumoperitoneum, and is a simple concept (see AFAST videos).[34] The free air, hyperechoic line, must be continuous with the peritoneal lining, another hyperechoic line, without an anechoic or black gap. Any black gap is gastrointestinal tract until proved otherwise. Postoperatively, it

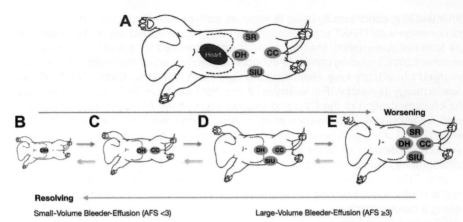

Fig. 5. The tracking of ascites may be accomplished by applying the AFAST AFS system. In (*A*) is shown the first 4 views of AFAST that make up the abdominal fluid scoring system. Total score and views that are positive and negative have clinical ramifications. The patient may be followed for being static (same score), worsening (increasing score B-E), resolving (decreasing score E-B). Moreover, the views that are positive may be clinically helpful as to source of bleeding or sepsis dependent on patient subset. (© 2021 Gregory R. Lisciandro.)

has been reported that dogs can have free air last as long as 3 weeks. Postoperative cases thus serve as a good model to practice identifying the enhanced peritoneal stripe sign. When free air obscures the SR view, the probe should be swept ventral to the risen air to acquire the view. Finally, a rule of thumb any time the sonographer is imaging the abdomen is that if a good image cannot be obtained, and the sonographer is used to the machine, then it is bone, stone, or air causing the imaging issue. A radiograph should be taken.

AFAST for Gastrointestinal Motility

The stomach/proximal duodenum and the jejunum may be observed for peristalsis, expecting 4 minute^{-1} to 5 minute^{-1} and 1 minute^{-1} to 3 minute^{-1}, respectively, if food is present in the canine gastrointestinal tract, helping detect ileus. With food absence, including intentional fasting, ileus occurs in normalcy and must be placed into clinical context.[35]

TFAST for Pneumothorax, the Lung Point, and Its Thirds Rule for Degree and Monitoring

The absence of lung sliding with A lines plus the finding of the lung point support the diagnosis of PTX best evaluated in standing/sternal. The TFAST PTX lung point thirds rule is as follows: upper third, trivial to mild; middle third, moderate; and lower third, severe; it serves as a tool for decision making (thoracocentesis and tube thoracostomy) and tracking for worsening, static, and resolving PTX (**Fig. 7**).[7,8,11,38,41]

Pearls for Imaging Lung Sliding

- Scatter the echoes. Place the rib in the center of the screen, called the 1-eyed gator sign, to bring out lung sliding, a trick discovered by the authors several years ago.[11,38,39]
- Ricochet the echoes. Change the angle of insonation from 90° to the lung line (surface) to more like 75° or by making the lung line less crisp and bright white

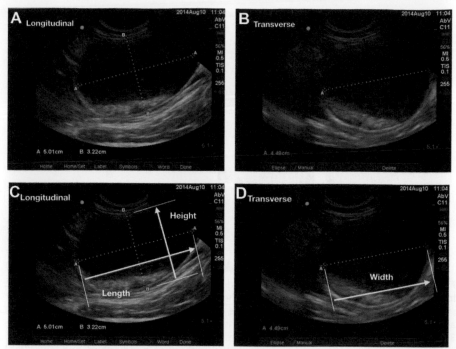

Fig. 6. Measurements of the urinary bladder may be taken at the AFAST CC view. In longitudinal, making the largest symmetric oval within that scanning plane without measuring into the trigone, length and height are measured and, in transverse, making the largest symmetric oval within that scanning plane, width is measured. Measurements in centimeters multiplied by 0.625 give an estimation of urinary bladder volume in milliliters. Over time with serial volume calculations, urine output may be estimated. (© 2021 Gregory R. Lisciandro.)

(hyperechoic) to gray and softer in appearance while still being able to identify the lung line.[11,39]

Reverse Curtain Sign

A newer strategy is to interrogate the transition zone curtain sign of the pleural and pericardial cavities at its caudodorsal extremity.[42,43] The pleural and abdominal cavities move in respirophasic synchrony in normalcy, whereas in PTX, they move in asynchrony, toward each other, and then away from each other. Paradoxic abdominal breathing also causes asynchrony (Gregory Lisciandro, unpublished data, 2020). Artifacts within the curtain should only be A-lines in PTX. Reverse sliding is an additional descriptor a similar phenomenon.[42,43]

TFAST Echocardiography

TFAST echocardiography views are from the right PCS view and include the left ventricular (LV) short-axis mushroom view for volume status and contractility, the LV short-axis LA to aortic (Ao) view for left-sided problems (increased LA filling pressures), the long-axis 4-chamber view for right-sided problems (increased RV filling pressures), and the long-axis LV outflow tract and Ao valves.[38,39,44–47] These views also serve as a screening test for cardiac-related soft tissue abnormalities because

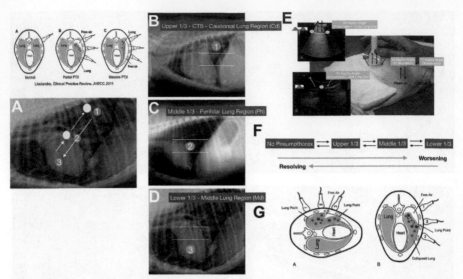

Fig. 7. TFAST composite for imaging lung and PTX. (*A*) The lung point, the location where lung recontacts the thoracic wall. This is searched for best and most accurately in standing or sternal position. In lateral positioning, probe positions are no longer gravity unequal (*G*) and a double-lung point can be present, that is, seeing the lung point at probe 1 and probe 3 in lateral recumbency. The fastest manner in which to search for the lung point, as shown in (*A*), as blue circles numbered 1 to 3 is to do the upper third, middle third, and lower third of the thoracic wall and then move dorsally to better define the exact location of the lung point (yellow circles). PTX can be tracked with recording and following the lung point location as (*B*) upper third, (*C*) middle third, and (*D*) lower third, which can be considered further as trivial to mild, moderate, and severe, respectively. (*E*) How the angle of insonation has an impact on observing for lung sliding by changing the angle of insonation from 90° to approximately 75° and placing the rib in the center of the screen, the one-eyed gator sign. In (*F*) is shown how the thirds rule is used for tracking. (© 2021 Gregory R. Lisciandro.)

the radiographic cardiac silhouette is unreliable.[48,49] Importantly, when the sonographer is unable to obtain its echocardiography views, the absence of wet lung during Vet BLUE rules out clinically relevant left-sided congestive heart failure, and absence of a fluid-intolerant (FAT) CVC and distended hepatic veins (tree trunk sign) rules out clinically relevant right-sided congestive heart failure.[11,18,27,38] These Global FAST fallback views allow an approach that often is easier (and faster) than echocardiography in the unstable patient.

TFAST-AFAST Diaphragmatico-hepatic View and Volume Status Using the Caudal Vena Cava

The CVC and hepatic veins are characterized at the TFAST-AFAST DH view as being fluid responsive (bounce), fluid intolerant (fat), and fluid starved or hypovolemic (flat).[8–10,25] The distention of hepatic veins, tree trunk sign, is nearly 100% specific for right-sided congestive heart failure and thus characterization of the CVC and hepatic veins may be used as a Global Fast non-echocardiography fallback view or as additional supportive evidence when interpreting right-sided echocardiographic findings.[18,25,27,29,30] Although the characterization of the CVC and hepatic veins generally trumps maximum height measurements (MHMs), MHMs may be used as well, with the rule that smaller dogs (<9 kg) should not have a CVC MHM of more than 1.0 cm and larger dogs (>9 kg) should not have a CVC MHM more than 1.5 cm.[8,9,25]

Vet BLUE and B-line Scoring

The B-line scoring system is the highest number of B-lines over a single representative intercostal space at each respective regional Vet BLUE view. The numbers of B-lines may be divided further into weak positives of 1, 2, and 3 and strong positives of greater than 3 and infinity (∞).[22,28,50] Vet BLUE B-line scoring at its regional views combines overall numbers and distribution of positive regional views to help rapidly develop a differential diagnosis that allows for tracking respiratory conditions as static, worsening, or resolving helping guide therapy (eg, loop diuretics, antibiotics, antifungal agents, and chemotherapy).[28]

Vet BLUE Visual Lung Language

The use of the echelon of Vet BLUE lung ultrasound signs, which includes dry lung (A-lines and lung sliding), wet lung (B-lines), shred sign (air bronchogram), tissue sign (hepatization of lung), nodule sign, and wedge sign (pulmonary thromboembolism [PTE]), helps assess and tract severity and response to therapy for respiratory conditions.[10,11,22,50–53] The signs of consolidation are dependent on the diagnosis (ie, congestive heart failure does not have nodules); however, the concept works for tracking progression of disease and response to therapy.

Other Point-of-Care Ultrasound Add-ons

Examples of the clinical utility of POCUS add-on examinations include focused ocular that may be used for optic nerve sheath diameter for intracranial hypertension; focused musculoskeletal for detecting fractures; focused diaphragm for abnormal diaphragmatic function; focused reproductive for such conditions as pyometra, uterine torsion, and testicular torsion; focused urinary tract for ureteral obstruction; and focused vascular for arterial and venous thromboembolic disease.

GLOBAL FAST FOR THE HS AND TS OF CARDIOPULMONARY RESUSCITATION, IMPORTANT PART OF BASIC LIFE SUPPORT

The Global FAST approach is used to rapidly determine if the patient has treatable forms of shock or cause for CPR by the veterinary Hs—hypovolemia/hypotension, hypokalemia/hyperkalemia, hypocontractility, hypertension, and heartworms (caval syndrome)—and Ts—trauma/hemorrhage, tamponade, tension PTX, thromboembolism, and toxin (**Table 1**).[4] Following return of spontaneous circulation, Global FAST becomes part of advanced life support and patient monitoring.[8]

Quick Rules of Thumb

- Hypovolemia—flat CVC (TFAST-AFAST DH view) combined with poor filling of the LV mushroom view (TFAST echocardiography)
  - Answer the question—Where is the leak in the tank? Do Global FAST for ascites, retroperitoneal fluid, pleural effusion, PCE, and wet lung.
  - Pitfall—at the Batman short-axis level of the TFAST echocardiography chart, when too low, ventral on the heart, and at the incorrect level, hypovolemia is mistakenly assessed.
- Hypokalemia/hyperkalemia—renal pelvic, ureteral, urinary bladder, and urethral distension at the respective AFAST SR and hepatorenal fifth bonus views and CC views. The feline urethra has considerable intra-abdominal length.

Table 1

Knowing Hs and Ts During Cardiopulmonary Arrest, Cardiopulmonary Resuscitation, and Advanced Life Support for Small Animals

The Hs	The Ts
Hypothermia	Tension PTX (TFAST and lung point)
Hypotension/hypovolemia (AFAST, TFAST, Vet BLUE, cavitary bleeds, and effusions)	Trauma, hemorrhage (AFAST, and AFS system, TFAST, Vet BLUE, and cavitary bleeds)
Hyperkalemia, hypokalemia (AFAST, urinary obstruction)	Thromboembolism (PTE) (TFAST, Vet BLUE)
Hypoglycemia	Tamponade (PCE) (TFAST and AFAST-TFAST DH view)
Hydrogen ion (acidosis)	Toxin, canine anaphylaxis (AFAST-TFAST DH view)
Hypocontractility (Dilated Cardiomyopathy [DCM]) (TFAST)	Tear, LA (TFAST, AFAST-TFAST DH view)
Hypertension (pulmonary hypertension) (TFAST)	
Heartworm disease/caval syndrome (TFAST)	Note: the Hs and Ts are rapidly evaluated for by physical examination, vital signs, venous (or arterial) blood gas, and the Global FAST approach

Modified by the author for veterinary medicine from AHA CPR Guidelines.

Courtesy of Dr Gregory Lisciandro, DVM, Hill Country Veterinary Specialists and FASTVet.com, Spicewood, Texas, and Point-of-care Ultrasound Techniques for the Small Animal Practitioner, Wiley ©2020, 2021.

- Hypocontractility—eyeballing the difference in left ventral size during systole and diastole (fractional shortening) or measuring the interval diameter of the LV on diastole.
  - Poor fractional shortening screens for DCM and also more transient myocardial stunning from sepsis, shock, or post-CPR that can help guide the use and tapering of inotropes (Video 2).
  - Pearl for double-checking the eyeball assessment—the internal diameter of the LV in diastole (as big as it will get) never should be more than 5 cm in any size dog (DeFrancesco, personal communication, 2017).
  - Pearl—DCM is rare in cats.
- Hypertension, pulmonary and systemic
  - Systemic—thickened LV walls and papillary muscles in dogs support chronic systemic hypertension. Hypertrophic cardiomyopathy is rare in dogs.
  - Pulmonary—an increased pulmonary artery-to-Ao ratio at the Mercedes-Benz sign level, flattening of the interventricular septum (top of the mushroom) at the LV short-axis mushroom view, and an enlarged RV (>1:2) (Videos 3 and 4).
- Heartworm, caval syndrome—the presence of intracardiac heart worms (Videos 5 and 6).
  - Pitfall—chordae tendinea can mimic heartworms. Freeze and roll the cine ball through frames to better differentiate between the 2 because heartworms are double-stranded, and their bodies appear like hyperechoic (bright white) equal signs

- Trauma/hemorrhage—AFAST, abdominocentesis, and fluid characterization through fluid analysis and cytology, and fluid scoring for semiquantitating volume.
  - Other sites for hemorrhage are screened for doing Global FAST grouped as follows:
    - Forgiving areas include the retroperitoneal space and pleural cavity where large volumes can remain clinically silent for prolonged periods of time before clinical signs.
    - Unforgiving areas of the pericardial sac and lung because large volumes are less possible, because cardiac function and ventilation are more rapidly affected
- Tamponade, cardiac—TFAST-AFAST DH view for the racetrack sign, and trans-thoracic views for the bull's-eye sign around the muscular apex of the heart from the right TFAST pericardial site view and the hammerhead view from the left TFAST pericardial site view.
  - Collapse of the right atrium and RV occur often creating a rippling effect to their walls (Video 7)
  - There are different degrees of cardiac tamponade so ask the question, Is the patient stable to determine the need for emergent pericardiocentesis?
  - A FAT-distended CVC and likely hepatic venous distention (tree trunk sign) are mandated for the obstructive shock from cardiac tamponade. Thus, if the CVC has a bounce or is flat in the presence of PCE, the problem causing collapse or weakness likely is somewhere else; so, do Global FAST.
- Tension PTX—use the TFAST thirds rule.
  - Pearl—directly and briefly inserting a needle to deflate the pleural cavity with or without a Heimlich valve arrangement is lifesaving. Using a finger from a glove through a large-bore needle serves as a quick and dirty temporary Heimlich valve.
- Thromboembolism, PTE—a wedge sign in non–gravity-dependent Vet BLUE views support PTE.[53] Other findings are an enlarged pulmonary artery at the Mercedes-Benz sign level and RV enlargement on the long-axis right TFAST echocardiography view. Consider other sites of arterial and venous thromboembolism.
- Toxin, canine anaphylaxis—gallbladder wall edema in the acute setting is due, as a rule of thumb, to canine anaphylaxis or PCE (or less commonly to other causes of right-sided heart failure).[12]
  - Flat small CVC supports and anaphylactic gallbladder
  - FAT-distended CVC, especially with distended hepatic veins (tree trunk sign) supports PCE and other causes of rights-sided heart failure
- Tear, LA rupture (Video 8)
  - PCE in a mitral valve disease dog
  - Classic thrombus in the PCE and a severely enlarged LA
  - Dachshunds and Shetland sheepdogs most common breeds (DeFrancesco, personal communication, 2017).
  - Pericardiocentesis uncommonly necessary
    - Treat for left-sided congestive heart failure, including pimobendan.
    - Most have relatively dry lung; do Vet BLUE and its B-line scoring to guide loop diuretic usage.
    - Most survive to hospital discharge; however, it is unpredictable how long patients will survive thereafter.

GLOBAL FAST FOR ADVANCED LIFE SUPPORT, MOVING BEYOND BASIC LIFE SUPPORT

Following the use of Global FAST for treatable forms of shock and the Hs and Ts of CPR, the Global FAST approach for patient monitoring, detailed previously, is used to direct fluid resuscitation and screen for complications to better direct care.[4,7,8] This Global FAST integrative approach provides evidenced-based information over traditional measures without ultrasound guiding decision making regarding the need for oxygen support (Vet BLUE), transfusion products (AFAST and abdominal fluid scoring [AFS]), thromboprophylaxis and thrombolytics (Vet BLUE wedge sign, and TFAST echocardiography), use of loop diuretics (Vet BLUE B-line scoring), vasopressors (Vet BLUE, CVC, and TFAST echocardiography), and inotropes (Vet BLUE, CVC, and TFAST echocardiography).[16]

GLOBAL FAST FOR STAGING PATIENTS

Staging patients is important for 2 major reasons: (1) to rapidly determine if diseases is localized versus disseminated and (2) to determine what the potential sampling sites are for a diagnosis (**Fig. 8**).[8] **Table 1** for a list of soft tissue abnormalities potentially detected during AFAST and its target organ approach

Common clinical questions that may be answered during Global FAST staging:

- AFAST
  - DH view—Are there obvious liver metastases (target lesions)?
  - SR and hepatorenal views—Are there any renal or retroperitoneal masses? Adjacent splenic and liver masses? Renal pelvic abnormalities?
  - SIU view—Are there any obvious splenic or midabdominal masses?
  - CC view—Is there any obvious urinary bladder mass? Caudal abdominal mass?
  - What is the AFS? Small-volume bleeder effusion versus large-volume bleeder effusion to help with decision regarding blood transfusion(s) and volume resuscitation.
- TFAST
  - Is there pleural effusion?
  - Is there PCE?
  - Is there any obvious intracardiac or intrathoracic mass?
- Vet BLUE
  - Are there any obvious lung nodules?
  - Any other lung surface abnormalities?

Consider a common practical case example for illustrative purposes.

As an example in a retrospective study looking at 432 cases of hemoabdomen in dogs, 422 were nontraumatic.[54] Only 86 of these 432 nontraumatic dogs were operated, or 20% of the study population. Those unoperated were euthanized, died, or left untreated. Considering the frequency of benign to malignant neoplasms in nontraumatic hemoabdomen, it seems plausible that many dogs with benign disease were disqualified from a surgical work-up. A reasonable explanation is that many dogs with hemoabdomen have a flash ultrasound of the abdomen (a quick sweep) or selective POCUS imaging with the determination of ascites, likely followed by abdominocentesis and possibly a sweep for a splenic mass. With all or some of this POCUS information, the client is presented with a continued work-up for a likely 25% to 33% probability of a benign tumor and a 67% to 75% probability of a malignant tumor.[55] With this painted picture, many dogs likely are euthanized or are treated palliatively without surgery.[54]

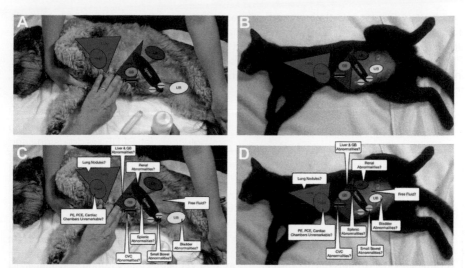

Fig. 8. Questions asked during staging with Global FAST. (*A, B*) Overlays of target structures evaluated during the Global FAST approach, including within the abdomen and thorax, including heart and lung. (*C, D*) Clinical relevant questions are on overlays for the staging of disease and conditions as being localized or disseminated. The Global FAST approach not only provides a means to quickly screen for local versus disseminated disease but also helps determine the diagnostic path, including the next best test(s). Moreover, by seeing the problem list with evidence-based information, treatment potentially is better directed. (© 2021 Gregory R. Lisciandro.)

Through the Global FAST approach, however, the dog may be staged for obvious liver nodules, pericardial and pleural effusion and lung nodules along the pulmonary DH at the AFAST-TFAST DH view, obvious cardiac-related masses during TFAST echocardiography, lung nodules during Vet BLUE. If the patient stages negative for obvious metastasis, then it should be considered a surgical candidate and this information should be presented initially to the owner. In cases of dogs (or cats) with no obvious metastasis or disseminated disease, a much different presentation can take place with the client, one of optimism and encouragement of pursuit of definitive surgical intervention.

GLOBAL FAST FOR DETERMINING SAMPLING SITES

As an example in the event that nodules or other forms of consolidation are found on Vet BLUE, Global FAST helps determine if disease is localized or disseminated and also may help locate more forgiving regions for sampling. If a cat had nodules or if neoplastic or fungal disease is likely suspected and the spleen is enlarged, a splenic aspirate may be less risky over a lung lobe aspirate. Moreover, lung masses found radiographically always should have Vet BLUE performed because there may be peripheral lung disease inapparent on radiographically that is obvious on Vet BLUE. This tells the clinician 2 things: (1) the disease is not localized but disseminated and (2) a lung lobe aspirate is something to consider diagnostically.

SUMMARY

Global FAST is low-impact, cost-effective, real-time information and rapid, radiation-sparing, point-of-care imaging that allows the veterinarian to see a problem list and thus better direct resuscitation and treatment and streamline the diagnostic plan. Its 15 views provide an unbiased set of data imaging points that prevent the common imaging mistakes of satisfaction of search and confirmation bias errors through selective POCUS imaging. Global FAST should be used as an extension of the physical examination on a daily basis for nearly all patients in the clinical setting and preempt all focused POCUS examinations.

CLINICS CARE POINTS

- Integrating Global FAST imaging findings prevents common image interpretation errors such as satisfaction of search error and confirmation bias error through selective POCUS imaging.
- Global FAST fallback views can be in combination with echocardiography or standalone when echocardiography is not possibly to assess the presence and absence of left- and right-sided congestive heart failure via Vet BLUE and characterization of the caudal vena cava and hepatic veins, respectively.
- Global FAST has an abdominal fluid scoring system, urinary bladder volume estimation formula, a TFAST thirds rule for pneumothorax, and Vet BLUE's B-line scoring system and visual lung language (including signs of consolidation) that have clear advantages over POCUS formats in people with no additional views.
- Global FAST may be used to determine if disease is localized or disseminated (staging) as well as a means to survey for potential diagnostic sampling sites.

DISCLOSURE

The authors are the owners of FASTVet.com, a private corporation that provides veterinary ultrasound training to practicing veterinarians. Ultrasound companies sponsor Global FAST Courses and include Oncura Partners, Universal Imaging, EI Medical, and Sound; and EI Medical and the Veterinary Medical Network have licensed Global FAST education materials. His spouse, Stephanie Lisciandro, DVM, is Medical Director at Oncura Partners, Fort Worth, Texas. The authors have no funding sources to declare for this article.

SUPPLEMENTARY DATA

Supplementary data to this article can be found online at https://doi.org/10.1016/j.cvsm.2021.07.011.

REFERENCES

1. Lisciandro GR. POCUS: introduction. In: Lisciandro GR, editor. Point-of-care ultrasound techniques for the small animal practitioner. 2nd edition. Ames, IA: Wiley Blackwell; 2021. p. 3.
2. Lichtenstein DA. Gallbladder. In: Lichtenstein DA, editor. Whole body ultrasound in the critically ill. London: Springer; 2010. p. 59–67.
3. Rozycki GS, Ballard RB, Feliciano DV, et al. Surgeon-performed ultrasound for the assessment of truncal injuries: lessons learned from 1540 patients. Ann Surg 1998;228(4):557–67.
4. Lisciandro GR. POCUS: global FAST-rapidly detecting treatable forms of shock, advanced life support, and cardiopulmonary resuscitation. In: Lisciandro GR, editor. Point-of-care ultrasound techniques for the small animal practitioner. 2nd edition. Ames IA: Wiley Blackwell; 2021. p. 729–55.

5. Perera P, Mailhot T, Riley D, et al. The RUSH exam: rapid ultrasound in shock in the evaluation of the critically ill. Emerg Med Clin Morth Am 2010;28(1):29–56.

6. Tavares J, Ivo R, Gonzales F, et al. Global ultrasound check for the critically ill (GUCCI) – a new systematized protcol unifying point-of-care ultrasound in critcally ill patinets based on clinical presentation. Emerg Med 2019;10(11):133–45.

7. Lisciandro GR, Armenise AA. Chapter 16: focused or COAST[3] - Cardiopulmonary Resuscitation (CPR), Global FAST (GFAST[3]), and the FAST-ABCDE Exam. In: Lisciandro GR, editor. Focused ultrasound for the small animal practitioner. Ames, IA: Wiley Blackwell; 2014. p. 269–85.

8. Lisciandro GR. POCUS: global FAST for patient monitoring and staging. In: Lisciandro GR, editor. Point-of-care ultrasound techniques for the small animal practitioner. 2nd edition. Ames IA: Wiley Blackwell; 2021. p. 685–728.

9. Cageside ultrasonography in the emergency room and the intensive care unit. Vet Clin North Am 2020;50(6):1445–67.

10. Lisciandro GR. Chapter 3: point-of-care ultrasound. In: Mattoon JS, Sellon R, Berry CR, editors. Small animal diagnostic ultrasound. 4th edition. St. Louis MO: Elsevier; 2021. p. 76–104.

11. Boysen SR, Lisciandro GR. The use of ultrasound in the emergency room (AFAST and TFAST). Vet Clin North Am Small Anim Pract 2013;43(4):773–97.

12. Lisciandro GR, Gambino JM, Lisciandro SC. Case series of 13 dogs and 1 cat with ultrasonographically-detected gallbladder wall edema associated with cardiac disease. J Vet Intern Med 2021;35(3):1342–6.

13. Ward JL, Lisciandro GR, Ware WA, et al. Evaluation of point-of-care thoracic ultrasound and NT-proBNP for the diagnosis of congestive heart failure in cats with respiratory distress. J Vet Intern Med 2018;32(5):1530–40.

14. Hall DJ, Shofer F, Meier CK, et al. Pericardial effusion in cats: a retrospective study of clinical findings and outcome in 146 cats. J Vet Intern Med 2007; 21(5):1002–7.

15. Lisciandro GR, Lagutchik MS, Mann KA, et al. Evaluation of an abdominal fluid scoring system determined using abdominal focused assessment with sonography for trauma in 101 dogs with motor vehicle trauma. J Vet Emerg Crit Care 2009;19(5):426–37.

16. Ollerton JE, Sugrue M, Balogh Z, et al. Prospective study to evaluate the influence of FAST on trauma patient management. J Trauma 2006;60:785–91.

17. Blackbourne LH, Soffer D, McKenney M, et al. Secondary ultrasound examination increases the sensitivity of the FAST exam in trauma. J Trauma 2004;57(5):934–8.

18. Nelson NC, Drost WT, Lerche P, et al. Noninvasive estimation of central venous pressure in anesthetized dogs by measurement of hepatic venous blood flow velocity and abdomen al venous diameter. Vet Rad Ultrasound 2010;51(3):313–23.

19. Lisciandro GR. Abdominal and thoracic focused assessment with sonography for trauma, triage and monitoring in small animals. J Vet Emerg Crit Care 2011;21(2): 104–22.

20. Lisciandro GR, Fosgate GT, Fulton RM. Frequency of ultrasound lung rockets using a regionally-based lung ultrasound examination named veterinary bedside lung ultrasound exam (Vet BLUE) in 98 dogs with normal thoracic radiographic lung findings. Vet Radiol Ultrasound 2014;55(3):315–22.

21. Lisciandro GR, Fulton RM, Fosgate GT, et al. Frequency of B-lines using a regionally-based lung ultrasound examination (the Vet BLUE protocol) in 49 cats with normal thoracic radiographical lung findings. J Vet Emerg Crit Care 2017;27(3):267–77.

22. Ward JL, Lisciandro GR, Keene BW, et al. Accuracy of point-of-care lung ultrasonography for the diagnosis of cardiogenic pulmonary edema in dogs and cats with acute dyspnea. J Am Vet Med Assoc 2017;250:666–75.

23. Lisciandro GR, Ward JL, DeFrancesco TC, et al. Absence of B-lines on Lung Ultrasound (Vet BLUE protocol) to Rule Out Left-sided Congestive Heart Failure in 368 Cats and Dogs. *Abstract*. J Vet Emerg Crit Care 2016;26(S1):S8.

24. Vezzosi T, Mannucci A, Pistoresi F, et al. Assessment of lung ultrasound B-lines in dogs with different stages of chronic valvular heart disease. J Vet Intern Med 2017;31(3):700–4.

25. Ferrada P, Attand RJ, Whelan J, et al. Qualitative assessment of the inferior vena cava: useful tool for the evaluation of volume status in criticall ill patients. Am Surg 2012;78(4):468–70.

26. Darnis E, Boysen S, Merveille AC, et al. Establishment of references values of the caudal vena cava by fast-ultrasonography through different views in healthy dogs. J Vet Intern Med 2018;32(4):1308–18.

27. Chou Y, Ward JL, Baron LZ, et al. Focused ultrasound of the caudal vena cava in dogs with cavitary effusions or congestive heart failure: a prospective observational study. PLoS One 2021;16(5):e0252544.

28. Murphy SD, Ward JL, Viall AK, et al. Utility of point-of-care lung ultrasound for monitoring cardiogenic pulmonary edema in dogs. J Vet Intern Med 2021;35(1):68–77.

29. Himelman RB, Kircher B, Rockey DC, et al. Inferior vena cava plethora with blunted respiratory response: a sensitive echocardiographic sign of cardiac tamoponade. J Am Coll Cardiol 1988;12(6):1470–7.

30. Tchernodrinski S, Arntfield R. Chapter 18: inferior vena cava. *In:* Point-of-care ultrasound, Edited by Soni NJ, Arntfield R, and Kory P. Elsevier: 2015; Philadephia PA, pp. 135-141.

31. Lisciandro GR. The use of the diaphragmatico-hepatic (DH) views of the abdominal and thoracic focused assessment with sonography for triage (AFAST/TFAST) examinations for the detection of pericardial effusion in 24 dogs (2011-2012). J Vet Emerg Crit Care 2016;26(1):125–31.

32. Lisciandro GR, Fosgate GT, Romero LA, et al. The expected frequency and amount of free peritoneal fluid estimated using the abdominal FAST-applied abdominal fluid scores in clinically normal adult and juvenile dogs. J Vet Emerg Crit Care 2021;31(1):43–51.

33. Lisciandro GR, Fosgate GT. Use of AFAST cysto-colic view urinary bladder measurements to estimate urinary bladder volume in dogs and cats. J Vet Emerg Crit Care 2017;27(6):713–7.

34. Kim SY, Park KT, Yeon SC, et al. Accuracy of sonographic diagnosis of pneumoperitoneum using the enhanced peritoneal stripe sign in Beagle dogs. J Vet Sci 2014;15(2):195–8.

35. Sanderson JJ, Boysen SR, McMurray JM, et al. The effect of fasting on gastrointestinal motility in healthy dogs as assessed by sonography. J Vet Emerg Crit Care 2017;27(6):645–50.

36. Quantz JE, Miles MS, Reed AL, et al. Elevation of alanine transaminase and gallbladder wall abnormalities as biomarkers of anaphylaxis in canine hypersensitivity patients. J Vet Emerg Crit Care 2009;19(6):536–44.

37. McMurray J, Boysen S, Chalhoub S. Focused assessment with sonography in nontraumatized dogs and cats in the emergency and critical care setting. J Vet Emerg Crit Care 2016;26(1):64–73.

38. Lisciandro GR, Lisciandro GR. Chapter 9: The Thoracic FAST[3] (TFAST[3]) Exam. In: Focused ultrasound for the small animal practitioner. Ames, IA: Wiley Blackwell; 2014. p. 140–65.

39. Lisciandro GR. POCUS: TFAST: Clinical Integration. In: Lisciandro GR, editor. Point-of-care ultrasound techniques for the small animal practitioner. 2nd edition. Ames IA: Wiley Blackwell; 2021. p. 337–88.

40. Ward JL, Lisciandro GR, Ware WA, et al. Lung ultrasound findings in 100 dogs with various etiologies of cough. J Am Vet Med Assoc 2019;255(5):574–83.

41. Lisciandro GR, Lagutchik MS, Mann KA, et al. Evaluation of a thoracic focused assessment with sonography for trauma (TFAST) protocol to detect pneumothorax and concurrent thoracic injury in 145 traumatized dogs. J Vet Emerg Crit Care 2008;18(3):258–69.

42. Hwang TS, Yoon YM, Jung DI, et al. Usefulness of transthoracic lung ultrasound for the diagnosis of mild pneumothorax. J Vet Sci 2018;19(5):660–6.

43. Boysen S, McMurray J, Gommeren K. Abnormal curtain signs with a novel lung ultrasound protocol in 6 dogs with pneumothorax. Front Vet Sci 2019;28(6):291.

44. Ferrada P, Evans D, Wolfe L, et al. Findings of a randomized controlled trial using limited transthoracic echocardiogram (LTTE) as a hemodynamic monitoring tool in the trauma bay. J Trauma Acute Care Surg 2014;76(1):31–7.

45. DeFrancesco TC. POCUS: heart: introduction and image acquisition. In: Lisciandro GR, editor. Point-of-care ultrasound techniques for the small animal practitioner. 2nd edition. Ames IA: Wiley Blackwell; 2021. p. 389–402.

46. DeFrancesco TC. POCUS: heart: abnormalities of valves, myocardium and great vessels. In: Lisciandro GR, editor. Point-of-care ultrasound techniques for the small animal practitioner. 2nd edition. Ames IA: Wiley Blackwell; 2021. p. 403–16.

47. Loughran KA, Rush JE, Rozanski EA, et al. The use of focused cardiac ultrasound to screen for occult heart disease in asymptomatic cats. J Vet Intern Med 2019; 33(5):1892–901.

48. Côté E, Schwarz LA, Sithole F. Thoracic radiographic findings for dogs with cardiac tamponade attributable to pericardial effusion. J Am Vet Med Assoc 2013; 243(2):232–5.

49. Guglielmini C, Diana A, Santarelli G, et al. Accuracy of radiographic vertebral heart score and sphericity index in the detection of pericardial effusion in dogs. J Am Vet Med Assoc 2012;241(8):1048–55.

50. Lisciandro GR, Lisciandro SC. POCUS: Vet BLUE: clinical integration. In: Lisciandro GR, editor. Point-of-care ultrasound techniques for the small animal practitioner. 2nd edition. Ames IA: Wiley Blackwell; 2021. p. 459–508.

51. Lisciandro GR, Lisciandro GR. Chapter 10: The Vet BLUE Lung Scan. In: Focused ultrasound for the small animal practitioner. Ames, IA: Wiley Blackwell; 2014. p. 166–88.

52. Kulhavy DA, Lisciandro GR. Use of a lung ultrasound examination called vet BLUE to screen for metastatic lung nodules in the emergency room. Abstract. J Vet Emerg Crit Care 2015;25(S1):S14.

53. Lisciandro GR, Puchot ML, Gambino JM, et al. The wedge sign: a possible lung ultrasound sign for pulmonary thromboembolism. J Vet Emerg Clin Care 2021; 34(4):356–61.

54. Lux CN, Culp WT, Mayhew RD, et al. Perioperative outcome in dogs with hemoperitoneum: 83 cases (2005-2010). J Am Vet Med Assoc 2013;242(10):1385–91.

55. Hammond TN, Pesillo-Crosby SA. Prevalence of hemangiosarcoma in anemic dogs with splenic mass and hemoperitoneum requiring a transfusion: 71 cases (2003-2005). J Am Vet Med Assoc 2008;232(4):553–8.

UNITED STATES POSTAL SERVICE® Statement of Ownership, Management, and Circulation
(All Periodicals Publications Except Requester Publications)

1. Publication Title
VETERINARY CLINICS OF NORTH AMERICA: SMALL ANIMAL PRACTICE

2. Publication Number
003 – 150

3. Filing Date
9/18/2021

4. Issue Frequency
JAN, MAR, MAY, JUL, SEP, NOV

5. Number of Issues Published Annually
6

6. Annual Subscription Price
$358.00

7. Complete Mailing Address of Known Office of Publication (Not printer) (Street, city, county, state, and ZIP+4®)
ELSEVIER INC.
230 Park Avenue, Suite 800
New York, NY 10169

Contact Person
Malathi Samayan
Telephone (Include area code)
91-44-4299-4507

8. Complete Mailing Address of Headquarters or General Business Office of Publisher (Not printer)
ELSEVIER INC.
230 Park Avenue, Suite 800
New York, NY 10169

9. Full Names and Complete Mailing Addresses of Publisher, Editor, and Managing Editor (Do not leave blank)

Publisher (Name and complete mailing address)
DOLORES MELONI, ELSEVIER INC.
1600 JOHN F KENNEDY BLVD. SUITE 1800
PHILADELPHIA, PA 19103-2899

Editor (Name and complete mailing address)
STACY EASTMAN, ELSEVIER INC.
1600 JOHN F KENNEDY BLVD. SUITE 1800
PHILADELPHIA, PA 19103-2899

Managing Editor (Name and complete mailing address)
PATRICK MANLEY, ELSEVIER INC.
1600 JOHN F KENNEDY BLVD. SUITE 1800
PHILADELPHIA, PA 19103-2899

10. Owner (Do not leave blank. If the publication is owned by a corporation, give the name and address of the corporation immediately followed by the names and addresses of all stockholders owning or holding 1 percent or more of the total amount of stock. If not owned by a corporation, give the names and addresses of the individual owners. If owned by a partnership or other unincorporated firm, give its name and address as well as those of each individual owner. If the publication is published by a nonprofit organization, give its name and address.)

Full Name	Complete Mailing Address
WHOLLY OWNED SUBSIDIARY OF REED/ELSEVIER, US HOLDINGS	1600 JOHN F KENNEDY BLVD. SUITE 1800 PHILADELPHIA, PA 19103-2899

11. Known Bondholders, Mortgagees, and Other Security Holders Owning or Holding 1 Percent or More of Total Amount of Bonds, Mortgages, or Other Securities. If none, check box ▶ ☐ None

Full Name	Complete Mailing Address
N/A	

12. Tax Status (For completion by nonprofit organizations authorized to mail at nonprofit rates) (Check one)
The purpose, function, and nonprofit status of this organization and the exempt status for federal income tax purposes:
☒ Has Not Changed During Preceding 12 Months
☐ Has Changed During Preceding 12 Months (Publisher must submit explanation of change with this statement)

PS Form 3526, July 2014 (Page 1 of 4 (see instructions page 4))   PSN: 7530-01-000-9931   PRIVACY NOTICE: See our privacy policy on www.usps.com

---

13. Publication Title
VETERINARY CLINICS OF NORTH AMERICA: SMALL ANIMAL PRACTICE

14. Issue Date for Circulation Data Below
JULY 2021

15. Extent and Nature of Circulation

		Average No. Copies Each Issue During Preceding 12 Months	No. Copies of Single Issue Published Nearest to Filing Date
a. Total Number of Copies (Net press run)		544	511
b. Paid Circulation (By Mail and Outside the Mail)	(1) Mailed Outside-County Paid Subscriptions Stated on PS Form 3541 (Include paid distribution above nominal rate, advertiser's proof copies, and exchange copies)	345	329
	(2) Mailed In-County Paid Subscriptions Stated on PS Form 3541 (Include paid distribution above nominal rate, advertiser's proof copies, and exchange copies)	0	0
	(3) Paid Distribution Outside the Mails Including Sales Through Dealers and Carriers, Street Vendors, Counter Sales, and Other Paid Distribution Outside USPS®	135	135
	(4) Paid Distribution by Other Classes of Mail Through the USPS (e.g., First-Class Mail®)	0	0
c. Total Paid Distribution (Sum of 15b (1), (2), (3), and (4))	▶	480	464
d. Free or Nominal Rate Distribution (By Mail and Outside the Mail)	(1) Free or Nominal Rate Outside-County Copies Included on PS Form 3541	48	31
	(2) Free or Nominal Rate In-County Copies Included on PS Form 3541	0	0
	(3) Free or Nominal Rate Copies Mailed at Other Classes Through the USPS (e.g., First-Class Mail)	0	0
	(4) Free or Nominal Rate Distribution Outside the Mail (Carriers or other means)	0	0
e. Total Free or Nominal Rate Distribution (Sum of 15d (1), (2), (3) and (4))	▶	48	31
f. Total Distribution (Sum of 15c and 15e)	▶	528	495
g. Copies not Distributed (See Instructions to Publishers #4 (page #3))	▶	16	16
h. Total (Sum of 15f and g)	▶	544	511
i. Percent Paid (15c divided by 15f times 100)		90.9%	93.73%

* If you are claiming electronic copies, go to line 16 on page 3. If you are not claiming electronic copies, skip to line 17 on page 3.

16. Electronic Copy Circulation

		Average No. Copies Each Issue During Preceding 12 Months	No. Copies of Single Issue Published Nearest to Filing Date
a. Paid Electronic Copies	▶		
b. Total Paid Print Copies (Line 15c) + Paid Electronic Copies (Line 16a)	▶		
c. Total Print Distribution (Line 15f) + Paid Electronic Copies (Line 16a)	▶		
d. Percent Paid (Both Print & Electronic Copies) (16b divided by 16c × 100)	▶		

☒ I certify that 50% of all my distributed copies (electronic and print) are paid above a nominal price.

17. Publication of Statement of Ownership
☒ If the publication is a general publication, publication of this statement is required. Will be printed in the NOVEMBER 2021 issue of this publication.   ☐ Publication not required.

18. Signature and Title of Editor, Publisher, Business Manager, or Owner

Malathi Samayan

Malathi Samayan - Distribution Controller

Date
9/18/2021

I certify that all information furnished on this form is true and complete. I understand that anyone who furnishes false or misleading information on this form or who omits material or information requested on the form may be subject to criminal sanctions (including fines and imprisonment) and/or civil sanctions (including civil penalties).

PS Form 3526, July 2014 (Page 3 of 4)   PRIVACY NOTICE: See our privacy policy on www.usps.com

Moving?

Make sure your subscription moves with you!

To notify us of your new address, find your **Clinics Account Number** (located on your mailing label above your name), and contact customer service at:

Email: journalscustomerservice-usa@elsevier.com

800-654-2452 (subscribers in the U.S. & Canada)
314-447-8871 (subscribers outside of the U.S. & Canada)

Fax number: 314-447-8029

Elsevier Health Sciences Division
Subscription Customer Service
3251 Riverport Lane
Maryland Heights, MO 63043

*To ensure uninterrupted delivery of your subscription,
please notify us at least 4 weeks in advance of move.

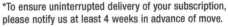